Principles of Laboratory Techniques and Methods

(Bioinstrumentation Techniques applied to B.Sc., M.Sc., Microbiology, Biotechnology, Bioinformatics, Biomedical, NET and JRF)

MEENA SRIVASTAVA
Reader & Head
Department of Zoology
M.P. Government P.G. College
HARDOI - 241 001 (U.P.) India

RAJESH SINGH YADAV
M.Sc. NET
Junior Research Fellow
Industrial Toxicology Research Centre
Mahatma Gandhi Marg,
LUCKNOW - 226 001 (U.P.) India

CBS

CBS Publishers & Distributors Pvt. Ltd.
New Delhi • Bengaluru • Chennai • Kochi • Mumbai • Pune
Hyderabad • Kolkata • Nagpur • Patna • Vijayawada

Principles of Laboratory Techniques and Methods

ISBN: 978-81-239-2685-8

First CBS Reprint: 2015

Published by:
Satish Kumar Jain for CBS Publishers & Distributors Pvt. Ltd.,
4819/XI Prahlad Street, 24 Ansari Road, Daryaganj, New Delhi - 110002
delhi@cbspd.com, cbspubs@airtelmail.in • www.cbspd.com
Ph.: 23289259, 23266861, 23266867 • Fax: 011-23243014

Corporate Office: 204 FIE, Industrial Area, Patparganj, Delhi - 110 092
Ph: 49344934 • Fax: 011-49344935
E-mail: publishing@cbspd.com • publicity@cbspd.com

Branches:
- ***Bengaluru:*** 2975, 17th Cross, K.R. Road, Bansankari 2nd Stage, Bengaluru - 70
  Ph: +91-80-26771678/79 • Fax: +91-80-26771680
  E-mail: cbsbng@gmail.com, bangalore@cbspd.com
- ***Chennai:*** No. 7, Subbaraya Street, Shenoy Nagar, Chennai - 600030
  Ph: +91-44-26681266, 26680620 • Fax: +91-44-42032115
  E-mail: chennai@cbspd.com
- ***Kochi:*** 36/14, Kalluvilakam, Lissie Hospital Road, Kochi - 682018
  Ph: +91-484-4059061-65 • Fax: +91-484-4059065
  E-mail: cochin@cbspd.com
- ***Mumbai:*** 83-C, Dr. E. Moses Road, Worli, Mumbai - 400018
  Ph: +91-9833017933, 022-24902340/41 • E-mail: mumbai@cbspd.com
- ***Pune:*** Bhuruk Prestige, Sr. No. 52/12/2+1+3/2,
  Narhe, Haveli (Near Katraj-Dehu Road Bypass), Pune - 411041
  Ph: +91-20-64704058/59, 32342277 • E-mail: pune@cbspd.com

Representatives:
- Hyderabad: 0-9885175004
- Nagpur: 0-9021734563
- Vijayawada: 0-9000660880
- Kolkata: 0-9831437309, 0-9051152362
- Patna: 0-9334159340

Printed at:
Neekunj Print Process, Delhi

Dedicated

With Love and Special Regards

to

our Parents

and

Teachers

Preface

The present book entitled **"Principles of Laboratory Techniques and Methods"** is aimed at presenting precise information on various Instruments for undergraduate and Postgraduate students of all Indian Universities. We have tried our level best to cover the syllabi of most Indian Universities recommended by UGC. The book has updated information on latest techniques and instruments used in life science laboratories like Genetic Engineering, Biotechnology, Microbiology, Forensic Science and cell culture.

Biology has made spectacular progress with the discovery of new tools and techniques. DNA Recombinant technology, DNA typing, cell culture, animal cloning and many other techniques have changed traditional biology in a revolutionary manner. Now a student of Biology can seek his career not only in the basic sciences, but also in many new branches like Forensic Science, Biotechnology, Bioinformatics, Environmental Science and Ecotoxicology etc. So it is the need of the present system that a student should have a better experience of instruments for working in advanced laboratories because without prior knowledge of various recent instruments it is not an easy task to handle them. Our intention, of writing this book has been mainly to develop the conceptual interest and curiosity in students.

As both the authors were associated with Forensic Science Laboratory, there was a good exposure to the Electrophoretic techniques, Chromatography, Spectroscopy and many other laboratory instruments. So this book is a concise account of their practical experience in the field. An effort has been made to represent all the instruments, their practical handling and techniques within the pages of a concise book. The book will also prove useful for Biotechnology, Biomedical and research students.

The contents have been dealt concisely and necessary illustrations. Tables and diagrams have been included to help the students.

Even though we have put in our best efforts to make the book error-free, some printing errors may have crept up, for which we express our regrets. We are looking forward to the valuable suggestions from our sincere readers especially students and teachers.

There are also references at the end of each chapter from which the required informations have been taken and will be helpful for future detailed study.

Authors

Acknowledgement

We express our esteemed profound sense of gratitude to Dr. Ramanand Prasad, Principal, M.P. Govt. P.G. College, Hardoi, for his evergreen inspiration, valuable guidance constant encouragement and support throughout the work.

We express our sincere thanks to Dr. Rajeev Kumar, Secretary, Higher Education, U.P. Govt., U.P. for providing us an innovative front in carrier advancement and sincere guidance.

We are greatly indebted to Dr. R.K. Baslas, Director, Higher Education, Directorate, Allahabad, for his triggering inspirations guidance and granting us permission to publish this book.

We owe our cordial thanks to Dr. J.R. Sethi, Director, FSL, Mahanagar, Lucknow for his kind cooperation and in providing us library facilities.

We would like to express our sincere gratitude to Dr. Ashok Verma, Reader, Zoology Deptt. Phaphamau, Allahabad, Dr. Archana Rajan, Reader, Botany Deptt. Govt. Degree College Harakh, Barabanki, Dr. Kiran Yadav, Reader Zoology Deptt., Dr. I.D. Singh, Dr. Kanchan Lata and all teachers of M.P. Govt. P.G. College Hardoi, for their continuous inspiration and timely valuable suggestions.

Our sincere thanks are due to Dr. R.B. Rayzada, Scientist, I.T.R.C ,Lucknow, Mrs. Seema Srivastava, Dr. A.K. Srivastava, C.F.S.L, Hyderabad, Dr. Rajesh Singh S.S.O. Police Forensic Science Laboratory, Jaipur and Mr. S.N. Yadav, S.S.A, F.S.L. Lucknow for their continued cooperation and valuable suggestions.

We would like to express our special thanks to Mr. B.K. Srivastava, Pranay, and Mansi for their sacrifice and cooperation without which this book would never have been published.

Last but not least we would like to show our appreciation for the esteemed Mohd. Asif, Nivedita Singh, Vinay Srivastava, Umesh Misra, Sandeep Verma, Akhilesh Pandey and S.S. Trivedi for their cooperation in making this task an easy and possible.

It gives us great pleasure to thank International Book Distributing Co. Lucknow, for agreeing to publish this book and whose help cannot be measured in mere words.

Dr. Meena Srivastava
Rajesh Singh Yadav

Contents

CHAPTER 1
Microscopy

1.1 A Journey to the Microscope

The present-day microscope started its journey during the first Century AD as "magnifying glasses" but apparently they were not used much until the invention of spectacles till the 13th century.

The earliest simple microscope was in the form of a simple tube with a plate for the object at one end and a magnifying glass at the other. In 1950, two Dutch spectacles makers Zaccharias Janssen and his son Hans discovered the forerunner of compound microscope by using a combination of several lenses in a hollow tube. In 1609, Galileo worked out the principles of lenses and made a microscope with a better focusing device.

Antony Van Leeuwenhoek of Holland (1632-1723), father of microscopy, used tiny lenses of great curvature which gave magnification up to 270 diameters. His microscope was used to observe bacteria, yeast, aquatic micro-organisms and blood cells for the first time. Later Robert Hooke, the English Father of microscopy, improved Leeuwenhoek's microscope. Van Leeuwenhoek used a single lens microscope, Hooke used a compound microscope.

Achromatic lenses for spectacles were developed by Chester Moore Hall, since 1729 Jan and Harmanus Van Deyl were the first to make small high power achromatic lenses, at the end of the 18th century. Carl Zeiss Jena produced its first oil immersion objectives in 1880, designed by Ernst Abbe, who was the Father of optical theory of microscopic lenses.

The first Stereoscopic-style microscope with double eyepieces and matching objectives was designed by Cherubin d'Orleans in 1671 but the instrument was actually a pseudostereoscopic system.

During the mid-19th century Francis Herbert Wenhon of London designed the first truly successful microscope. He used an achromatic prism to split the light beam at the rear of a single objective.

The first modern Stereomicroscope was introduced in the United States by the American Optical Company in 1957 named the "Cycloptic". Bausch and Lomb in 1959 introduced a Stereo-Zoom with cutting edge advancement.

Phase Contrast Microscope was invented by Dutchman Zernike in 1934. This microscope is a modified form of compound microscope which has the capacity to visualize the transparent object. Living cells may be observed by this microscope.

The Electron Microscope was co-invented by Germans, Max Knoll and Ernst Ruska in 1931. The object as small as an atom may be viewed from this microscope. It can magnify an object up to 1 million times. There is a serious drawback in Electron Microscope, since no living specimen can survive under its high vacuum.

Table 1.1. Milestones in the Journey to the Microscope

Scientist	Year	Achievements
Arabian Alhazen	(962 – 1038 C.E.)	Described the actions of the lenses in his treatise on optics.
Roger Bacon	(1214-1292 C.E.)	Referred to the concepts and uses of lenses in his scientific works
Antony Van Leeuwenhoek	1623	Invented Compound Microscope
Talboot	1839	He invented Polarizing Microscope
Ernst Leitz	1873 C.E.	Introduced microscope with revolving nose piece for objectives
August Kohler	1880 C.E.	Told about the optimum spacing for the light and condenser which would produce sharp images
Gerd Binning and Heinrich Rohren	1980	Invented Scanning Tunneling Microscope to provide 3D image and surface structure.
Katherine Blodgett	1917 C.E.	Developed micro-coatings which allowed her to develop non-reflecting invisible glass
Max Knoll and Ernst Ruska	1931 C.E.	Built the first Electron Microscope
Ernst Ruska	1933 C.E.	Increased magnification of electron microscope to levels higher than a compound light microscope
Max Knoll et.al	1942	Invented Scanning Electron Microscope
Fritz Zernike	1953	He invented the Phase Contrast Microscope

1. 2 Introduction

Microscopy is a technique by which investigations are made on fine details of an object which are not visible to the naked eye. The human eye possesses limited resolving power so they are unable to distinguish the object smaller than 0.1mm (100 μ in size). Moreover, the living cells are transparent in ordinary light and cannot be distinguished among their various cellular components. To overcome these problems, the biologist of the past investigated various methods of staining and magnifying the cells and their components. This was made possible by using combination of various types of lenses. These lenses could magnify the minute object up to a particular limit. Therefore many lenses combined together to form an instrument known as Microscope. (Gr. Micros = small; Skopeis = to see, to view)

1.3 Properties of Light

As all types of Microscopes function on the principle and properties of light, so in order to understand the principle and mechanism of image formation, one should have the basic idea of properties of light. A brief description of the same is given as follows:-

- Light is the form of energy which makes objects visible to our eyes. It propagates as electromagnetic waves with a speed of 3.0×10^8 m/ sec in vacuum.
- It travels straight in homogeneous medium.
- It lies in the visible region of electromagnetic spectrum from 4000 A° to 8000 A°.
- It can emit electrons from metal surface and produce photoelectric effect.
- It exhibits the phenomena of refraction, reflection, interference, diffraction and polarization.

When light ray passes through a medium, due to absorption, its amplitude reduces and diminishes its intensity.

Light wave travels in straight line in the form of photon energy. The distance between two peaks is **wavelength** while strength of energy of brightness is known as amplitude. Different source of light produce light of different wavelength and amplitude. Similarly light rays of different wavelength produce different colours. The **frequency of light** is defined as the number of waves produced per/sec, which remains constant (Fig. 1.1).

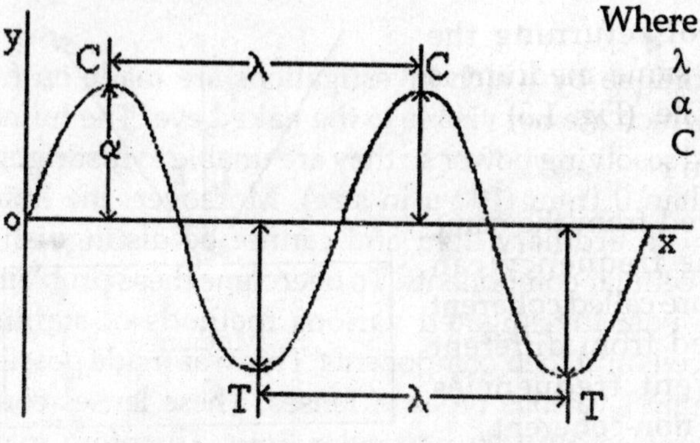

Where -
λ = wave length
α = amplitude
C = crest

Fig. 1.1. Traveling of Light wave

Whenever a light ray passes through one transparent medium to another, it deviates from its original path, and is known as **refraction of light**. The angle at which the ray deviates from its path, is known as the angle of refraction. (Fig. 1.2)

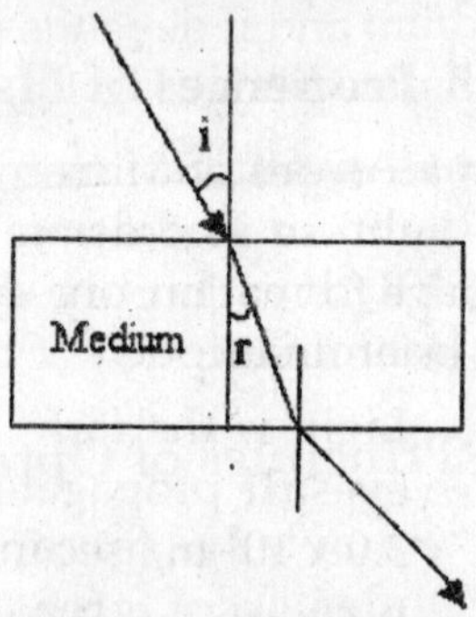

Fig. 1.2. Refraction of light

$$\frac{\sin i}{\sin r} = \text{Constant}$$

If the angle of incident is i and the angle of refraction is r, then

Where sin i = angle of incident
sin r = angle of refraction

In the process of refraction, speed, wavelength and intensity of light changes while frequency remains unchanged. The refractive index of a medium depends on the ratio of sin value of angle of incidence and angle of refraction. The refractive index is of great importance in the microscopy because

- Design of the lens
- Material of the lens
- Density of the material
- Angle of incidence

All the above factors should be in compatible range. Higher the density of the medium greater the value of refractive index.

The phenomenon of returning the incident ray in the same medium is known as **reflection** i.e. (Fig. 1.3)

$$\sin i = \sin r$$

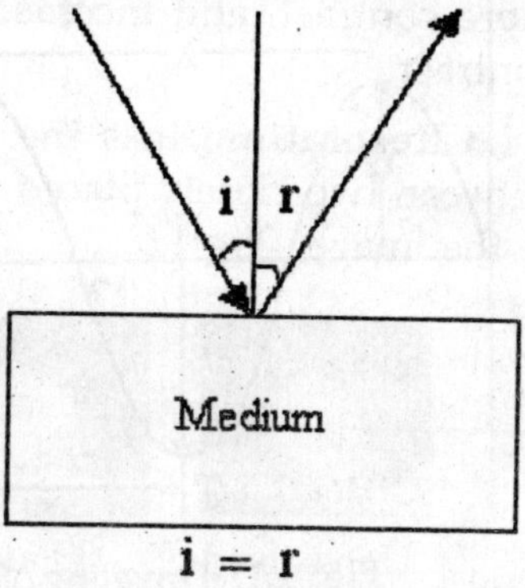

Fig. 1.3. Reflection of light

The light rays radiated from the same source having same frequency can firmly hold together are called **coherent** but the rays radiated from different source have different frequencies cannot do so, called **non-coherent**.

In **absorption** the intensity of light is reduced when passed through a medium and it depends on the density of the medium. (Fig 1.4)

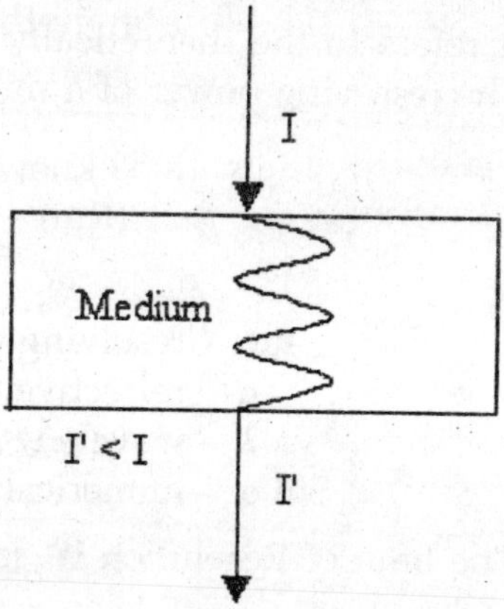

Fig. 1.4. Absorption of light

Light Amplification by Stimulated Emission of Radiation is known as **LASER**. It is highly coherent and monochromatic.

1.4 Principles of Optics

The knowledge of optics and its principles is of great importance because they are practically applied in different kinds of microscopes and other optical instruments. Some of the important optical principles are given as follows:-

1.4.1 Magnification

The Microscope enlarges or magnifies the image of an object and changes the ratio of image size to actual size. A magnification of "100 x" means the image is 100 times bigger than the actual object. Details of the object are visible only if resolution and contrast are in appropriate ratio.

1.4.2 Contrast

It is defined as the ratio of intensity between image and its background. It also distinguishes variation in brightness and colour. If the aperture of the lens is small the scattering of light produce more contrast, and increase in numerical aperture diminishes the contrast.

1.4.3 Resolution: It is the ability of a microscope to distinguish between two closely placed points. It provides clarity and sharpness to the image. (Fig 1.5)

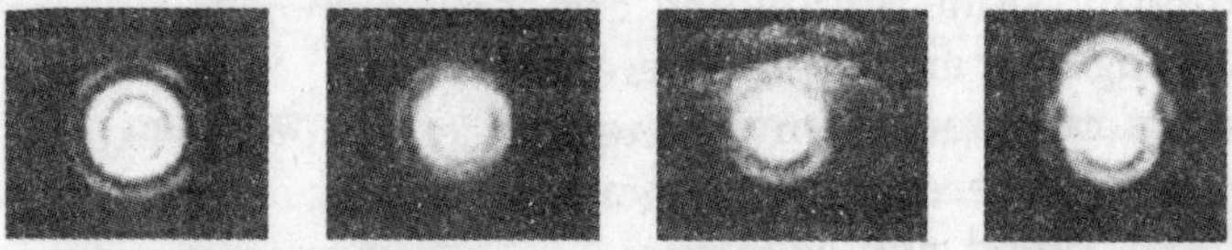

Unresolved   Partially Resolved   Resolved

Fig. 1.5. Resolution between two closely related points

1.4.4 Resolving Power

It refers to the theoretically calculated capacity of the instrument. The resolving power of a microscope may be expressed as follows:-

$$(Rm) = \frac{2\mu \, Sin\, \alpha}{\lambda}$$

Rm - resolving power of microscope
μ- refractive index of the medium
λ - wavelength of light illuminating the object
Sin α - numerical aperture

The limit of Resolution is reciprocal to the resolving power:

$$d\ min = \frac{\lambda}{2\mu \, Sin\, \alpha}$$

d min - minimum resolvable distance between two points
μ- refractive index of the medium
λ - wavelength of light illuminating the object
Sin α - Numerical aperture

The resolving power of a microscope can be increased by using light of shorter wavelength and achromatic lenses. The value of d min is a little more than 0.1μ which is the minimum possible distance and is distinguished between two points.

The above formulae is known as **Abb's Relationship.** High resolution may be achieved by changing the wavelength of illuminating radiation, refractive index and the numerical aperture.

1.4.5 Numerical Aperture

Numerical aperture = n sin α

Where n = refractive index of the medium between cover slip and front lens of the objective. This medium may be air, water or oil.

α = angle between the optical axis of the lens and outermost limit of light ray that reaches the lens.

Since the microscopes are made up of lenses or combination of lenses, so the knowledge of lenses and their properties is essential to understand the working of a microscope.

1.4.6 Lens

A lens is a homogenous transparent medium (such as glass) bounded by two curved surfaces or one curved and one plane surface. (Fig. 1.6)

Mainly two types of lenses are used in microscopes

1. Concave lens (diverging lens)
2. Convex lens (converging lens)

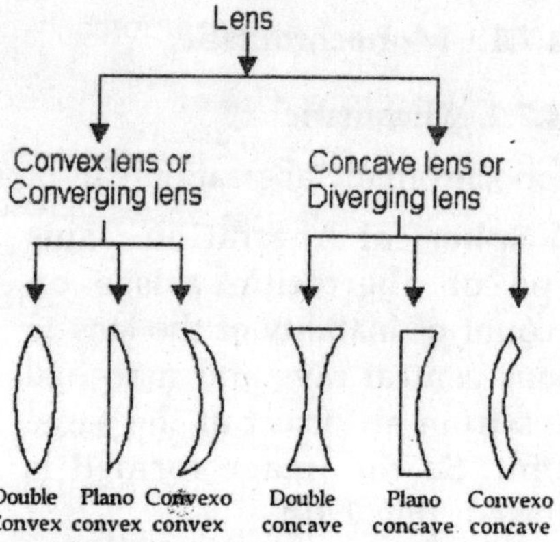

Fig.1.6. Type of Lenses

The nature size and position of image formed depends on the position of object and lens. In convex lens, if object is placed at 2F the image formed will be inverted equal and real. (Fig 1.7)

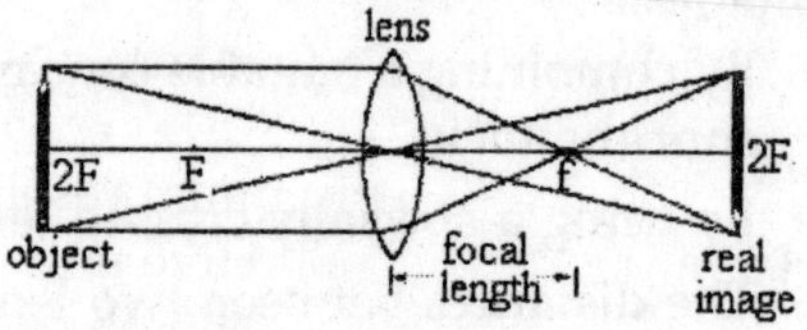

Fig.1.7. Formation of real image by Convex lens

If object is placed between lens and focus (F) its image will be straight, magnified and virtual. (Fig 1.8)

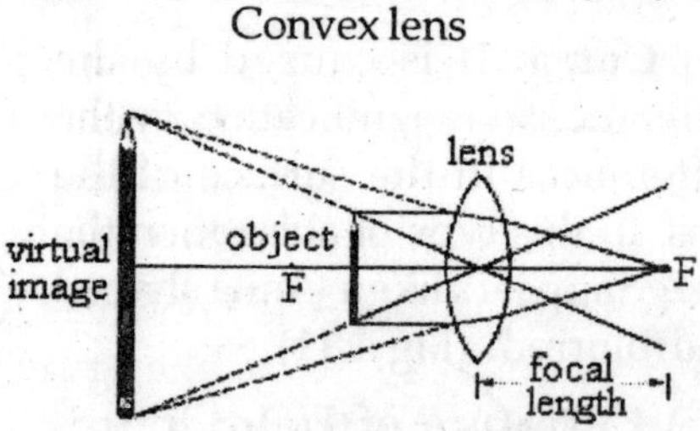

Fig. 1.8. Formation of virtual image

In concave lens, if object is placed between infinity and lens its image will be straight, virtual and diminished. (Fig 1.9)

1.4.7 The Aberration of Lenses

The defect in lenses on account of which, it does not form a white point image of a white point object is defined as aberration. These aberrations do not arise from manufacturing defects but they are inherent or they are transferred in perfectly made simple lens.

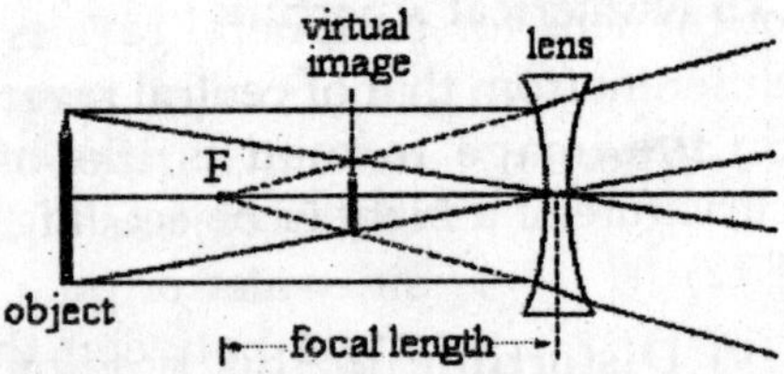

Fig. 1.9. Formation of virtual image by Concave lens

There are two types of aberrations in lenses.

1.4.7.1. Monochromatic

1.4.7.2. Chromatic

Monochromatic aberration can be divided into five categories

(i) Spherical Aberration : This type of aberration arises on account of inability of the lens to focus central rays and marginal rays from an object at the same point. So the image formed is blurred. (Fig 1.10)

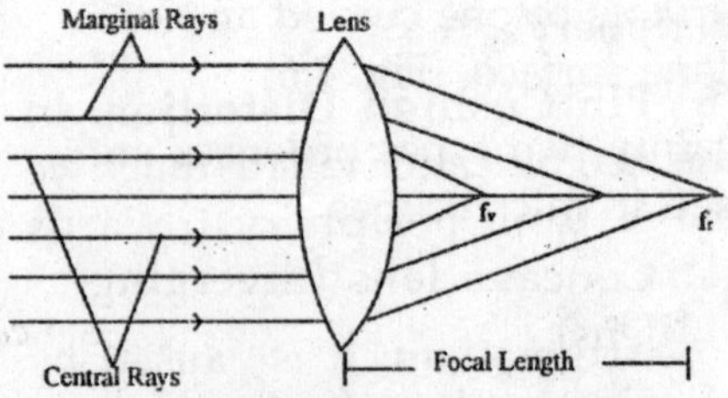

Fig. 1.10. Spherical Aberration

This defect can be removed by adopting the following techniques:-

- By combining a suitable concave lens with convex lens, so as to shift the focus.
- By using a specially crossed lenses.
- The distances between two lenses must be

$$d = f_1 = f_2$$

(ii) Coma: It is caused by the difference in magnification by the differences in the surface of the lens. In this type of aberration the image appears like a Coma shaped and blurred. (Fig 1.11)

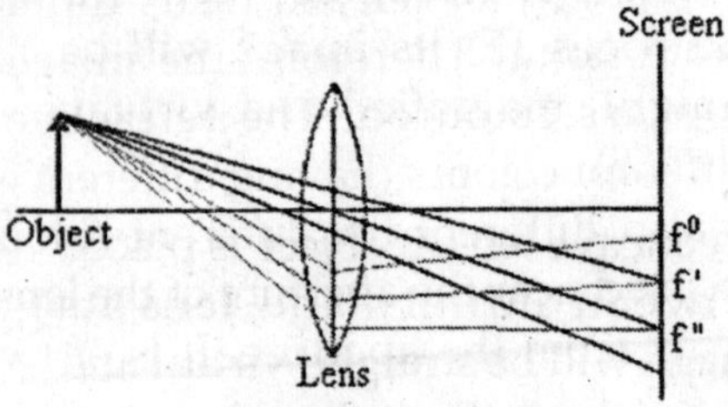

Fig. 1.11. Coma

(iii) Curvature of Field: In this type of aberration, the focal length of the lens for peripheral rays is different from that of central rays. So the image formed is like a curvature of a planner object. (Fig 1.12)

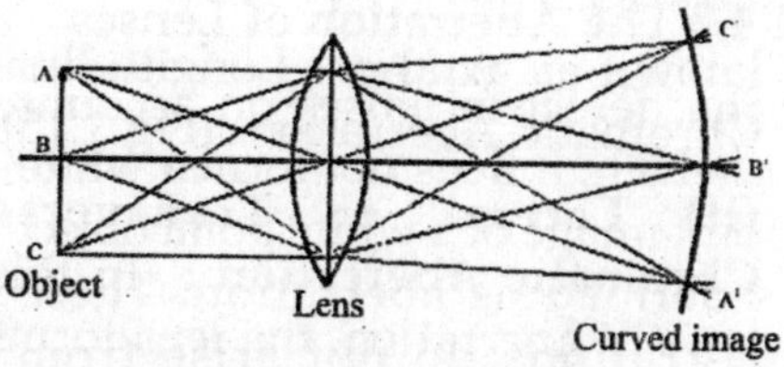

Fig. 1.12. Curvature of Field

(iv) Distortion: In this type of defect the lens exhibits variation in magnification as a function of distance from the center of view field in which the image formed is not only distorted but also curved. It is of two types : (Fig 1.13)

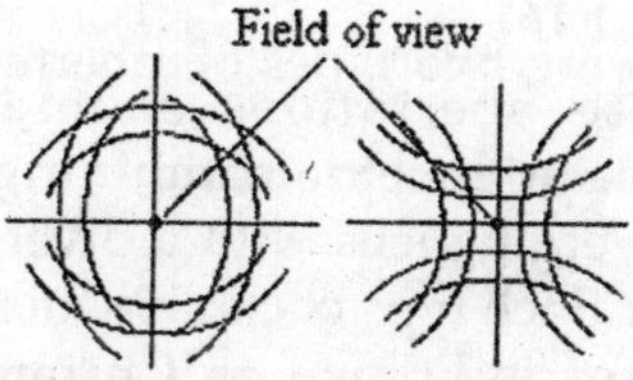

Fig. 1.13. Barrel and Pin cushion distortion

(a) Barrel Distortion: In this magnification falls as quick we move from center towards periphery.

(b) Pin Cushion Distortion: In this magnification falls as quick we move from periphery towards center.

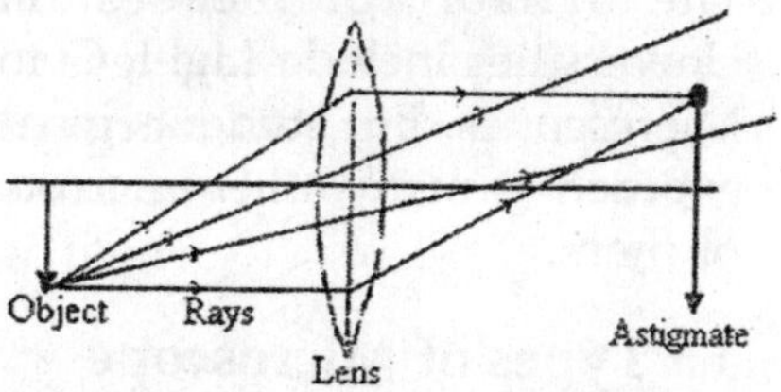

Fig. 1.14. Astigmatism

(v)Astigmatism: It is caused by imperfect spherical nature of lenses. The focal length of lens in two orthogonal directions become different and so we cannot see the object in two orthogonal directions clearly and simultaneously. (Fig 1.14)

This defect is directional and removed by using cylindrical lens in a particular direction.

1.4.7.2. Chromatic aberration: This type of defect arises on account of inability of lens to focus different colours of white light at the same point. Therefore, the image of an object seen in white light appears coloured. The refractive index of a lens is different for different colours (having different wavelength). Hence its focal length is also different for different colours ($f_r > f_v$). So the violet rays are focused near the aperture of the lens where-as the red rays are focused away from the aperture. It is of two types:-

(i) Longitudinal Chromatic Aberration: In this type of aberration,the lens forms images of different colours at different positions. So it is known as axial or Longitudinal Chromatic Aberration. (Fig 1.15)

(ii) Lateral or Transverse Chromatic Aberration : In this type of aberration, the lens forms images of different colours and different sizes. So it is known as Lateral Chromatic Aberration. (Fig 1.16)

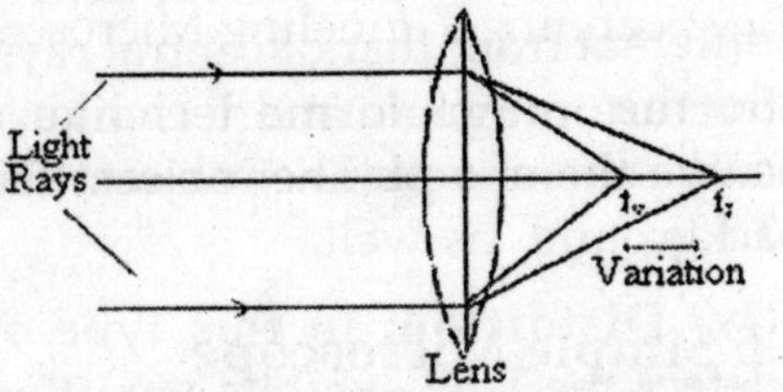

Fig. 1.15. Longitudinal Chromatic Aberration

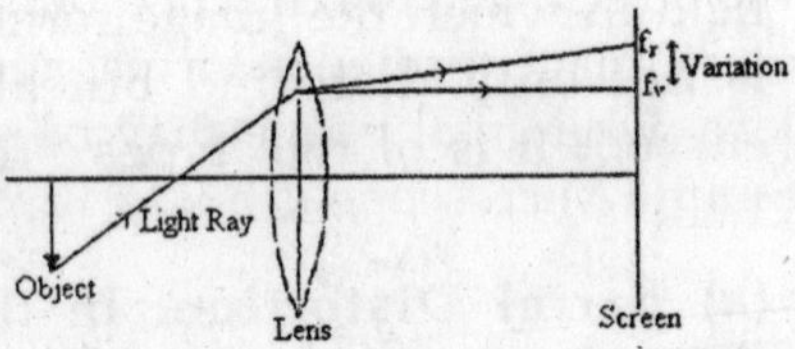

Fig. 1.16. Lateral Chromatic Aberration

These aberrations should be corrected by combining a converging lens with a diverging lens. Such type of combinations of lenses is known as **Chromatic Doublets.**

The Syllabi of most Indian Universities include Light, Compound, SEM, TEM and Fluorescence Microscopes. But students in research laboratories and Institutes are exposed to many other microscopes. So an effort is made to cover all of them.

1.5 Types of Microscope

- Simple Microscope
- Light Microscope
  - (i) Dark Field Microscope
  - (ii) Bright Field Microscope
- Compound Microscope
- Phase Contrast Microscope
- Polarizing Microscope
- Interference Microscope
- Fluorescence Microscope
- Stereoscopic Microscope
- Comaprison Microscope
- Confocal Microscope
- Oil Immersion Microscope
- Electron Microscope
  - (i) Scanning Electron Microscope
  - (ii) Transmission Electron Microscope

- Scanning Tunneling Microscope

Structure principle and technique of use will enable the students to handle them well. The account will also provide a sound theoretical background as well.

1.6 Simple Microscope

Simple Microscope is also known as magnifying lens. It is an important tool in examining the documents and macro organisms. It enlarges the objects due to refraction of light from air to glass and again to air. Here image formed is virtual and can be seen by looking through the lens, while real image may be seen directly. Magnification range of Simple Microscope is 5 x to 10 x (i.e. 5 times to 10 times) (Fig. 1.17)

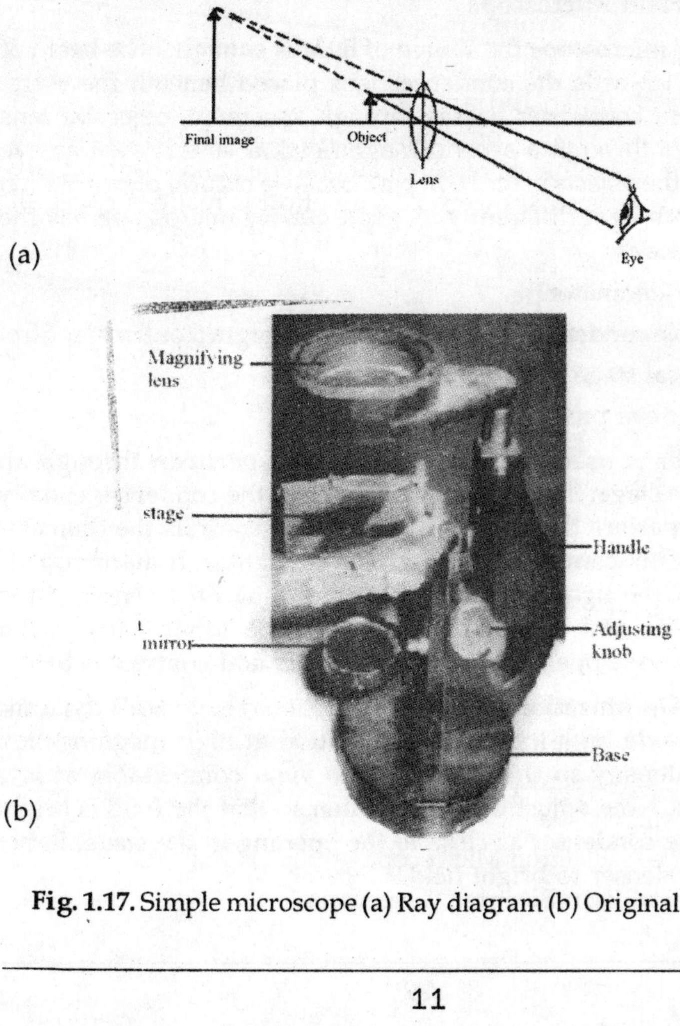

Fig. 1.17. Simple microscope (a) Ray diagram (b) Original photograph

1.7 Light Microscope

The Light Microscope, is so called because it detects small objects by using visible light. It is the most common Microscope, invented by **Antony Van Leeuwenhoek of Holland (1632 - 1723),** a Dutch scientist. He ground pieces of glass into lenses and made a microscope with a magnification of 150 - 300 times. It has lenses and depends on light for their magnification. While observing any tiny object, we desire to meet the following challenges.

- To obtain sufficient contrast
- To find the focal plane

Types of Light Microscope

1.7.1. Bright Field Microscope

In this type of microscope the source of light is sunlight. The beam of light focused towards the condenser lens placed beneath the stage. This light from condenser passes through specimen, objective lens and to the eye through a second magnification lens known as eye piece. We see the objects in the light path because natural pigmentation or stains absorb light differently. A good quality microscope has the following features.

- Built-in illuminator
- Adjustable condenser with aperture diaphragm (contrast) control
- Mechanical stage
- Binocular eye piece

The condenser is used to focus light on the specimen through an opening in the stage. In bright field microscope the condenser usually contains an aperture diaphragm, a device that controls the diameter of the light beam coming up through the condenser. If diaphragm is nearly closed, the light comes straight up through the center of the condenser lens and contrast is high. On the other hand if the diaphragm is wide open the image is brighter and contrast is low.

1.7.1.1. Light Optimization: A light source should have wide dynamic range, to provide high intensity illumination at high magnification and lower intensity so that the user can view comfortably at low magnification. Now adjust the illumination so that the field is bright and adjust the condenser as close to the opening in the stage. Better to set the condenser to bright field.

- Start with the aperture diaphragm stopped down (High contrast).
- Now focus, locate and center the specimen.
- Starts with the lowest magnification objective lens
- For observing unstained specimen, use dark field mode or starts with high contrast (aperture diaphragm closed down)
- Now bring stage and objective together
- Now bring the specimen in focus
- After focusing the specimen, adjust contrast and intensity of illumination and adjust sufficient area of viewing.

1.7.1.2 Using the Bright Field Microscope

There should always be a cover slip on the specimen specially when we are using high magnification because higher magnification lens cannot focus through a thick glass slide, so very thin cover slip is used.

- Adjust the specimen slide manually with the help of holder clips
- Position the specimen, with the help of mechanical stage without touching it.

(i) Adjustment of eye piece and focus

Monocular vision is very simple to adjust but binocular eye pieces are much more difficult to adjust and are more sensitive to light and details. In binocular microscope look with the appropriate eye into the fixed eye piece and focus with the microscope focus knob then adjust the eyepiece.

(ii) Selection of objective lens

Generally 4 x objective lens is known as scanning lens and is used to locate the specimen.

Next use 10 x objective with 10 x ocular to get 100 x magnification. Typically high magnification lenses i.e. 40x and 100 x are used exclusively with oil to get best resolution.

Magnification should be step by step. Every time with higher power objective, refocusing and re-centering the specimen is required. Higher magnification lenses must be physically closer to the specimen itself.

(iii) Adjustment of illumination for the selected objective lens

When magnification is raised, the area of illuminated specimen becomes smaller and less light reaches the eyes so image darkens. Thus with higher magnification illumination should be increased.

1.7.1.3. Significance of Bright Field Microscopy

This type of microscopy is best to view stained or naturally pigmented specimens, but living specimens like bacteria, non-photosynthetic Protista or Metazoans may not be viewed in bright field microscope.

1.7.1.4. Application

Bright field microscopy is used for the study of:-

- Slides of stained bacteria (1000 x)
- Thin film of blood stains (400 x, 1000 x)
- Wet mounts, unstained pond water (40 x, 100 x, 400 x)
- Protists, algae and other microscopic plant materials (40x, 100 x, 400x)

1.7.2 Dark Field Microscopy

In dark field microscope the condenser of ordinary microscope is replaced by a dark field condenser. To view specimen in dark field, an opaque disc is placed underneath the condenser lens. So no direct light enters the objective, only light reflected or deflected from the specimen, enters the objective. Therefore the object appears bright and the background remains dark. It gives us better resolution than that of bright field viewing (Fig 1.18).

A higher intensity light is required because only reflected light reaches the objective. At low magnification (up to 100 x) the instrument may be set up, so that the light is reflected towards the viewer rather than passing through the object directly towards the viewer. To set dissecting microscope for Dark Field viewing the specimen should be placed over the opening

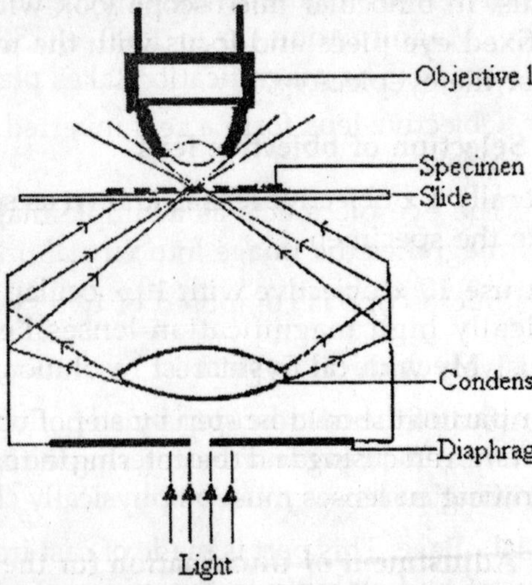

Fig. 1.18 Schemetic diagram of Dark Field Illumination

so that the light reflects only from surface. Cell suspension, flora and fauna of pond water may be observed well in dark field microscope. Instead of protists, metazoans, algae and other microscopic organisms are clearly visible in dark field microscope. At 100 x bacteria are visible.

1.7.2.1 Application

- To observe the object in liquid sample, debris and cell.
- To observe minute dust particles.
- To observe cell suspension and tissues.
- In initial examination of cell suspension such as yeast, bacteria, small protists etc.
- Cheek or vaginal epithelial cells, chloroplast, mitochondria and blood cells.
- Initial observation at low power of pond water samples, soil infusions etc.
- Motility of microorganism may be viewed in their cultures.

1.8 Compound Microscope

It is also known as bright field compound microscope or student microscope. It is the most commonly used microscope in the laboratory. In this microscope two lenses are used. One is eye piece and the other is objective. They are mounted on a hollow tube. The objective lens is close to the object and upper lens is known as eye piece. Magnification up to **1500 x** (1500 times) is possible by this microscope. The magnification takes place in two steps:-

1. Objective lens form a real inverted and magnified image of the object.
2. The eye piece acts as a simple magnifying glass which further magnifies the image into virtual image.

This microscope is composed of two systems (Fig. 1.19).

1.8.1 Mechanical System

This part of the microscope is made of objects which holds the optical system and provide a better shape to the instrument. It has the following parts:-

1.8.1.1 Base: This part is made of cast iron/ steel and provides a firm support and stability to the microscope. Generally it is horse shoe shaped.

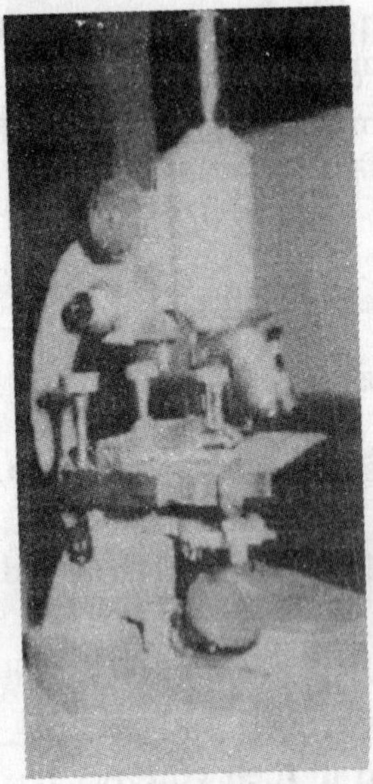

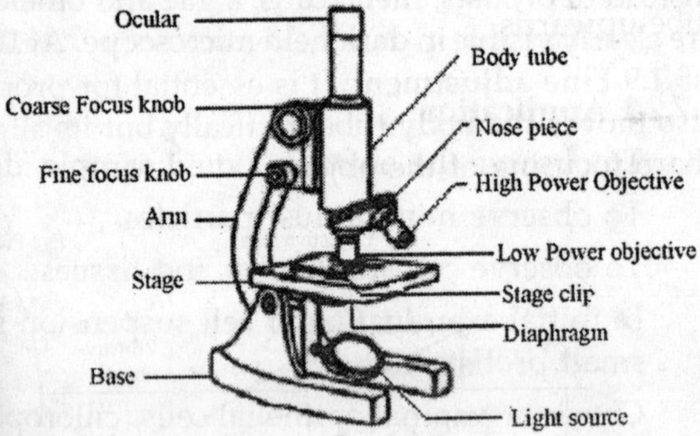

Fig. 1.19. Different parts of a compound microscope

1.8.1.2 Mirror: The mirror is fitted below the stage. It has concave and plane surfaces adhered back to back. It may be turned to any degree on its axis in order to reflect light beam to the objective lens.

1.8.1.3 Stage : It is a rectangular platform with its side attached to the arm. It holds the slide which admits light from the mirror through the condenser. A pair of clips are fitted on the stage which holds the slide in position over the stage.

1.8.1.4 Arm : It is a sort of handle which is movable and helps the viewer during observation. It supports the body tube and coarse adjustment.

1.8.1.5 Body tube: It bears objective lens at the lower end and eye piece at the upper end. Both objective and eye piece are placed at proper working distance. It possesses a rack and pinion arrangement to adjust the object for proper view.

1.8.1.6 Nose piece: In this part low and high power lenses are fitted.

1.8.1.7 Condenser: It is fitted between the mirror and stage. It is used for focusing light and adjusting the intensity of illumination.

1.8.1.8 Coarse adjustment: It helps in rapid focusing of the object. It is attached to the body tube. It moves the body tube vertically to adjust the proper distance from the object. The knob of coarse adjustment is large and its clockwise movement brings the body tube downwards, while its anti-clock-wise movement brings the body tube upwards.

1.8.1.9 Fine adjustment: It is essential for proper image formation. It also moves the body tube vertically but its slight revolution helps in sharp focusing of the object.

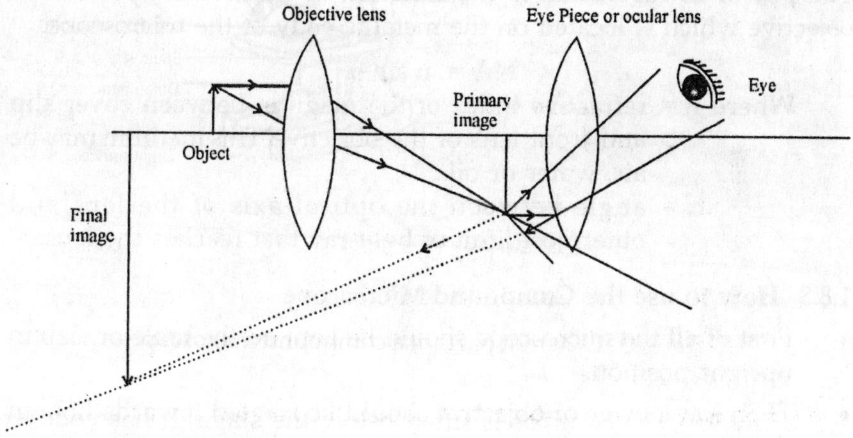

Fig. 1.20. Ray Diagram of working of compound microscope

1.8.2 Optical System

It consist of two series of lenses (Fig. 1.20).

1.8.2.1 Eye Piece or Ocular: This is the lens lying at the top of the body tube. It magnifies the real image formed by the objective. Thus we may observe a virtual image. Usually the distance between eye and virtual image is 250 mm, which is a normal view distance of the human eye. Eye piece lenses are loosely attached and may be replaced by lower or higher magnification. The eye pieces are generally 5 x, 6 x, 10 x, 15 x, 20 x, etc.

1.8.2.2 Objective: They are attached with the rotary noise piece. They also have lenses of different magnifications i.e. 10 x, 40 x, 45 x, 100 x and oil immersion. The greatest magnification obtained is 10 x 100 = 1000x. The quality of objective depends on:–

- Numerical aperture
- Magnification
- Focal length

- Working distance

All the above factors in appropriate ratio give the best resolution. 100 x objective is used with oil immersion. Actually light rays passing from object to objective lens are refracted away from perpendicular to cover slip, as they enter into air. But if oil of about same refractive index is placed between cover slip and objective lens, all the rays will enter the lens giving maximum numerical aperture and resolution.

The power of resolution is the function of numerical aperture of objective which is located on the metallic body of the microscope.

$$NA = n \sin \alpha$$

Where n = refractive index of the medium between cover slip and front lens of the objective. This medium may be air, water or oil.

α = angle between the optical axis of the lens and outermost limit of light ray that reaches the lens.

1.8.3 How to use the Compound Microscope

- First of all the microscope should be kept on the table or slab in upright position.
- Then low power of objective should be rotated towards hole in the stage.
- By using coarse adjustment, raise the body tube 2.5 - 3.0 cm above the stage.
- Now pass the light by opening the diaphragm of the condenser.
- Adjust the light rays through the hole by using plane mirror.
- Now put the specimen slide on the stage above the hole and observe through the left eye.

1.8.4 Focusing the Microscope

- Put the slide on the stage
- Bring the body tube in contact of cover glass with the help of coarse adjustment.
- Now view through eye piece and raise the body tube till the object becomes visible.
- Now focus the image with fine adjustment.

If object has to be focused under high power, first focus it under low power than replace it with high power. At high power, fine adjustment should be used for sharp focusing.

1.8.5 Care and precautions

A compound microscope should be handled with all care and precautions. Some of them are given as follows:-

- Take out the microscope from its case by holding its arm with one hand and support the base with the other hand.
- Do not lift the microscope carelessly with one hand.
- Now place the microscope on working table to prevent its accidental fall.
- Clean the lens surface and other parts of microscope with the help of soft cloth or lens paper before and after use.
- Avoid the tilting of microscope, keep it in upright position.
- While focusing light on object do not allow the direct sun rays to strike the mirror.
- Use plain mirror for natural daylight and concave for artificial light.
- The material to be observed should be properly mounted and covered with coverslip.
- Objective should not touch the coverslip.
- The 100 x objective lens should never be used without oil.
- After use, make the objective free and transfer it into its box to keep it in its position.

1.8.6 Application

- Compound microscope is widely used in bacteriology, biological and medicinal field.
- It can resolve the object as small as 5000A°.
- It is used to observe the histological slides of plant parts and animal tissues.
- To observe the formation of spindle in mitotic and meiotic cell division.
- To observe the algae, fungi, bacterial cell and their spores.
- To study the stomata in leaves and vascular bundle in their cells

1.9 Oil Immersion Microscopy

For the study of bacteria and other microorganisms oil immersion is used to get best resolution and higher magnification. **Robert B. Tolles (1824–1833)** used oil immersion objectives and invented an improved model which was termed as oil immersion microscope.

1.9.1 Basic Principal

When light passes from a material of one refractive index to material of another refractive index as from glass to air or from air to glass it bends. Light of different wavelength bends at different angles resulting in poor resolution of image. To overcome this difficulty a drop of oil (cedar wood oil or paraffin oil) with same refractive index (as glass) is put between cover slip and objective lens. This eliminates two refractive surfaces (i.e. air.) Thus a magnification of 1000 x or greater may be achieved with good resolution (Fig. 1.21).

1.9.2 Handling of Oil Immersion Microscope

For use of immersion oil, the objective lens must be designed specifically for the purpose.

- First focus the area of specimen to be observed with the dry lens.
- Place a drop of immersion oil on the cover slip over the target area.
- Carefully lower the oil immersion lens into the place.

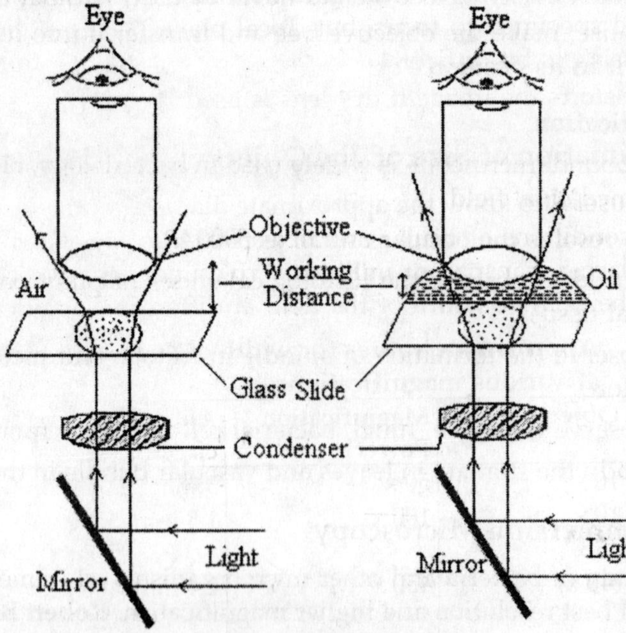

Fig. 1.21. Schematic representation of dry objective and oil immersion microscopy

- Carefully bring the lens in contact with cover slip.
- Now move the lens away from the specimen till best resolution is achieved.

When an object is bacteria or micro-organisms (1 - 2 micrometer in diameter) and it is fixed or dead we use oil immersion to get best resolution and better magnification.

1.9.3 Application

- Study of fixed and dead micro-organisms (bacteria, protozoans etc.)
- Study of individual bacteria in fixed condition.
- To study the details of striation of skeletal remains and muscles.

1.9.4 Limitation of Oil Immersion Microscope

- Oil must stay in contact during observation.
- A wet mount must be very secure to use oil.
- Oil immersion lenses are used only with oil but it is not applicable with dry lenses (400x lens).
- Lenses of very higher magnification must be brought very close to the specimen to focus, but focal plane being very shallow, focussing is bit difficult.
- Oil distorts the image if dry lens is used.

1.10 Estimation of Size of the Object with Microscope

It is quite useful to know the approximate diameter of the field under different conditions of ocular and objective. It is suggested that the student place a transparent millimeter rule under the objective and estimate the relative width of the field at different magnifications.

Table 1.2. Approximate values for width of the field of view seen at various magnifications

Ocular lens	Objective lens	Magnification Power	Approximate width of circular area viewed
5 x	10 x	50 x	3 mm (3000 μm)
10 x	10 x	100 x	1.5 mm (1500 μm)
10 x	45 x (40 x)	450 x	0.4 mm (400 μm)
10 x	Oil immersion 90 x (100 x)	900 x	0.15 mm (150 μm)

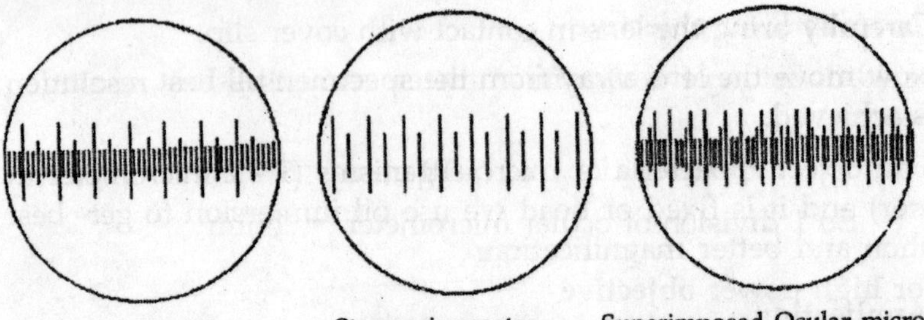

Ocular micrometer
A

Stage micrometer
(Scale 10μm = 0.1 mm)
B

Superimposed Ocular micrometer
over stage micrometer
C

Fig. 1.22. (A) Ocular micrometer (B) Stage micrometer (C) Superimposed ocular micrometer over stage micrometer

1.11 Micrometry

Micrometry is the measurements of an object by using the microscope. For this purpose ocular micrometer serve as a scale. An ocular micrometer consist of 100 divisions marked with 0-10.

This 1mm (1000 μm) distance is encircled and mounted by cover glass. Thus each division of stage micrometer is equal to 0.01mm or 10 μm. The distance of each division of stage micrometer becomes correspondingly enlarged under high power and oil immersion objective of the microscope (Fig. 1.22).

1.11.1 Procedure

- Place the ocular micrometer on the circular shelf. Now there will be seen scale lines of ocular micrometer in sharp focus.
- Mount the stage micrometer on the microscope stage and bring its scale in the center of microscopic field under a sharp focus.
- Adjust the scale of ocular micrometer and stage micrometer in such a way that the lines of the former superimpose up on the latter. Adjust in such a way that lines of the two coincide at one end of the microscopic field. Thus we may count how many division of ocular Micrometer support are equal to how many divisions of stage micrometer.
- Calculate the value of 1 division of ocular micrometer for different objective in the following way.

  Since 100 division of stage micrometer = 1 mm = 1000 μm

  So 1 division of stage micrometer = 0.01mm = 10μm

(i) For low power objective

Suppose 40 division of ocular micrometer = 60 division of stage micrometer

i.e.. 60 x 10 mm = 600µm

So 1 division of ocular micrometer = 15µm

(ii) For high power objective

Suppose 16 division of ocular micrometer = 6 division of stage micrometer

i.e. 6 x 10 mm = 60µm

So 1 division of ocular micrometer = 3.75µm

(iii) For oil immersion objective

Suppose 10 division of ocular micrometer = 2 division of stage micrometer

i.e.. 2 x 10 mm = 20µm

So 1 division of ocular micrometer = 2µm

- Replace the stage micrometer with the slide bearing microorganism whose measurements are to be taken e.g. total length of the chain of bacteria covers 18 division of ocular micrometer when examined.

1.12 Phase Contrast Microscopy

Phase contrast microscope was invented by **Fritz Zernike in 1953**. It is also a type of light microscope. Living, unstained and transparent objects are very difficult to view, as most of details of living cell is undetectable in bright field microscopy because there is too much contrast between structure with similar transparency. Also there is least or no pigmentation. However various organelles show wide variety in their refractive index. Thus they are distinguished under this microscope.

In order to understand the phase contrast microscopy, phase relationship of the wave should be understood. If light wave passes through the material of higher refractive index its amplitude is not affected, but a change in phase or retardation occurs. But if the same wave travels through a thicker object, its retardation is more prominent. This retardation is directly proportional to the differences between the refractive index of the object and surrounding medium and thickness of the object. Again if light wave passes through absorbent material, it shows both retardation and decrease in intensity.

1.12.1 Principle

The light from highly refractive structures bends further away from the center of the lens than light from less refractive structures and arrive about quarter of a wavelength out of phase. Light from most object passes through the center of the lens as well as to the periphery. If the light from an object to the edge of an objective lens is retarded a half wavelength and light to the center is not retarded at all, then the light rays are out of phase by half wavelength. At the time of image into focus these rays cancel each other (Fig. 1.23 & 1.24).

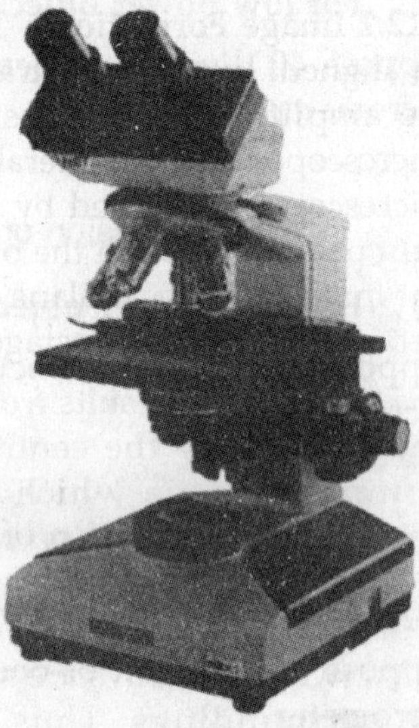

Fig. 1.23. Phase Contrast Microscope

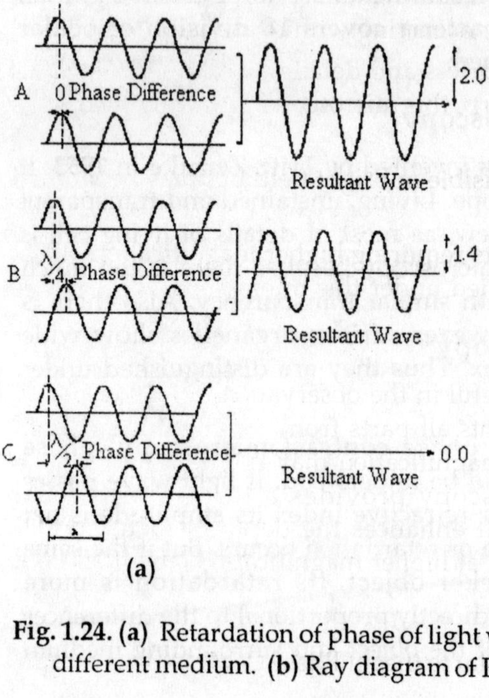

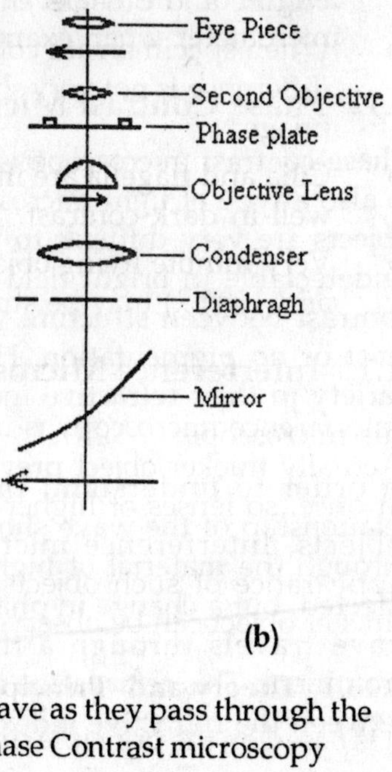

Fig. 1.24. (a) Retardation of phase of light wave as they pass through the different medium. **(b)** Ray diagram of Phase Contrast microscopy

1.12.2 Image Formation: To use phase contrast, the light path must be aligned. In phase contrast microscope the small phase differences are amplified and intensified so that they are detected. In this microscope the most lateral light passing through the objective of the microscope is retarded by ¼ wavelength with respect to the central light passing through the object. It is done by an annular phase plate put in the back focal plane of the objective. An annular diaphragm is also placed in the sub-stage condenser.

The phase effect results from the interference between the geometric image given by the central part of the objective and the lateral diffracted image which has been retarded or advanced to ¼ wavelength, negative or bright contrast is produced as a result of addition of two sets of rays. In this condition the object appear brighter than the surroundings. On the other hand positive contrast results when two sets of rays are subtracted. The object appears darker than the surroundings. Thus minute changes in the object due to interference of rays changes the amplitude and is responsible for image formation.

1.12.3 Advantages and Application of Phase Contrast Microscopy

- This Microscopy is very useful for the study of living cells, cell culture and other events, occurring within the cell.
- When specimen are colourless and details are so fine that colour difference is not very sharp, this microscope gives bright contrast image.
- Cilia and flagella are invisible in bright field but may be studied well in dark contrast.
- Very minute living objects requiring higher magnification (400 x and 1000 x) may be studied under this microscope.

1.13 Interference Microscopy

Interference microscopy is useful in the observation of thicker object. Actually thicker object prevents all parts from coming into focus all at once, so lenses of higher magnification may not be used for such objects. Interference microscopy provides a three-dimensional appearance of such objects. It enhances the depth of focus so that thicker object can be observed at higher magnification (about 1500 x).

1.13.1 Theory and Principle

It is based on the principle similar to that of Phase Contrast Microscope.

Here the light from the incandescent source is passed through a polarizer, vibrates in a single plane. This beam of light is then split-up into two beams with the help of semi-reflecting mirror/prism. One beam is sent through the object, other bypasses the object. The beam passing through the object is retarded, both the beams are recombined with the help of mirror. (Fig 1.25)

This interference of the beams makes the object visible or distinguishable. At optimum contrast, we can get distinct, three-dimensional image of the object.

1.13.2 Application

- By using interference microscopy we can measure dry weight of cellular structure, thickness of the object, water contents etc.
- Small or continuous changes in refractive index may be elected.
- Edges of the cell or nucleus may be viewed under this microscope.
- This microscope enhances the depth of focus so that thicker specimen can be observed at higher magnification.

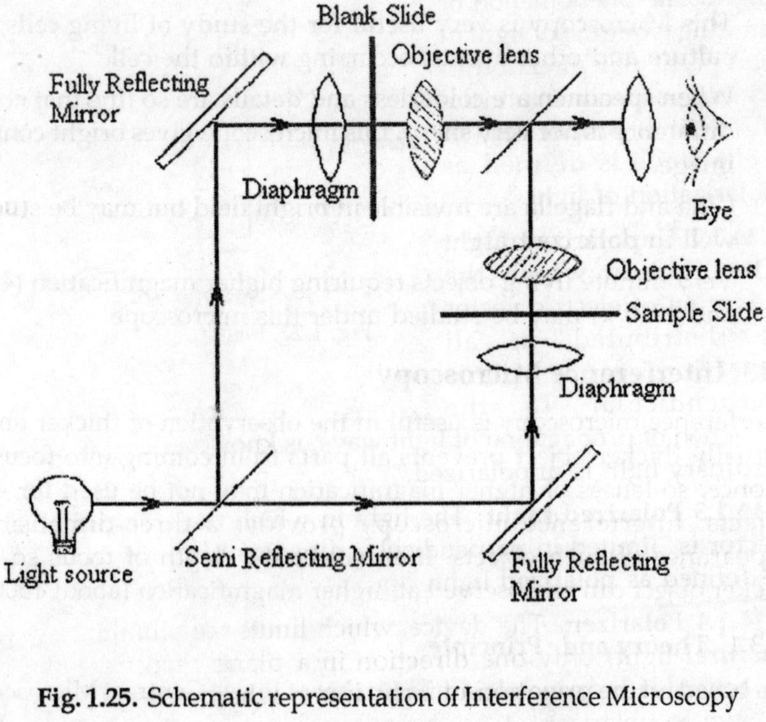

Fig. 1.25. Schematic representation of Interference Microscopy

1.14 Polarizing Microscope

Polarization Microscope was invented by **Talboot in 1839.** It differs from the ordinary microscope in having two additional devices known as polarizer and analyzer, both may be prepared from Polaroid film or Nicol film of calcite. The Nicol prism polarizer is mounted below the substage condenser and analyzer above the objective lens of the microscope (Fig. 1.26).

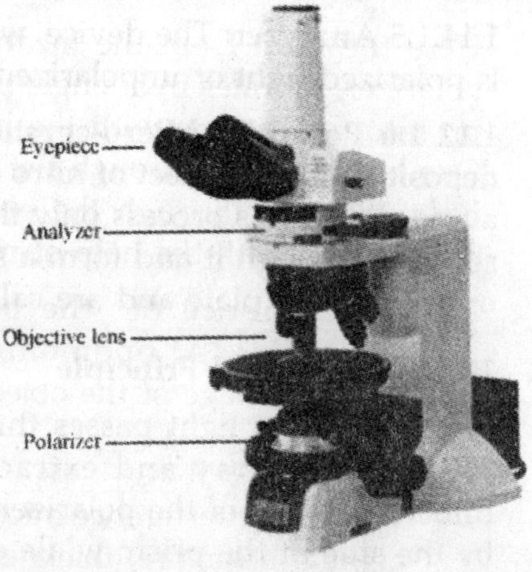

Fig. 1.26. Polarization Microscope

It is important to know the salient features of light in order to understand the working of polarizing microscope.

1.14.1 Salient Features of Light

1.14.1.1 Polarization of Light: The phenomenon of limiting vibration of light in one particular direction in a plane perpendicular to the direction of propagation of light wave is defined as polarization of light.

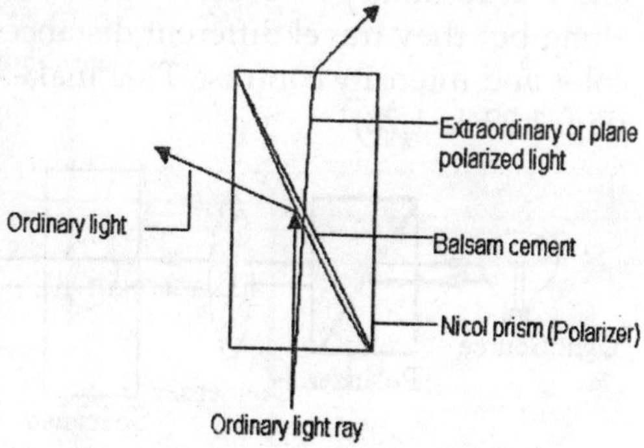

Fig. 1.27. Principle of Polarization Microscope

1.14.1.2 Unpolarized Light The light in which the vibration of electric vector is distributed in all direction in a plane perpendicular to the direction of propagation of light wave, is known as unpolarized light. Ordinary light is unpolarized.

1.14.1.3 Polarized Light The light in which the vibration of electric vector is limited in perpendicular direction of propagation of light, is defined as polarized light.

1.14.1.4 Polarizer: The device, which limits the vibration of light in (natural light) only one direction in a plane perpendicular to the direction of propagation of light wave, when passed through it, is known as polarizer.

1.14.1.5 Analyzer: The device, which detects whether any given light is polarized light or unpolarized light, is known as analyzer.

1.12.1.6 Polaroid: Micro-crystal of iodo- sulphate or quinine are deposited on thin sheet of nitro cellulose and then squeezed through a fine slit. In this process only the crystals having axis parallel to the slit pass through it and form a sheet. These sheets are kept between ordinary glass plate and are called polaroid.

1.14.2 Theory and Principle

When ordinary light passes through Nicol prism it splits into two rays ordinary ray and extraordinary ray. Both rays strike the cemented plane of the polarizer obliquely. Ordinary ray is reflected by the side of the prism while extraordinary ray passes through the prism with little deviation. It is plane polarized light (i.e. vibrate in one direction). Now this light when it enters through specimen splits again into ordinary and extraordinary ray but both are polarized and traveling in the same direction at different velocities. Further these rays enters into the analyzer and are broken up into ordinary and extraordinary rays. Here again only extraordinary ray continues along but they travel different distances and thus cause interference, color and intensity contrast. That makes the specimen distinguishable (Fig. 1.27 & 1.28).

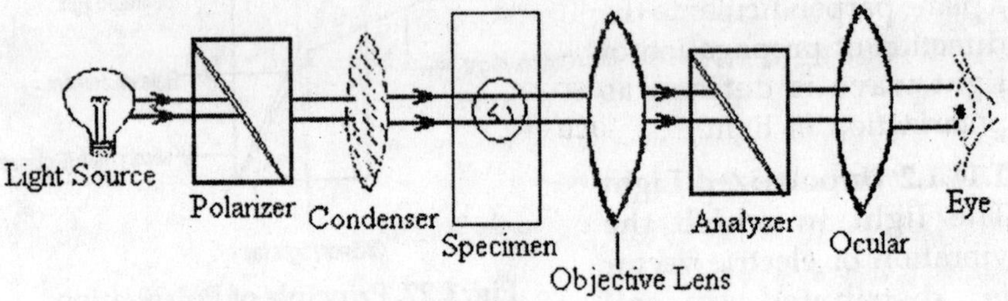

Fig. 1.28. Different components of a Polarization Microscope

1.15 Fluorescence Microscopy

Fluorescence Microscope was introduced by **Coons in 1941**. There are many substances which emit light of their own known as natural fluorescent substance e.g. starch, cellulose few fat and protein etc. but the substances which are not naturally fluorescent may be made fluorescent by using fluorescent dyes. It involves the use of U.V. light and quartz condenser in place of ordinary condenser because it does not absorb U.V. light.

1.15.1 Theory and Principle

Certain compounds which are fluorescent, they absorb light energy of shorter wave length e.g. UV light and re-emit the light of longer wavelength like visible light. This phenomenon is called fluorescence and is used in fluorescence microscopy. Fluorescence may be produced at any wavelength and fluorescent light is always of longer wavelength than the absorbed exciting light, and thus it is not monochromatic.

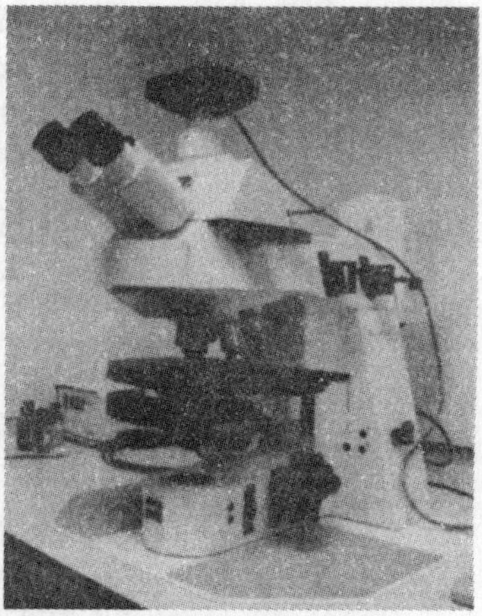

Fig. 1.29. Fluorescence Microscope

1.15.2 Instrumentation

The fluorescent microscope is an ordinary microscope equipped with two special filters. A primary filter (excitation) is placed in-between the light source and specimen. This filter transmits radiation with desired wavelength that matches the fluorescing material.

The second filter is known as barrier filter placed between specimen and eye. This filter separates the much brighter and excitation wavelength light from reaching viewer's retina and allows only the light of lower energy and long wavelength. Thus fluorescing material becomes visible in the microscope as a shine against dark background. (Fig 1.29 & 1.30)

The arrangement of optical components in a fluorescent microscope are as follows :-

1. Illumination source
2. Collector lens
3. Excitation filter
4. Sub stage mirror (Dichromic mirror)
5. Field lens and diaphragm
6. Condenser
7. Specimen (fluorescent)
8. Objective lens
9. Barrier filter (Long wave length filter)

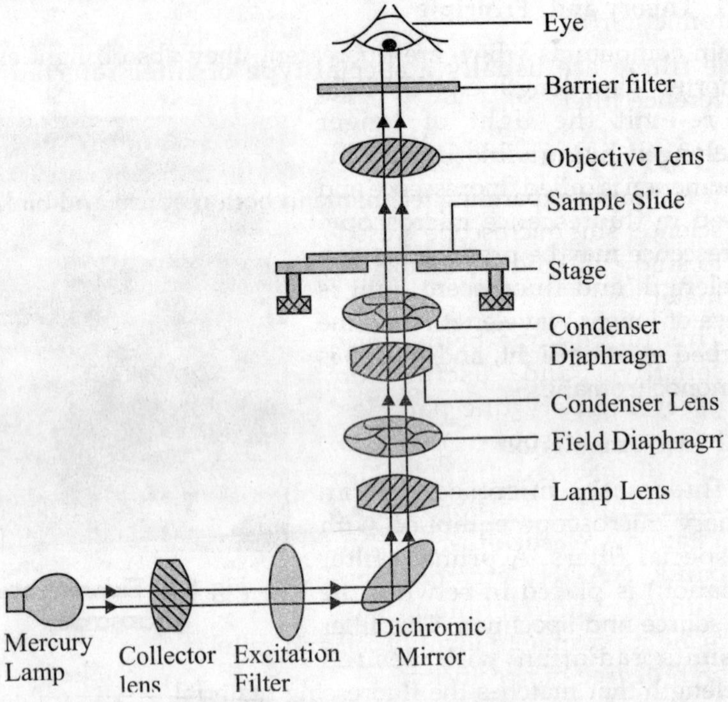

Fig. 1.30. Ray Digıaıı ur Fluorescence Microscope

10. Ocular lens
11. Observer eye or camera

The UV light is obtained from lamp source. It falls on excitation filter through collector lens. Excitation filter allows only the light of required wavelength through it. This light reaches the specimen through reflector and condenser lens and cause fluorescence in the specimen. Another filter called barrier filter is placed beyond objective lens. It allows only light of larger wavelength.

Since the image is formed entirely by light emerging from the specimen, fluorescent object appears as a bright image in an uniformly dark background.

Excitation Filter: In order to select the excitation wavelength, an excitation filter is placed in the excitation path just prior to the dichromic mirror.

Emission Filter: For selecting the specific wavelength of the light emitted from the sample an emission filter is placed beneath the dichromic mirror.

These filters are usually a special type of filter referred to as interference filter.

1.15.3 Application

- It is a rapid expanding technique in both medical and biological science. This microscope is used to study all kinds of biological materials.
- This microscope being very sensitive and useful for observing very fine particles and very thick objects may also be observed. Instead of collagen fiber, Porphyrin, Vitamin A, elasticnfiber, protein band, $NADH_2$ etc. may be studied. This technique has made it possible to identify cell and cellular components with a high degree of specificity.

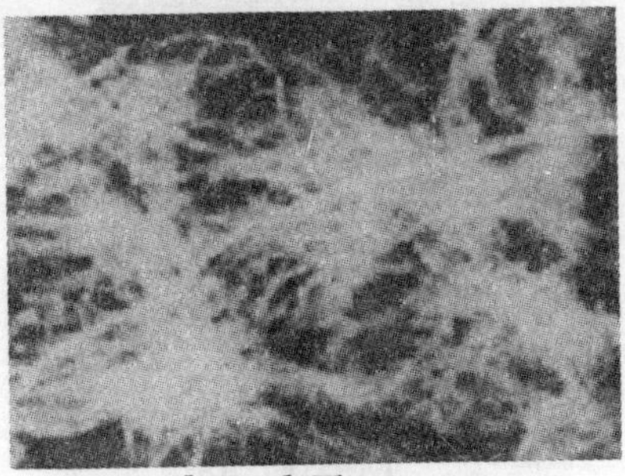

Image through Fluorescence Microscope

- Certain antibodies and diseases, impurities in inorganic material can be detected with the help of fluorescence microscope.
- This technique is useful in the investigation of structural abnormalities in materials (cracks, pores, welds) and confirming presence of adhesives in cemented applications.
- This microscope is widely used for sample analysis of various forensic exhibits e.g. ink, biological fluids, drugs etc.
- This microscopy is very useful in diagnostic analysis of microbiology in which bacteria are combined with labelled antibodies (fluorescent dyes).

1.16 Stereoscopic Binocular Microscope

This microscope was designed by **Greenaugh in 1897** and commonly known as dissecting binocular microscope. It is very useful for low magnification and fine mounting. The peculiar feature of this microscope is that it provides three dimensional (3D) visualization of the object. So, it is used for the examination of certain physical evidences in forensic science e.g. disputed documents, fibres etc. It provides magnification of 10 x to 25 x.

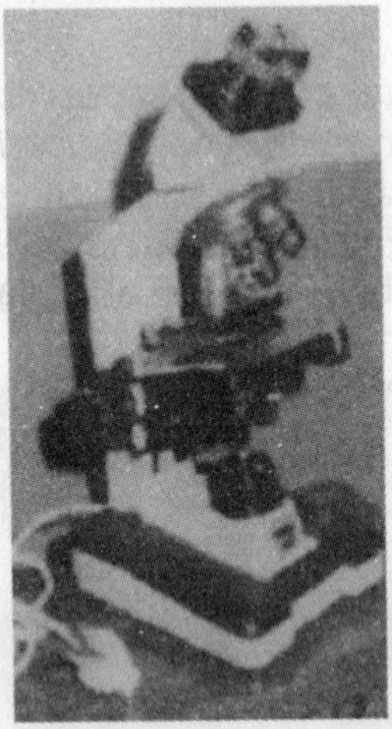

Fig. 1.31. Stereoscopic Microscope

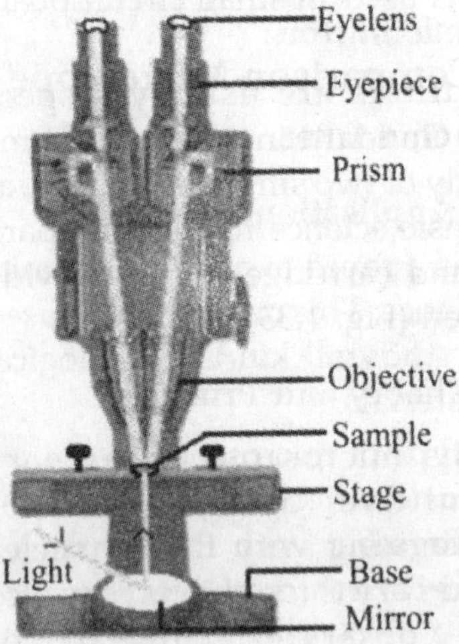

Fig. 1.32. Different components of Stereoscopic Microscope

1.16.1 Theory and Principle

The stereoscopic microscope is light illuminated but it is designed differently and serves for different purposes. Actually there are two eye pieces which serves as a complete microscope. Both the eye pieces are mounted at an angle of 15° to 16° and provide different viewing angles to the right and left eye. This microscope provides greater working distance and depth of field. Both the qualities are inversely co-related with resolution. The higher the resolution (magnification) the smaller the depth of field and working distance. It has a magnification up to 100x. The resolution is maximally in the order of an average of 10x objective in a compound microscope, and often much lower (Fig. 1.31 & 1.32).

Both objective and eyepieces focus on the same area of object, but from different angles. Prism mounted between each objective and eyepiece helps to form erect image. It provides stereoscopic view of the object due to reflected light.

1.16.2 Uses of Stereomicroscope

- It is used to study the surface of solid specimen.
- Used for closed work such as sorting.
- Used for dissection of smaller animals, insects etc.
- It is also very useful in microsurgery.
- It is used in watch making and repair.

- It is used in small circuit board manufacture and repair.

1.17 Comparison Microscope

Calvin Goddard invented the comparison microscope. Sometimes in the study of two similar specimen, a comparison is required, especially in forensic science for the comparison of striation and pin mark on bullet and cartridge. It can provide 1000 times greater image of the specimen (Fig. 1.33).

1.17.1 Theory and Principle

In this type of microscope two compound microscopes are joined together with the help of a series of mirrors. Objective lenses are joined independently giving separate view of the standard and sample specimen. When the viewer observes through eyepiece, a circular field divided into two equal halves by a fine line is visible. Comparison specimens are mounted on the right and left halves of the field of the stage and observer can view both of the specimens together at right and left half of the field

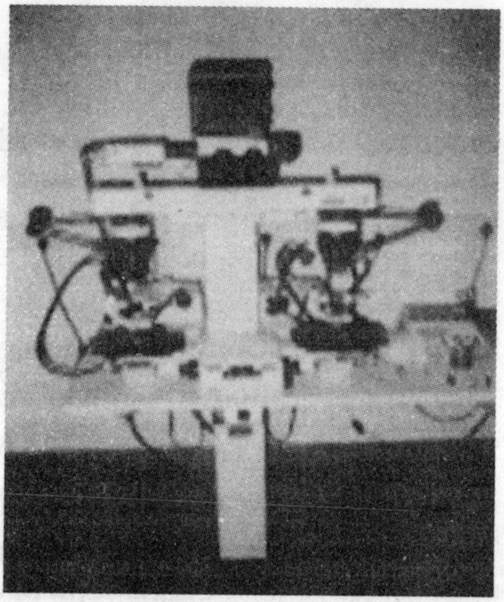

Fig. 1.33. Comparison Microscope

This type of microscopy provides fine and comparative details of the specimen.

1.17.1 Application

This type of microscope is basically used in forensic science laboratory for the following purpose:-

- Comparison of striation and pin mark on the bullet and cartridge respectively.
- Comparison of glass fragments, paint chips, cut marks etc.
- Comparison of nail striation.
- Comparison of morphological feature of hair and fibers.

- Comparison of known and unknown insects, small animals and plant materials.

1.18 Confocal Microscopy

Confocal microscopy is a very useful tool for the study of living cells, cell organelles as well as fixed tissue and cells. At very low resolution, confocal microscopy can produce a three-dimensional (3D) image of fluorescent tagged gene products to determine their distribution in the cell during different stages of cell cycle. Such information allows detailed study of cell and organelle biology.

1.18.1 Basic Principle

In confocal microscopy, scattered, reflected or fluorescent light is eliminated from the out of focus plane by keeping the illumination, specimen and detector at the same focus, so they are confocal. The source of illumination is Laser rays which provide faster scanning. When a Laser beam of monochromatic light is condensed as a small spot, it is scanned by mirror and image is formed on computer screen.

1.18.2 Types of Confocal Microscope

There are basically two forms of confocal microscope :

1.18.2.1 Confocal Laser Scanning Microscope (CLSM)

1.18.2.2 Multiphoton Laser Scanning Microscope (MPLSM)

These two forms are very similar at the illumination side. MPLSM is more sensitive than CLSM because all the light generated to make an image is sent directly to the photon multiplier tube. But in CSLM there is a pin hole required to select the light from the focus plane. In this there is considerable loss of signal in the optics required to direct the light to the pin hole.

MPLSM gives sharper image than CLSM because of the lack of extraneous light and improved geometry of detection. In MPLSM the photon multiplier tube can be placed very close to the specimen whereas CLSM has all the intervening optics and the pin hole.

1.18.3 Basic Methodology

In this microscope LASER* is used to provide excitation of light. It reflects off a dichromic mirror then hit on two scanning mirrors, these mirrors scan the LASER across the sample. In the sample the dyes get

---

* LASER-(Light amplification by stimulated emission of radiation).

fluoresce and emit light that is descanned by the same scanning mirrors. The emitted light passes through the dichromic mirror and is focused on to the pin hole that is measured by a detector (i.e. Photo multiplier tube) attached to the computer. Instead of complete image we can observe only one point of the sample. (Fig 1.34)

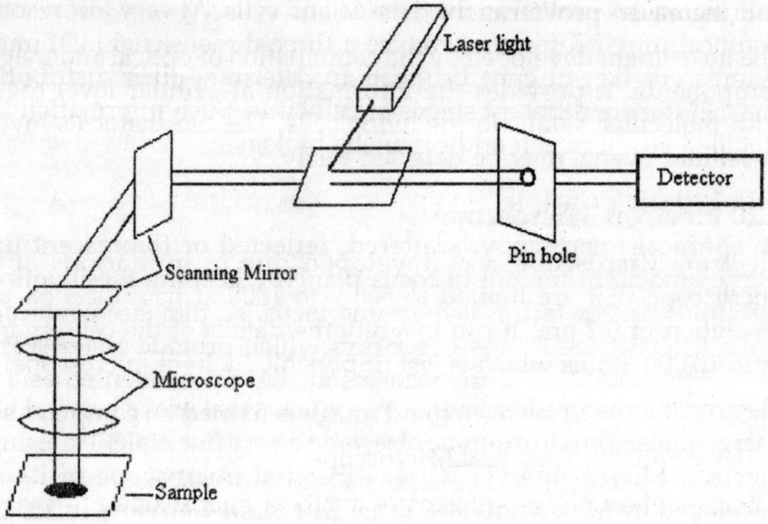

Fig. 1.34. Schematic Representation of Confocal Microscope with their Different Parts

1.18.4 Application of Confocal Microscopy

- This microscopy is very useful for visualization of cellular protein, lipids, nucleic acids and other cell organelles.
- This microscopy is very useful for watching the cellular protein binding with substrate in real time with sub micrometer.
- The state of ionic fluctuation e.g. Ca or Mg within the cell may be observed.
- It provides three dimensional (3D) image of the sample due to scanning of very thin section.

1.19 Magnetic Resonance Microscopy

With the advancement of tools and techniques in biological sciences, Confocal or Optical microscopy and Magnetic Resonance Microscopy have become an important tool for cellular research. Actually optical microscopy requires only the expression or uptake of fluorescent labeled molecule for detection. But magnetic resonance microscopy provides quantitative information like metabolic concentration, chemical shifts, spin coupling and diffusion constant etc. Such types of quantitative estimations are useful in the detection of cellular events such as tumor formation, programmed cell death (apoptosis) necrosis and increased proliferation.

The instrument developed by the combination of optical and magnetic components. It provides the information at cellular level together with molecular details in the living cells. The biochemicals involved in cellular events may be detected easily.

1.20 Electron Microscope

Electron Microscope was developed due to limitations of light microscope that are limited to 500 x to 1000 x magnification and a resolution of 0.2 μm. It can magnify the details of the cell organelles upto 10,000 x plus which is just impossible by light microscope.

Electron microscope is scientific instruments that uses a beam of highly energetic electrons to examine objects on a very fine scale. Transmission Electron Microscope (TEM) was the first microscope of its kind, developed by **Max Knoll** and **Ernst Ruska, in Germany in 1931.** The first scanning electron microscope (SEM) was developed in **1942.**

Electron Microscope uses a focused beam of electrons instead of light to image. In TEM the charged particle i.e. a stream of electrons is formed by the electron gun and accelerated towards the specimen using a positive electrical potential. This stream is confined and focused using metal aperture and magnetic lenses into a thin focused, monochromatic beam. This beam is focused on to the sample using magnetic lenses. Interaction occurs inside the irradiated sample, affecting the electron beam. These interactions and effects are detected and transformed into an image, which may be taken on photographic plate. There are two types of Electron Microscope depending on the type of analysis and quality of image formation.

1.20.1 Transmission Electron Microscope

In this type of microscopy electrons are transmitted through the specimen and the differential scattering of electrons are viewed on a fluorescent screen or a photographic plate. In this the image is formed by using electron beam instead of light beam.

1.20.1.1 Principle

In this type of microscopy a large area of specimen is illuminated by a homogenous beam. The emerging beam is refracted by a system of imaging lens to form a real and magnified image on photosensitive plate. Here the specimen or matter is radiated with high velocity particles (electrons). The wavelength of particle radiation is as follows:-

$$\lambda = h / mv$$

Where h = Plank's universal quantum number
m = mass of the particle
v = velocity of the particle

The resolution power of TEM is 0.025A° but practically it is 2.5A°.

1.20.1.2 Image Formation

In electron microscope the scattering of electrons depend on the atomic numbers of the atoms present in the object. Most of the atoms that constitute the biological structures e.g. C, H, N, O are of low atomic number. Therefore, to increase the contrast, heavy atoms such as Osmium tetra oxide and lead ion, which act as electron stains are employed that combine selectively with certain region of the specimen and is responsible for image formation.

1.20.1.3 Instrumentation

In TEM there is an electron source at the top of the microscope (not at the bottom), an air tight iron cast, one meter long column is attached for vacuum creation in it. It allows to follow down the electron. Vacuum pumps are placed below and behind the column.

Different components of the microscope are arranged as follows:-

(i) Electron gun
(ii) Electron lens
(iii) Specimen
(vi) Image forming system

(i) **Electron gun** : In TEM illumination system consists of **electron beam** or **cathode**. It is a small tungsten wire maintained at 2500K by 2W of AC or DC power. Its functions are as follows:-

- A positive electrical potential is applied to the anode.

- The tungsten wire is heated in order to produce the electrons.
- The electrons are then accelerated by the positive potential down the column.
- A negative electrical potential (-500 V) is applied to the whenelt cap.
- Electron move towards the anode.
- A collection of electrons occurs in the space between the filament tip and wehnlet cap. This collection is called space charge.
- Electrons at the bottom of the surface charge (nearest the anode) can exit the gun area through a small hole in the whenelt cap.
- These electrons then move down the column and help in image formation.

(ii) **Electron Lenses :** All the lenses are magnetic or electron lenses from the condenser to objective. Negatively charged electrons are deflected by electromagnetic field. So only positive lenses are possible in TEM. Lenses of very short focal length are constructed by concentrating the magnetic field on axis. Actually these are circular electromagnets capable of producing precise circular magnetic field in a specified region. The field acts like an optic lens having the same focal length, angle of divergence and errors. They are used to focus and steer electron in an electron microscope.

(iii) **Specimen :** It allows the proper placement of specimen in electrical path. The thickness of the specimen should be 2-10 $\mu g/cm^2$ i.e. the specimen should be ultra thin. The electron stains are heavy metal salts such as vanadium, lead, uranium, osmium etc. that combine with specific site of cell organelles. The specimen is embedded in epoxy resin which is very hard and has same elements as that of specimen. Specimen is supported by very thin (about 20 nm thick) electro translucent film of low atomic number, which itself is supported by a grid of gold, palladium or copper.

(a) **Sample Preparation:** Sample viewed under electron microscope may be prepared by the following way (Fig. 1.35):

1. **Cryofixation :** In this method specimen is freezed very rapidly at liquid nitrogen temperature (-196°C)so that all the water forms vitreous (non- crystalline) ice. It is the best method for specimen preservation but not applied for all specimens.

2. **Fixation :** In fixation, to make sample more realistic it is treated with chemicals such as Glutaraldehyde- for hardening, Osmium teteraoxide - for stabilizing protein and lipids etc.

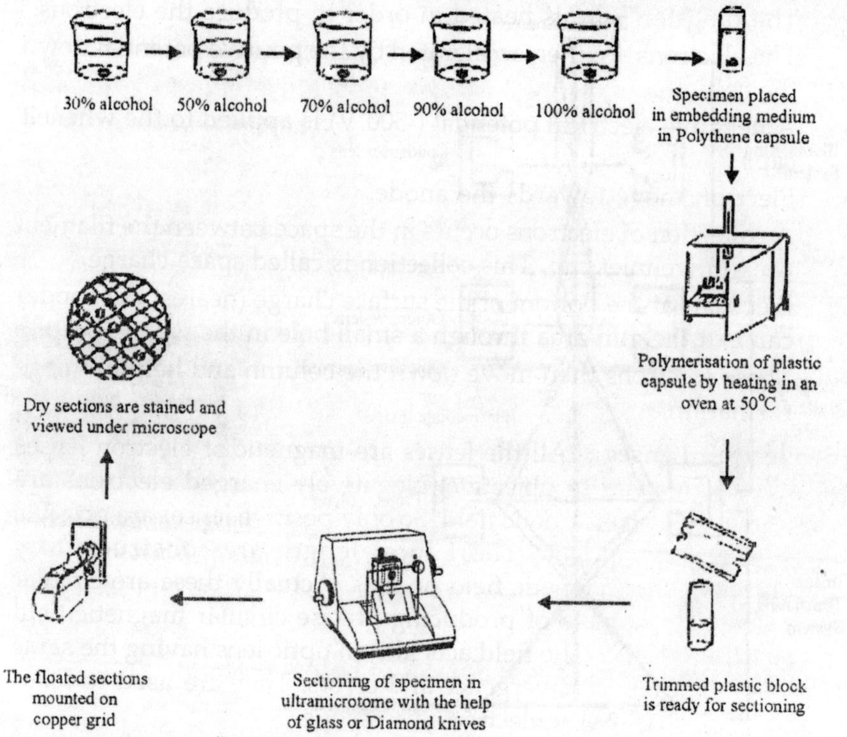

Fig. 1.35. Sample preparation for Transmission Electron Microscopy

3. Dehydration: To remove all the water from the specimen it is passed through different grades of ethyl alcohol or acetone. Acetone has an advantage over ethanol that it does not react with OsO_4, remains in the tissue. The common procedure of dehydration is as follows:-

1. Wash the tissue
2. 30 % alcohol ---- 8 - 10 minutes
3. 50 % alcohol ---- 8 - 10 minutes
4. 70 % alcohol ---- 8 - 10 minutes
5. 90 % alcohol ---- 8 - 10 minutes
6. 100 % alcohol ---- 8 - 10 minutes

4. Embedding: Embedding materials (resin) is used to support the tissue for sectioning. It includes Araldite, Epon, Methacrylate etc. Embedding is most commonly done in polythene capsule and it is placed in an oven for 12 hrs at 50° C for polymerization.

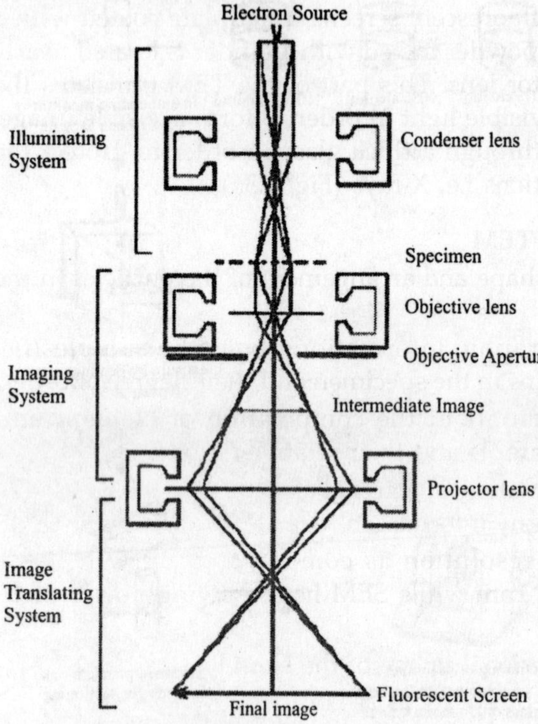

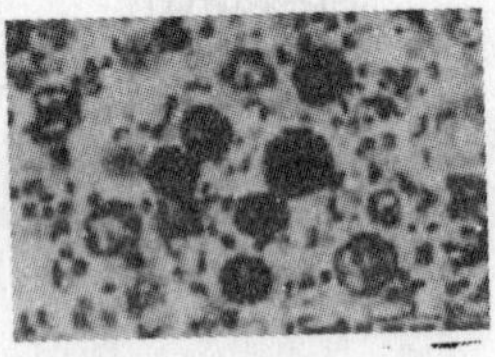
Image through Electron Microscope

Fig. 1.36 Different Components of an Eletron Microscope.

5. Sectioning: The thin slices of specimen may be obtained by sectioning it in ultramicrotome, containing diamond or glass knives. Then it is placed in 10-20% acetone where it floats in the form of a ribbon. After that it is mounted on copper grid.

6. Staining: Staining is used for reflection of electron in specimen which give contrast between different structures. Stains contain heavy metal such as lead and uranium.

7. Ion beam milling: It is used to produce electron transparent membrane in a specific region of the sample. It is done by firing it with ions (gallium ions) or spray with organic materials (collodion).

(vi) Image Forming System: Electron transmitted through the specimen enter the objective and form image. An objective lens of 100x in combination of intermediate lens of 25x is used. The final image is projected by a projector lens. The voltage of current running through the lens control the magnification. The magnification of image depends on position of fluorescent screen. A flat plate coated with a thin layer of fluorescent powder mixed with a binder is located nearly 30 cm below the projector lens. This part of the TEM translates the energy of electron into visible light in order to form a visible image. The image is observed through a thick glass in order to protect the eye from harmful radiations i.e. X-rays (Fig. 1.36).

1.20.1.4 Application of TEM

- It reveals the size, shape and arrangement of the particles in the specimen.
- It gives crystallographic information about the sample (i.e. arrangement of atoms in the specimen and their degree of order)
- It gives information about the composition of element and compound in the sample and their relative ratios.
- It allows the examination of internal structure of the cell while SEM does not give any information regarding internal structure.
- TEM has a better resolution as compared to SEM. It has a resolving power of 1nm while SEM has resolving power of 10 nm.
- It provides 2 dimensional image of the sample.
- TEM has greater depth of focus as compared to SEM.

1.20.2 Scanning Electron Microscopy

SEM was first constructed in **1960 by Knoll et al.** It produces the magnified image by using electron instead of light. The beam of electrons from tungsten filament are formed into very fine probe, this electron beam scan the surface of the object resulting in emission of secondary electron due to excitation of primary electron beam. These scanning electrons are collected by positively charged grid and signals are sent to the cathode tube of monitor. It is a comparatively new instrument and has a different principle than that of electron microscope.

1.20.2.1 Theory and Principle

SEM visualize the structure by bombarding the specimen with a scanning electron beam and then by collecting slow moving secondary electrons that are generated by specimen. These are collected, amplified and displayed on the computer screen. In the electron microscopy electrons are focused on the specimen from electron gun by using a positive electrical potential. As these electron beam strike on the specimen several types of signals are produced. Some of the

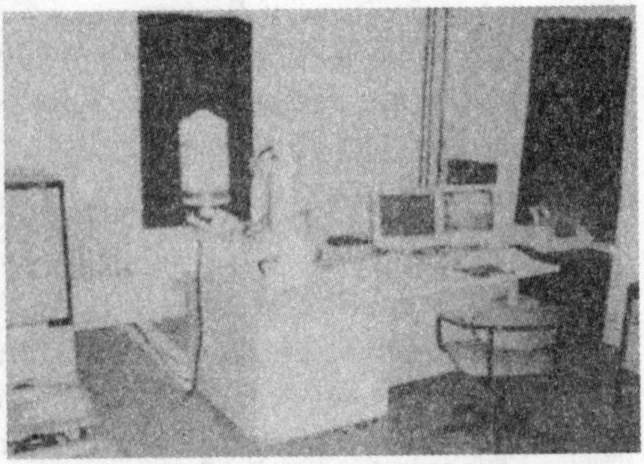

Fig. 1.37. Scanning Electron Microscope

electrons are bounced back and are called backscattered electrons but some collide with the orbital electron in the atom of the specimen resulting in the production of secondary electrons from the specimen. At the same time due to rearrangement of the electron characteristic X-rays are produced. Secondary electrons are detected to obtain the image of the specimen. It reflects the surface topography of the specimen (Fig. 1.37).

1.20.2.2 Specific features

SEM is characterized by a great depth of focus and permits a direct observation of a surface of even a bulky specimen. SEM occupies the magnification in the range of **20 x to 20,000 x.** The specimen up to 15 mm in diameter and 10mm in thickness can be examined by using this technique. It provides resolution of **3.5 nm to 10 nm**.

1.20.2.3 Instrumentation

Scanning Microscope is composed of various systems and devices for the proper investigation of the specimen. It includes the following parts (Fig. 1.39):-

(i) Electron Gun: A thermionic electron gun is used in electron microscope. It is composed of wehnelt cap and filament. The filament (cathode) is heated until a stream of electrons is produced. A positive electrical potential is applied to the anode to accelerate electrons and make electron beams. A collection of electrons occurs in the space between the filament tip and wehnelt cap. This collection is called space charge. The electrons at the

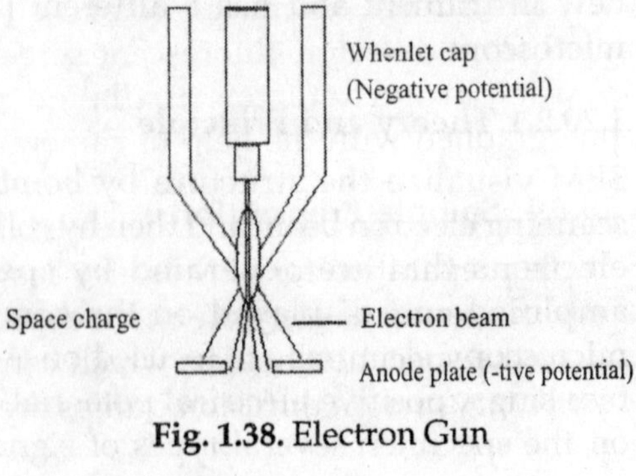

Fig. 1.38. Electron Gun

bottom of the space charge (nearest to the anode) can exit the gun area through the small (<1mm) hole in the wehnelt cap for producing image. (Fig 1.38)

(ii) Electromagnetic Lens: Electronagnetic lens consists of condenser lens and objective lens. The function of these lenses is to reduce the electron gun into electron probe and this electron probe is irradiated on to the surface of specimen to form surface view of the specimen.

(iii) Astigmatism correction device : It has two sets of electromagnets each with a pair of four poles and corrects the electron probe into true roundness for obtaining a clear and sharp image. Due to astigmatism blurred image is formed.

(iv) Scanning system: It is composed of a deflector coil to deflect electron vertically and horizontally, to operate over the surface of specimen and the scanning circuit. It controls magnification by changing the scanning width over the surface of specimen and also the scanning speed.

(v) Specimen Stage: Specimen stage can move the specimen placed in vacuum in high precision so as to allow the observation of each specific position of specimen.

(vi) Vacuum system : This system consists of oil rotary pump for roughing, oil diffusion pump for high vacuum evacuating and circuit to control the vacuum sequence. It evacuates the chamber in order to avoid scattering of electron beam. This system is fully autonomous.

(vii) Detector: It is composed of scintillator and photo multiplier tube. The signal intensity of secondary electron and backscattered electron emitted from specimen are converted to intensity of light by scintillator, and then converted into electrical signal and amplified with photomultiplier tube. This amplified signal is sent to the recorder.

(viii) Recording System: It is composed of control circuit for electrical signal from detector, fluorescent screen and camera. The image is obtained from detector displayed on fluorescent screen and photographed with the help of camera for recording purpose.

1.20.2.4 Sample Preparation

Sample preparation for SEM is also easy and much simpler than that of the conventional electron microscope. Specimen is mounted on the end of the specimen holder, which can be removed through the air lock. Rotary and oil diffusion pumps are used to evacuate the system.

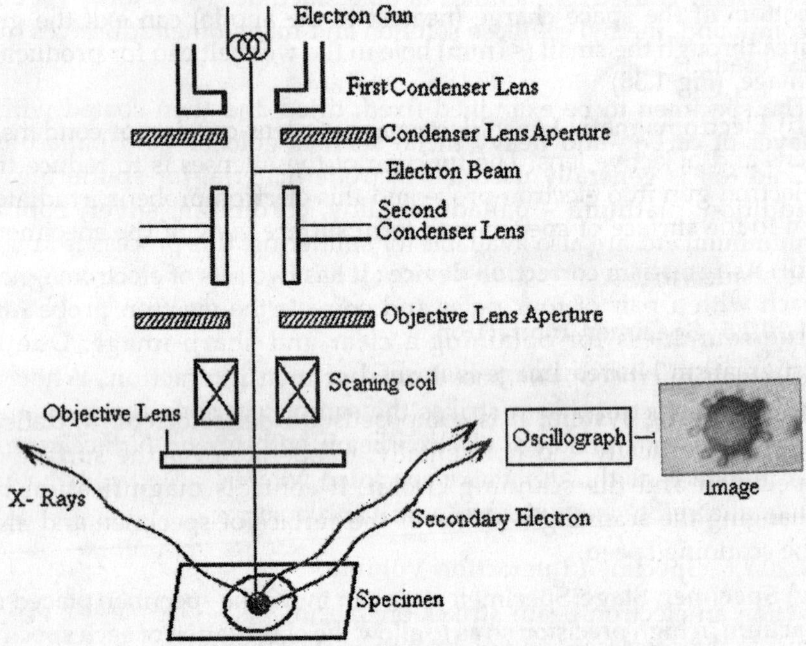

Fig. 1.39. Schematic Representation of Scanning Electron Microscope

The specimen can be shifted or rotated by X,Y axis and rotation control about the center of the field of view and can be therefore viewed from various sides. To study under electron microscope the sample should be prepared by taking the following points into consideration.

- The specimen should be shaped so as to fit the specimen holder.
- The specimen should be secured firmly in the specimen holder.
- The conductivity between the specimen and specimen particle should be proper.

After a proper treatment sample may be examined under the microscope. The sample to be examined may be radioactive, wet sample, magnetic material or gas-absorbing specimen. These types of samples contaminate the inside of the instrument column and also may cause astigmatism and deviation of electron probe in the magnetic field so that satisfactory micrographs cannot be obtained. Therefore it requires the cleaning up of the microscope each time it is used. For securing the specimen to the mount, conductive paint such as silver or carbon is used. Sometimes double sided adhesive tape, vacuum compound, methyl cellulose solution and many other adhesives may be used.

The specimen to be examined fixed, dried and then coated with a layer of carbon and heavy metal such as gold or gold palladium. Gold foil is generally used as electrode material for sputtering. In addition, platinum - palladium alloy, chromium, silver, copper, aluminum etc. are also available for sputtering; this process is known as shadowing.

1.20.2.5 Specimen Interaction

Electron microscopy is based on specimen interaction. When an energetic electron beam strikes the sample, various reactions may occur. The interaction of electron beam with upper surface reveals examination of thick or bulky specimen whereas reaction at bottom side allowed to examine thin or foil specimen.

1.20.2.6 Specimen Interaction Volume

When an electron beam strikes on specimen the interaction occurs inside the specimen volume known as specimen interaction volume. This volume depends on the following factors:-

- Atomic number of the material being examined. Higher the atomic number, more the absorption of electrons and hence smaller interaction volume.
- Higher the voltage greater the penetration into the sample. Thus increasing the interaction volume.
- Greater the angle of incidence for electron beam the smaller is the interaction volume.

1.20.2.7 Signal Obtained by Specimen

(i) Secondary Electrons: Electrons emitted from the specimen surface are low energy electrons, known as secondary electrons. Emission is different depending on the composition and surface structure of the specimen.

(ii) Backscattered Electrons: Electrons are backscattered from the specimen and have almost the same energy as that of incident electrons. These allow to obtain information from the inner parts of the specimen.

(iii) Transmitted Electrons: Electrons transmitted through a thin specimen are known as transmitted electrons. A scanning electron microscope provides a transmitted electron image of less chromatic aberration and allowing contrast enhancement.

(vi) **X-Rays :** X-rays emitted from specimen may be used for elements detection present in the sample.

1.20.2.8 Application

- It provides surface view of specimen formed by scattering of secondary electrons from its surface.
- It provides three dimensional structure of the specimen.
- It is used for various elements such as Pb, Sn, Sb, Bi in Gun Shot Residue.
- To observe the hair scaling patterns.
- It is also useful for examining various physical evidences such as soil, mineral, paint chips, glasses etc.
- It is used to observe the surface view of nucleus, mitochondria, ribosomes, cell membrane, chromatin fibres, nucleic acid etc.

Table: 1.3. Comparison of the Light and Electron Microscope:

Light Microscope	Electron Microscope
Easy to handle	Typical to produce electron beam
Small and portable	Large and require special room
Sample may be prepared easily	Sample may be prepared through a complex process
Vacuum is not required	Vacuum is required
Sample viewed in their natural colour	All images seen in black and white
Magnification Range up to 2000 x	Magnification Range over 500,000 x
Specimen can be living or dead	Only dead specimen can be seen
Stains are required to make the cell visible	The specimen stained with heavy metal like Osmium etc.

1.21 Scanning Tunneling Microscope

The Scanning tunneling microscope (STM) is also a type of electron microscope, that provide three dimensional image of the specimen. STM scan the surface structure of the specimen from a fixed distance. STM was invented by **Gerd Binning** and **Heinrich Rohren** in **1980** and got Nobel Prize in **1986**. It shows the magnification of more than

Table 1.4. Comparison of Various Microscopes

Type of Microscope	Total Magnification	Resolution	Source	Medium	Basis of Contrast	Application
Bright field	1000 x	200 nm	Visible light	Air	Absorption of light	To study prepared slide, stain bacteria, smear blood stain, wet mount
Dark field	1000 x	200 nm	Visible light	Air	Reflection of light	Examination of cell suspension, motility of specimen may be view.
Compound microscope	1500 x	200-500 nm	Visible light	Air	Absorption of light	Used in biological, bacterialogical and medicinal field.
Oil immersion microscope	1500 x	100-200 nm	Visible light	Oil	Absorption of light	To study the individual bacteria, details of striation in skeleton.
Phase Contrast	1500 x	100-200 nm	Visible light	Air	Absorption & retardation in intensity of light	To study the cilia and flagella, and micro-organism in their culture
Interference microscopy	1500 x	100-200 nm	Visible light	Air	Interference of light	To measure the dry weight of cellular structure
Polarizing microscope	1000 x	100 x	Polarized light	Air	Polarization of light	To analyze ultra structure of the cell and measure thickness of the object.
Fluorescence microscope	1500 x	100-200 nm	U V light	Air	Fluorescence of light due to presence of dyes	To study all kind of biological materials, collagen fibers, Vit A, protein band etc.
Confocal microscope	500-1000x	100 nm	LASER	Air	Emission of light from specimen containing dyes.	To visualize cellular protein, lipids, nucleic acid and other cell organelles. It provides 3 dimensional image.
Transmission electron microscope	5,00,000 x	1 nm	Electron beam	Vacuum	Transmission of electron through specimen	To visualize internal structure of the cell. It gives 2 dimensional image
Scanning electron microscope	20,000 x	3.5 - 10 nm	Electron beam	Vacuum	Scattering of secondary electron from specimen	It provides surface view and used in elemental analysis. It gives 3 D image

100 million. Such a high magnification enables us to view the surface of an atom. Actually electrons, which surround the surface atoms, project a short (tunnel) distance from the surface.

1.21.1 Theory and Principle

STM has a very fine needle probe having only the atom on its tips. This probe is lowered towards the surface of the specimen. A small voltage is applied between the tip of the probe and the specimen. When electron clouds of the probe touch the surface atoms, electron flow through a narrow channel in the clouds. Thus, by moving the probe tip back and forth over the surface, the arrangement of the atoms and its motion is recorded. This motion of the electron create a 3D image of the surface atoms, which is to be analyzed by computer. The surface map so obtained is displayed on a computer monitor and may be plotted on paper.

1.21.2 Application

- It provides high resolution and three dimensional view of specimen.
- It is used to observe surface structure of viruses and DNA macromolecules.

References

Bastiaens, P.I. and Squire, A., (1990); Trends in Cell Biology (21) 48–52.

Bradbury, S., (1967); The Evolution of the Microscope. Pergmon Press, London.

Carr, K.E., (1971); Application of Scanning Electron Microscopy in Biology. int. Rev. Cytology, 30 :183

Dubey, R.C., Maheswari, D.K., (1999); A Text book of Microbiology. S. Chand. & Co. Ltd., New Delhi.

Gander, R., (1969); Photomicrographic Technique, Hafner Publishing Company, New York.

Haggis, G.H., (1966); The Electron Microscope in Molecular Biology. John Wiley & Sons, New York.

Harris JR., (1991); Electron Microscopy in Biology - A Practical Approach. Oxford: Oxford University Press.

Kay, D.H., (1965); Technique for Electron Microscopy. Blackwell Oxford.

McClung, C.E., (1939); Handbook of Microscopical Technique, New York, Hoeber.

Nunn, R.E., (1970); Electron Microscopy, Preparation of Biological Specimen. London, Butterworth.

Pantin, C.F.A., (1946); Notes on Microscopical Technique for Zoologist, Cambridge Univ. Press.

Ross, K.E.A., (1967); Phase contrast and Interference Microscopy for Cell Biologist. Arnold, London.

Semwogerere, S., Weeks, E.R., (2005); "Confocal Microscopy" published in the Encyclopedia of Biomaterials and Biomedical Engineering, Taylor and Francis.

Singh, M., (1999); Instrumental Technique, 4th edition.

Slayter, E.M., (1970); Optical Methods in Biology. John Wiley & Sons, New York.

CHAPTER 2

Photomicrography

The term "Photography" was first coined by **Sir John Herschel** in 1930. "Photo" means light and "graphy" means writing or drawing. Thus photography is combination of two scientific processes i.e. "Optical" and "Chemical" Optical part includes microscope and camera while chemical part includes developer, hypo, fixer and stop bath etc.

2.1 History of Photography

Technique of photography is very old and started before 1600 yet there are few milestones in the invention of photography.

S. No	Name of Inventor	Contribution
1.	Robert Boyle (1600)	Proved that Silver Chloride turns dark when exposed to air.
2.	Angelo Sala (1700)	Observed that powder of Silver Nitrate turns black in sunlight
3.	Johann Heinrich Schulze (1727)	Discovered that certain liquids change colour when exposed to light
4.	Louis Daguerre (1829)	Discovered the method of developing photographic plate in half an hour.
5.	William Henry Fox, Talbot (1844)	Developed "Calotypes" photography in which a number of positive films may be developed on photographic paper
6.	Frederic Scott Archer (1851)	Introduced the wet "Collodion" process of photography in which exposure time was reduced to only 2-3 seconds.
7.	Archer (1852)	Developed "Ambrotype" photography i.e. development of direct positive pictures.
8.	Dr. Richard Maddox (1871)	Used Gelatin coated plates instead of glass, which led to the development of the dry plate.
9.	George Estman (1884)	Introduced flexible celluloid film
10.	Herman Vogel	Developed a process whereby film becomes sensitive to green light
11.	Eadweard Muybridge	Started the motion picture photography

2.2 Introduction

In microscopic study of animals plants, microorganisms, cells, documents and many other materials, we need their actual figure and documentation. Which may be achieved only through photography. Actually photography represents the facts regarding scientific examination of aforesaid materials. Photography shows logical sequence and documentation of the material in desired plane.

Photomicrography is widely accepted for detailed study of materials. In scientific explanations, classroom demonstration and research documentation, there is a great need of photography. Photomicrography is the use of microscope in photographing the object. The device includes microscope, illumination source and camera.

Photography through microscope is proceeding from film to digital in order to get best resolution. The quality of photomicrograph (sharpness, brightness, contrast, etc.) depend upon the quality of microscope.

2.3 Photography

The word "Photography" means to write or draw with the help of light. It is an art of obtaining actual picture or photograph of an object. Image is created by exposing film to light sensitive film. Picture creating device is a "Camera". It receives the reflected light from an object. Which reaches to focusing lens forming an image.

2.4 Photomicrography

Photomicrography is the technique of taking image of very small object with the help of compound microscope or stereomicroscope. Compound microscope reveals a real and minute detail of an object. This technique is useful in handwriting for comparison of forgery, signature, sequence of strokes, alternations and nature of ink. A 35 mm SLR camera is commonly used for the purpose. Photomicrography provides an image having uniform illumination over the whole field of view. The contrast and resolution of image depends upon the following factors i.e.-

- Filter quality
- Film quality
- Lens aberrations
- Dirt and debris

- Fungus on lens
- Handling mistakes

Photomicrography involves two steps

1. Optical operation
2. Chemical operation

Optical operation includes following devices:

2.4.1 Microscope

The choice of suitable microscope is an important task to get quality image. Generally compound microscopes are used. Stereomicroscopes require light lamp for better illumination. In case of trinocular microscope, its third eyepiece is used to mount the camera. It should have following qualities –

- The eyepiece diameter should be the same as that of camera lens.
- The microscope should have the ability to change the magnification to obscure different sized objects
- It should be of best optical quality.

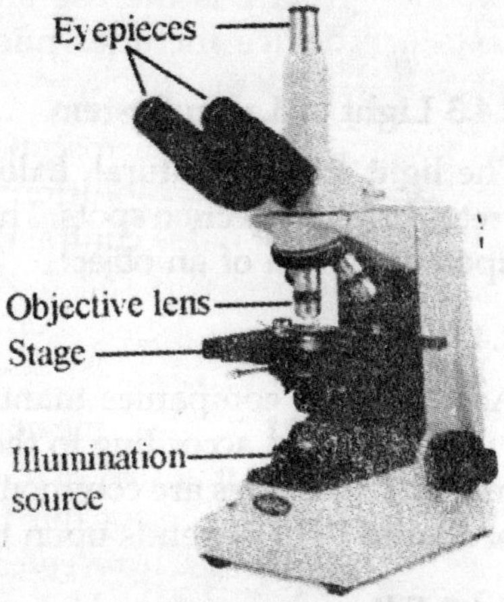

Fig. 2.1. Trinocular Microscope.

2.4.2 Camera

Any SLR camera may be used for photomicrography. It may be 35 mm or digital but its lens system should be removable. A good camera should possess following qualities.

- The camera should have a socket. Adaptor should have a socket mount for the camera at one end and attachment to the microscope at the other.
- Camera should have the device for attachment of its lens to the eyepiece of the microscope.
- Diameter of the lens of camera should be equal to or less than the diameter of the microscope eyepiece.
- It should have an internal zoom.
- It should have a manual control speed, focus and flash.

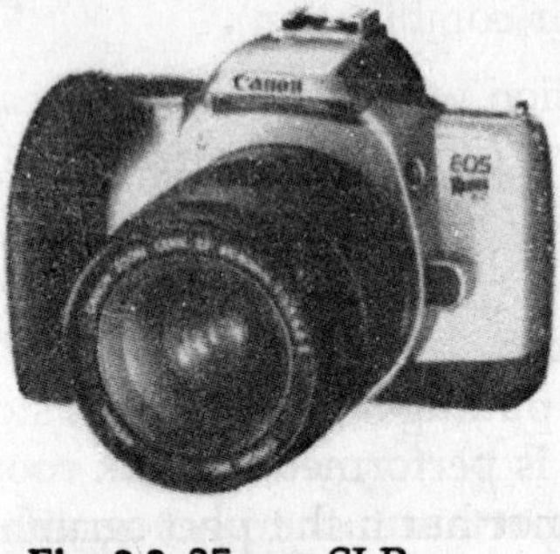

Fig. 2.2. 35 mm SLR Camera

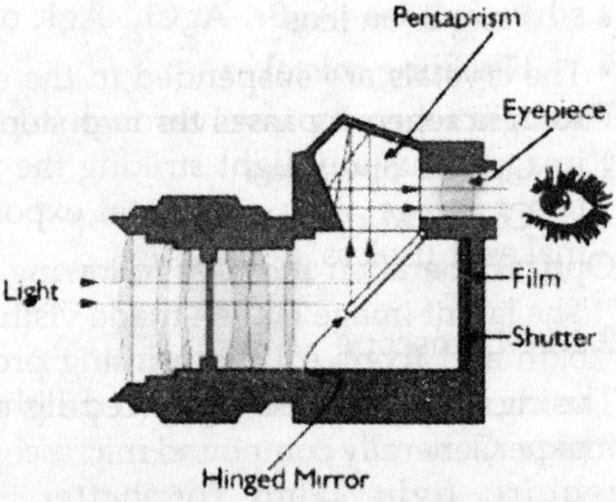

Fig. 2.3. Working of SLR Camera

2.4.3 Light or Lamp System

The light may be natural, halogen or an electric bulb it should not create bright reflection spots. The intensity and colour of light depends upon condition of an object.

2.4.4 Film

A number of companies manufacture the photomicrographic film, which are used according to the need. There are 24 x 36 mm, 60 x 60 mm or 4 x 5 inches are commonly available format of a film. Exposure of film to light depends upon the intensity of light.

2.4.5 Filters

Filters are circular or square pieces of glass placed in front of the camera. They allow only desired spectrum to reach the film e.g. green filter allows only green light to pass through but does not allow the complimentary colours red or blue to pass. They are absorbed. Filters are used to contrast during image capture. They control the optical aberrations and increase resolution by restricting illuminating wavelength. Visible-light transmission region for Kodak wratten colour filter is used for contrast and resolution control in black and white photomicrography. A number of filters are used for colour photomicrography i.e. colour compensating filters, neutral density filters, ultraviolet light restriction filters and heat absorbing filters.

2.4.6 Photographic or Printing Paper

Photographic paper is supporting medium coated with light sensitive emulsion. The emulsion is very important component consisting of silver halides (AgBr, $AgCl_2$, AgI_2 or their combination).

The crystals are suspended in the emulsion with gelatin. They react to light when it passes through a lens or a camera. It creates a latent image. Thus any light striking the photographic paper will create a latent image. Any accidental exposure to light will fog it and will makes it useless.

The latent image is then made visible by putting it in developer, stop bath and fixer. All the printing process is performed in dark room using only dim red light (red light do not harm the photographic paper).

2.4.7 Photo Capture or Taking the Photograph

The process of taking the picture is as follows –

- Attach the camera to microscope eyepiece and turn its switch on
- Switch on the light (lamp)
- Now focus the camera and set it to infinity press the focus button until a clear broad zone appears.
- Put the object or slide on platform of microscope under objective lens.
- Focus on the object with the microscope's focus adjustment, using the camera's LCD to see the changes in focus unless the resolution and sharpness are achieved.

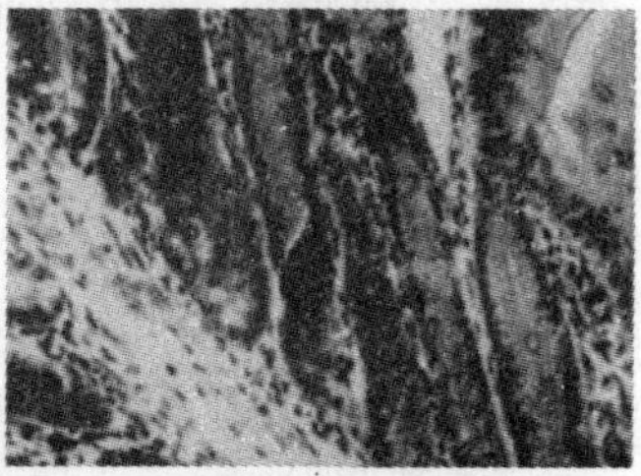

Image through Photomicrography

- For fine focussing and smaller details, use camera digital zoom.
- Now turn it off before taking the picture.
- Now make adjustment to light and exposure control.
- These adjustments are different for different objects. Faster shutter speed i.e 1/20 of a second is sufficient for histological slides.
- After setting everything check the position and plane of the object once again and click with the help of lead.
- Wait for click sound and adjust for another photograph similarly.
- After reel is finished, detach the camera from the microscope and take out the reel in dark room for further developing process.

2.4.8 Development of Film/reel

- Load the reel/film in developing chamber in dark room
- Fill it with developer
- Put the reel in developer for about 3-4 hours shaking it well.
- Take out the reel and wash it well with water and clip for drying.

Now this negative film is ready for printing.

2.4.9 Positive photograph preparation

- First put the photographic paper on platform under the enlarger and negative under the lens of enlarger.
- Focus the image and adjust the sharpness and size.

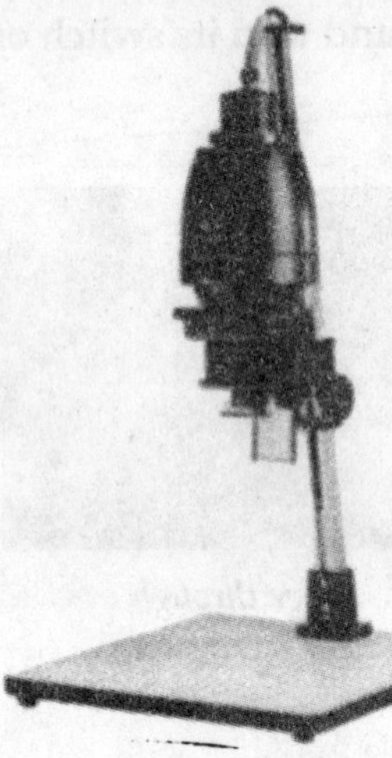

Fig. 2.4. Enlarger

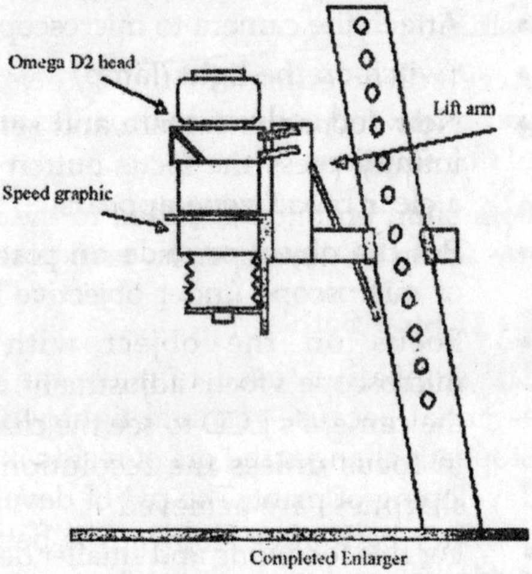

Fig. 2.5. Diagrammatic Representation of Enlarger.

- Now strike the light for 1-3 seconds (according to need) and shut the slit.
- Repeat the process for another negative, and proceed for positive printing.

Printing of picture is done in dark room which requires developer, stop bath and fixer.

2.4.10 Developer

Developer has following components :

- Developing agents
- Preservative
- Accelerator
- Restrainer
- Water

Developer has reducing agents such as metal and hydroquinone in ionized condition in solution. They provide electrons to silver ions (in silver halides) reducing them to atoms of metallic silver.

Preservative sodium sulphite and potassium metabisulphite and potassium metabisulphate is used to protect developing agent from oxidising.

Accelerator enhances the rate of development. Borax, sodium carbonate and sodium hydroxides are used as accelerator to raise the pH of solution.

Potassium bromide is added to the solution as **restrainer.** It reduces the action of developer on unexposed part of paper.

2.4.11 Stop Bath

The stopbath is used to make the developer inactive. This step is essential because residual light will cause continues development. Stopbath changes the pH of residual developer and checks the further developing of print. The pH of developer is always more than 7. Use of water bath after stopwath is better as it dilutes out the residual developer and make it inactive.

2.4.12 Fixing

Fixing is the last step after the development of picture. It removes the undeveloped silver halide grains. The print (picture) is treated with a solution of sodium thiosulphate (Hypo) which forms a soluble compound with silver halide $Ag^{+} + 2(S_2O)_3) \rightarrow Ag\ (S_2O_3)_2$. Then fixing in hypo removes unexposed and undeveloped silver halide grains from emulsion of photograph paper. These areas then become transparent as film.

Lastly the print is treated with running water (by putting into a tray) to remove the traces of hypo.

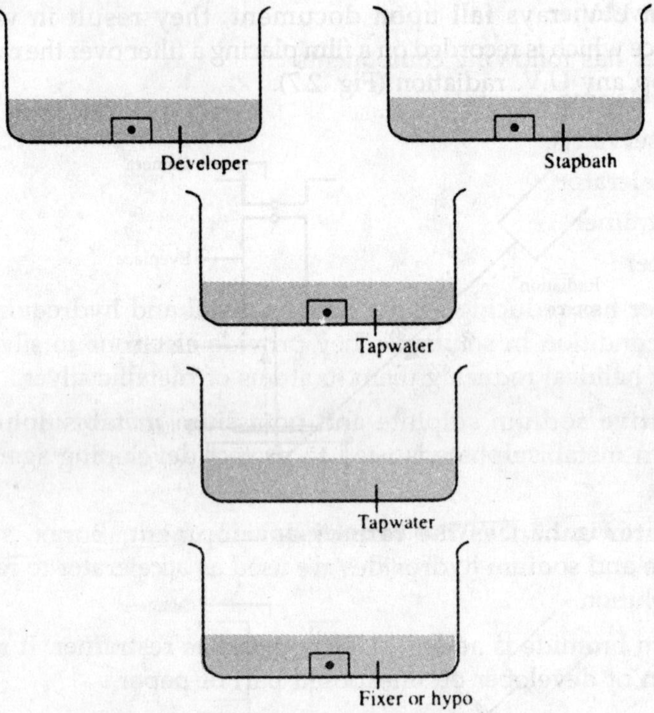

Fig. 2.6. Steps for Developing the Picture.

After developing the picture (printing) photomicrographs are glazed by putting them in glazer for 15 minutes. Then they are taken out and cut in demand size.

2.5 Ultraviolet Photography

This type of photography is used to examine the questioned documents specially in making faded documents visible, detecting traces of inks, dyes or stains. It is of two types.

a. Topographic study by UV rays (direct photography)

It involves ultraviolet radiation and a screening filter for visible radiation. In this wratten 18-A filter is used which prohibits the visible radiations and allows only UV radiation which are recorded by the film.

b. Fluorescent photography

In this type of photography all the UV radiation are stopped by a filter and only visible fluorescence reach to the camera. Wratten 18-A filter is placed over the U.V. source which stop visible rays and allows only U.V. rays to pass through it.

When U.V. rays fall upon document, they result in visible fluorescence which is recorded on a film placing a filter over the camera lens to stop any U.V. radiation (Fig. 2.7).

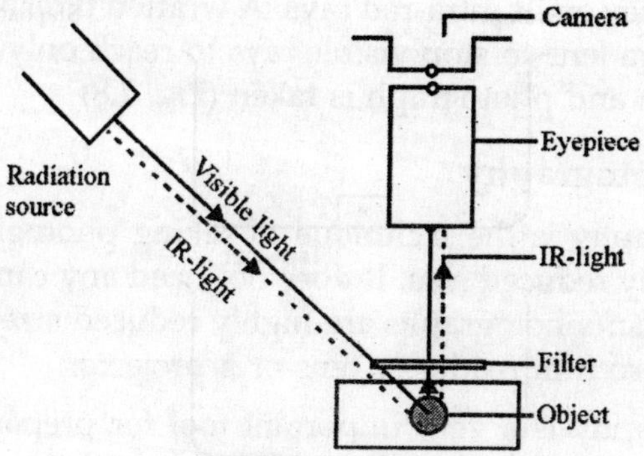

Fig. 2.7. UV-Visible Photographic Technique

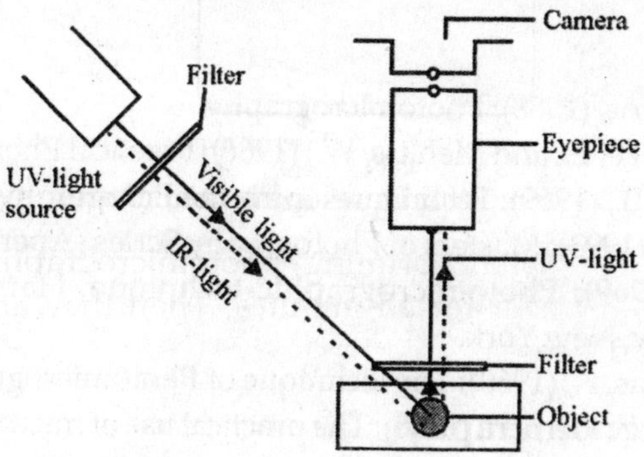

Fig. 2.8. Infra Red Photographic Techniuqe

2.6 Infrared Photography

Infrared photography is very useful for the examination of sealed envelopes, ink differentiation, pigments, detection of erasures obliterated writing and writing of charred documents. It is of two types:

a. Infrared reflective photography

In this technique, a high speed infra - red film is used. Infra - red rays are projected on the object and photographs are taken by placing wratten filter No. 87 over the camera lens which allows only infra-red rays.

b. Infrared luminescent photography

This technique is used in comparison of dyes, pigments and ballpoint pen inks. In this photography, a corning glass filter 9780 is placed in front of light source to stop infra-red radiation. When these rays fall on an object, they emitt infra-red rays. A wratten filterNo 87 is placed over the camera lens to stop visible rays to reach only infra-red rays pass to camera and photograph is taken (Fig. 2.8)

2.7 Microphotography

Microphotography is the technique of taking photographs of large object in greatly reduced size. It does not need any camera or optical instrument. Microphotographs are highly reduced size of an object it requires a micro film reader or lens or a projector.

Microphotography is a very important tool for preparing microfilm of documents, photographic plates, slides and other materials. These film are made visible by projector. Few decades back, research literature and documents were used to send as microfilms.

References

Allem, Roy Morris, (1958); Photomicrography

Bergner, J., Gelbke, E., and Mehliss, W., (1966); Practical Photomicrography.

Brain, Edward, B., (1969); Techniques in Photomicrography.

Evans, Walker, (1993); Masters of Photography Series (Aperture).

Gander, R., (1969); Photomicrographic technique. Hafner Publishing Company, New York.

Lawson, Douglas, F., (1960); The technique of Photomicrography.

Needham, George Herbert, (1958); The practical use of microscope including Photomicrography.

Schaefer, John, P., (1998); Basic Techniques of Photography, Book 2 (Little Brown and Company)

Smith, Robert, F., (1982); Microscopy and Photomicrography.

CHAPTER 3
Spectroscopy

3.1 Introduction

Spectroscopic technique is used for the analysis of pharmaceutical and biomedical materials. The technique involves measurement of absorption spectrum of the sample. Thus spectroscopy is defined as the interaction between material and electromagnetic radiation. Previously it was believed that light travels in a straight line but some important phenomenon like interference, refraction, diffraction etc. could not be explained. Later it was proved by various theories that light travels in wave form. There are various forms of electromagnetic radiations such as ultra violet, visible, infra red, X- Rays, radio waves, cosmic rays etc. The study of spectroscopy relates to emission and absorption spectra of the matter. An emission spectra is produced by the excitation of atom of the element. Excitation may be due to heat or electrical energy. Electron moving to lower energy level releases radiations which are analyzed with the help of spectroscope as emission spectrum. To understand the phenomenon of spectroscopy, one should know the basic principle of electromagnetic radiation and light spectra.

3.2 Electromagnetic Radiation

Electromagnetic radiation may be produced by changing electric and magnetic field simultaneously which act at right angle to each other and also perpendicular to the direction of electromagnetic wave (Fig. 3.1).

3.2.1 Properties of Electromagnetic Radiations

- These waves are transverse in nature

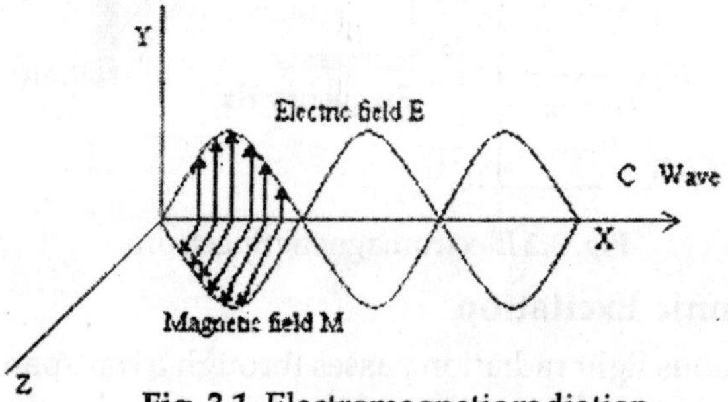

Fig. 3.1. Electromagnetic radiation

- They can propagate in vacuum also.
- They may produce optical effects.
- They can be polarized.

3.3 Electromagnetic Spectrum

Complete electromagnetic radiation consist of γ rays, X-rays, ultraviolet-visible, infra-red, microwaves and radiowaves. If all of them are arranged according to their increasing wavelength and decreasing frequency, γ rays will be at 10^{-4} nm while Radiowaves will be at 10^9 nm. The visible region of the spectrum extend between violet and red colour (3800A° - 7600A°) known as VIBGYOR, below the visible region is ultraviolet region (200 - 400 nm) and above the visible region is Infra-red region (0.78μ-500μ). Cosmic rays have shorter wave length hence highly energetic, while radio waves have longer wavelength, hence less energetic. (Fig 3.2)

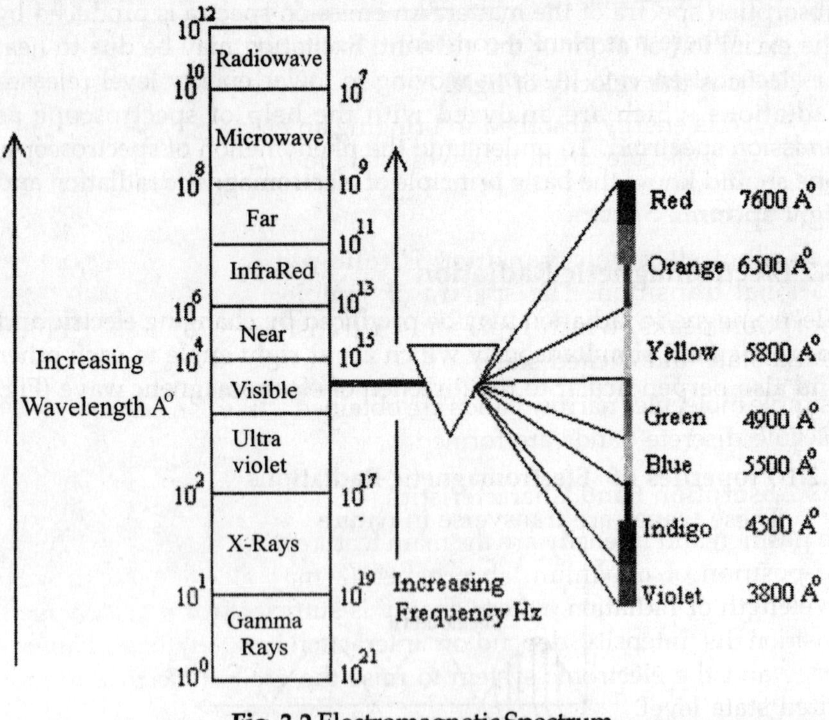

Fig. 3.2 Electromagnetic Spectrum

3.4 Electronic Excitation

When continuous light radiation passes through a transparent material or organic compound a portion of the light may be absorbed. The residual radiation when passes through a prism yields a spectrum which is known as absorption spectrum.

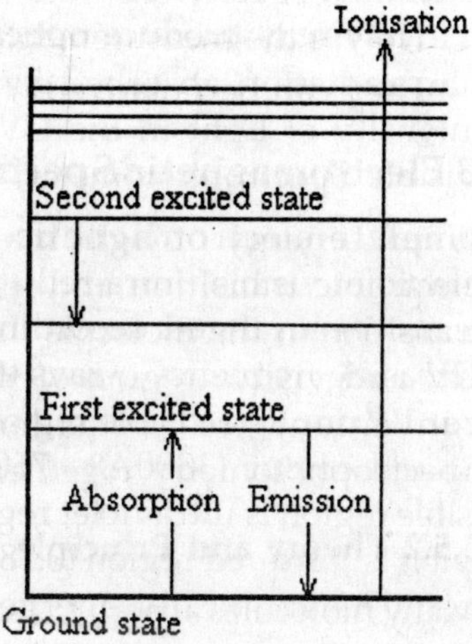

Fig. 3.3. Electronic Excitation

A molecule can only absorb radiation of certain frequency. As a result of absorption of energy, atoms or molecule pass from a state of low energy (the initial or ground state) to a state of higher energy (the excited state). It is found that the electrons of the component atom are excited (Fig. 3.3).

The relationship between the energy absorbed in electronic transition is expressed by the following equation.

$$E = h\nu = hc/\lambda$$

Where h is plank's constant

c is the velocity of light

E is energy absorbed in bringing an electronic transition in a molecule from its lowest state to higher state.

3.4.1 Electronic Spectra

In an atom electronic transition is followed by vibrational and rotational transition. The spectra of sample molecule consist of absorption peaks, which represents a transition in the electronic ground state and excited state.

In simple molecules narrow bands are obtained while in more complex molecule discrete bands are formed.

3.4.2 Absorption Band Characteristics

The position and intensity are the main feature of an absorption band. The position of maximum absorbance (λ max) correspond to the wavelength of radiation, whose energy is sufficient for an electronic transition. Its intensity depend on interaction between the radiation energy and the electronic system to raise the ground electron to an excited state level.

3.5 UV – Visible Spectrophotometer

3.5.1 Introduction

This technique is actually Electronic Spectroscopy because it includes excitation of electrons from lower energy level to higher energy level. It involves the measurement of UV (190 - 380 nm) or visible (380 - 800 nm) radiation absorbed by the electrons of solution. The ratio of intensity of light in the UV - Visible region is measured by UV-Visible Spectrophotometer.

When energy of light matches with that required to induce an electronic transition and its associated vibrational and rotational transition in the molecule then the absorption of light occurs in both UV and visible region of the electromagnetic spectrum. It is thus convenient to consider the techniques of UV-Visible Spectrophotometry together.

3.5.2 Theory and Principle

Many molecules absorb UV – Visible light. The absorbance of a solution increases as attenuation of the beam increases. Absorbance is directly proportional to the path of length, (I) and the concentration (C) of the absorbing species (Fig. 3x.4).

The intensity of the absorption is governed by two fundamental laws of absorption known as Beer and Lambert's Law.

3.5.2.1 Beer and Lambert's Law

When a beam of light passes through a transparent sample cell containing a solution of an absorbing substance the intensity of light reduces.

This is due to :-

1. Reflection of the inner and outer surface of the cell
2. Scattering by particle in solution
3. Absorption of light by molecule in the solution

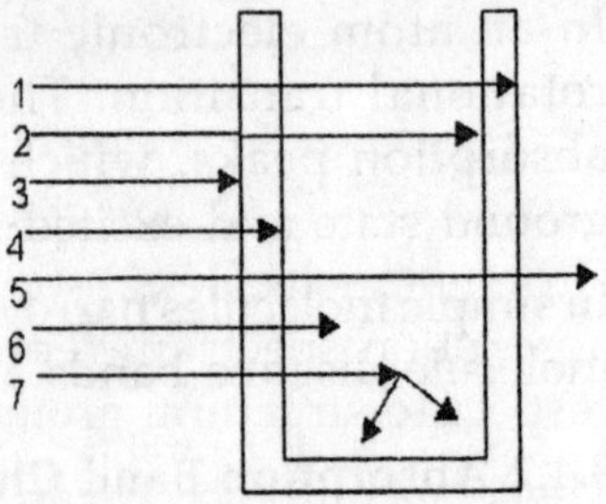

Fig. 3.4. The Reduction of the Intensity of Light by Reflecting Absorption and Scattering.

Since it is not possible to directly measure the amount of radiation absorbed by a partially transparent substance, it may be measured by calculating the difference in intensity between the original and transmitted radiations falling on the sample.

$$I_{absorbed} = I_0 - I_T$$

Where I_0 is the original intensity falling on to the cell

I_T is the reduced intensity transmitted from the cell

Beer and Lambert's Law is a combination of two Laws, also known as Bouguer's law.

(i) Beer's Law: When a ray of monochromatic light passes through an absorbing medium, its intensity decreases exponentially as the concentration of absorbing material increases.

$$\text{Intensity (I)} = \frac{1}{\text{concentration of absorbing medium}}$$

(ii) Lambert's Law: When a ray of monochromatic light passes through an absorbing medium, its intensity decreases exponentially as the length of absorbing material increases.

$$\text{Intensity (I)} = \frac{1}{\text{length (b) of absorbing medium}}$$

The Beer Lambert's law is the combination of two laws each dealing separately with the absorption of light related to the concentration of the absorbing substance.

$$A = \log_{10} I_o/I_T = abc$$

Where I_o - Incident radiation
I_T - Transmitted radiation
a - Absorptivity
b - Length of absorption path
c - Concentration of absorbing atom
A - Absorbance

Different molecules absorb radiation of different wavelength and the absorption spectrum represent a number of absorption bands with respect to structural groups present within the molecule.

The Transmittance T can be expressed as –

$$T = I_T / I_o$$

Where I_T is the intensity of transmittance radiation
I_o is the intensity of incident radiation

and the % Transmittance is

$$\%T = 100\, I_T / I_o$$

If the value of T = 100 it means there is no absorption of radiation (i.e. transparent substance) whereas the 0 value of T represents an opaque substance in which complete absorption takes place.

The intermediate values of Absorbance (A) can be expressed as-

$$A = \log_{10}(1/T)$$
$$= \log_{10}(I_o/I_T)$$

3.5.2.2 Conditions of Beer and Lambert's Law

- Radiation should be monochromatic and of narrow wavelength range
- Absorbing species must be homogenous i.e. free from all ionization, dissociation or association of the solute.
- Solution should not be too concentrated

3.5.3 Instrumentation

When the light of certain intensity and frequency range passes from a sample, the % transmittance of light radiation is measured by an instrument known as spectrophotometer (Fig. 3.5 & 3.6).

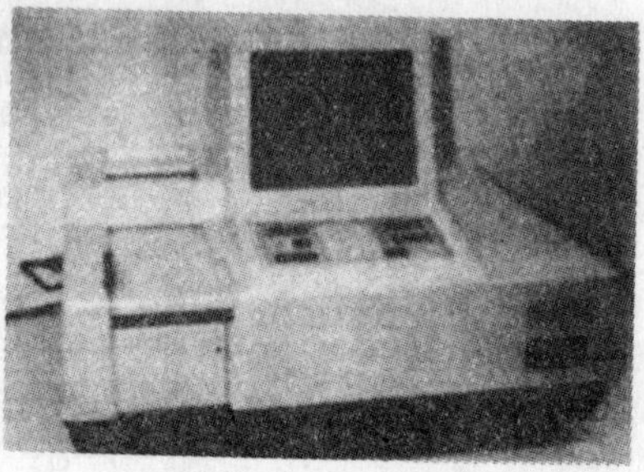

Fig. 3.5. UV Visible Spectrophotometer

The UV–Visible Spectrophotometer mainly consist of the following parts:–

1. Radiation source
2. Monochromator
3. Sample cell
4. Detector
5. Data output and recording device

3.5.3.1 Radiation Source

The radiation source is deuterium lamp used for the Ultraviolet region and always has a wavelength range of approximately 190 – 450 nm. For the visible region, tungsten filament bulb is used and has wavelength range from about 330 to 850 nm. The condensing mirror is rotated manually to focus the light omitted from either source into the entrance slit of the monochromator.

3.5.3.2 Monochromator

It is a device for isolating monochromatic (homogenous) or narrow bands of radiant energy from the source. It will allow to pass radiant energy of particular wavelength. Quartz prism was used in earlier

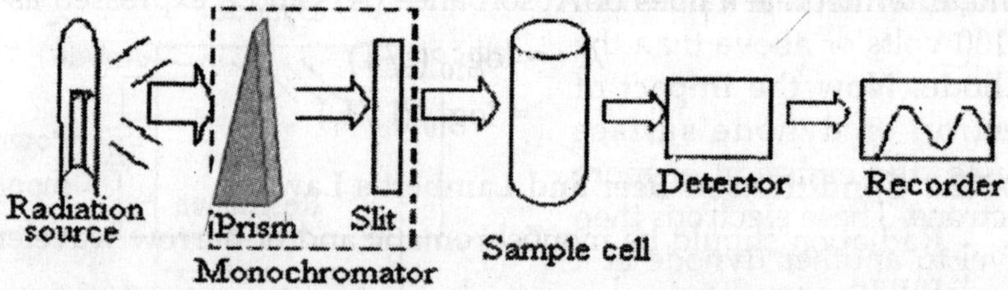

Fig. 3.6. Schematic Representation of UV Visible Spectrophotometer

photometer but now they are completely replaced by diffraction grating. It mainly contains two parts

- Slit
- Dispersion media (prism or grating)

The purpose of monochromator is to separate the light of different wavelength produced by the light source and isolate the particular light of interest.

3.5.3.3 Sample or Reference Chamber

Pyrex glass in visible region is satisfactory material for a sample cell but below 350nm wavelength (for UV region) quartz i.e. glass of pure silicon dioxide must be used. The beam of monochromatic light entering the sample area becomes more concentrated as they pass through the area towards the detector. The photomultiplier tube of the detector area are protected from exposure to excessively bright light by automatic shutters that seal the detector area when the sample area is opened.

3.5.3.4 Detector

The detector measures the quantity of radiation that passes through the sample by converting it to an electric signal. The most common detector used are vacuum photocells. These are based on photoelectric effect. The signal is obtained when a photon of sufficient energy strikes the metal surface, causes the ejection of an electron. This is determined by quantitative measurement of the amount of light passing through the instrument by means of detector.

Another type of detector used is photo multiplier tube (PMT). It resembles the photocell except that the electron emitted from cathode do not go to anode directly but hit an intermittent anode called dynode, which is at a potential of 100 volts or above than the cathode. Now the impact of electron or dynode surface causes the emission of more electrons. These electrons then travel to another dynode at a potential of 100 volts or so than the first dynode. In this way they acquire considerable kinetic energy.

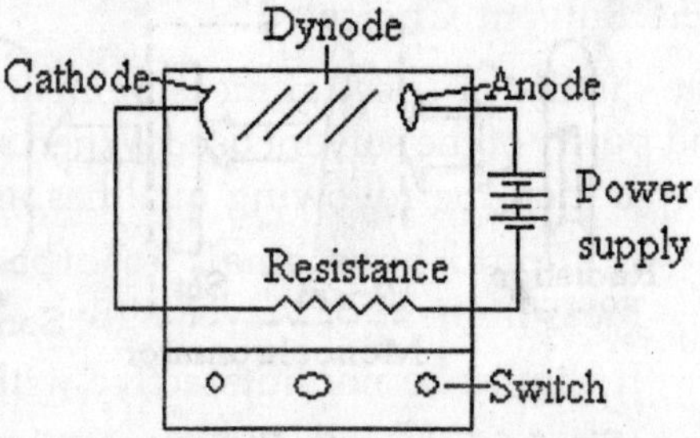

Fig. 3.7. A Typical Photomultiplier tube

Now each secondary electron causes emission of more electrons from secondary dynode and so on. A typical photomultiplier has a dozen dynode in sequence, so that the emission of single electron from cathode causes emission of multiple electrons from final dynode, which are finally collected by the anode. The photomultiplier thus act as vacuum photo cell with built in high gain amplifier (Fig. 3.7).

Table 3.1. Some Chromophores and the approximate wavelength at which they absorb the radiation

Chromophore	System	λ max (nm)
Ether	- O -	185
Amine	$-NH_2$	195
Nitrile	$-C \equiv N$	160
Ethylene	$-C = C$	190
Ketone	$>C = O$	195
Aldehyde	- CHO	210
Carboxyl	- COOH	200 – 210
Nitro	$-NO_2$	210
Benzene	$-C_6H_6$	184

3.5.3.5 Data Output and Recording Device

The sample signal output device can be an analog absorbance or transmittance meter where the data can be read, recorded and processed. Some spectrophotometers have microprocessor for control and monitoring of the instrument operation. These instruments provide an interface to a computer along with software to control instrumentation operation and also enables a numerical printout of the absorbance spectrum.

3.5.4 Solvent Choice

The quality of spectral measurement is directly affected by the type and purity of the solvent used. When selecting a solvent for the sample preparation the following qualities are taken into consideration.

- It should have small absorbance in the spectral region of measurement of wavelength.
- It should be non-interactive with solute.
- It should be compatible with the cuvette material (sample cell)
- It should not absorb UV - radiation

Each solvent has a cutoff wavelength (corresponding to about 10% transmittance) and this varies with solvent purity. The solvent should not be used with measurement below its cutoff wavelength. The cutoff point equivalent to 10 % transmittance for some of the spectroscopic solvent given in the table is as follows:-

Table 3.2

Solvent	Wavelength in (nm)
Water (Distilled)	190
Acetonitrile	190
Isooctane	195
Cyclohexane	210
Ethanol	210
Hexane	210
Methanol	210
Ether	220
Sodium hydroxide	225
Chloroform	245
Benzene	280

3.5.5 Sampling Technique

Usually any transparent solid, liquid or gaseous sample can be used for analysis. The microliter or microgram amount of sample is sufficient for detection.

The following points should be considered while preparing the sample.

- An appropriate high purity transparent solvent must be chosen.
- Aqueous system often requires the use of appropriate buffer system.

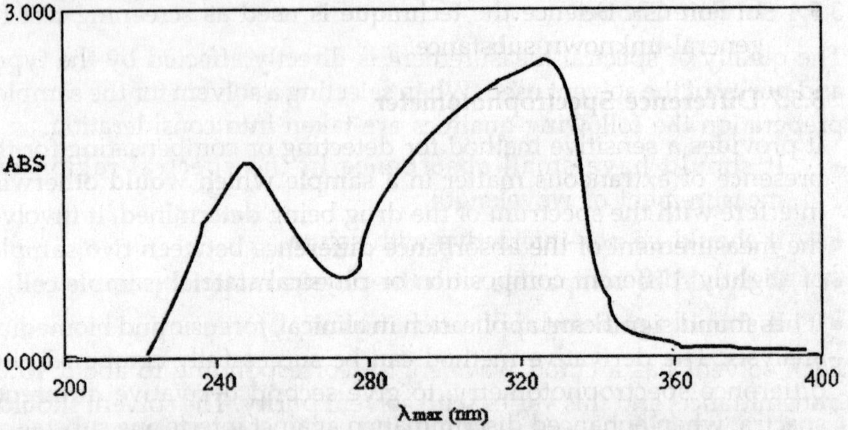

Fig. 3.8. UV Visible Spectra of Diazepam

- Sample clean up (isolation of analyte from interfacing species) may be required.
- Turbid sample should be filtered to reduce the light scattering.

Table 3.3. Some Benzodiazepine Derivatives and their respective Wavelength

Benzodiazepine Derivatives	λ max (nm)
Clonazepam	279 - 350
Diazepam	242, 285 - 360
Flurazepam	235- 283 - 362
Lorazepam	236- 283 - 366
Oxazepam	244- 289 - 358

3.5.6 Application

UV – Visible Spectrophotometry is often used as a quick and inexpensive method for identification of certain classes of material substances containing chromophores.

- It is used in quantitative analysis of the substance like bulk drugs or biological extracts.
- It is a useful technique for preliminary examination of explosive materials such as Nitrobenzene, TNT, RDX, HMX, Tetryl etc.
- The determination of drugs and metabolites in body fluids.
- In the ink examination.
- Examination of various fibers.

- In Forensic Science the technique is used as screening test for general unknown substance.

3.5.7 Difference Spectrophotometer

It provides a sensitive method for detecting or compensating for the presence of extraneous matter in a sample which would otherwise interfere with the spectrum of the drug being determined. It involves the measurement of the absorbance difference between two samples of slightly different composition or physical state.

It has found significant application in clinical, forensic and biomedical analysis. The derivative method can be successfully combined with difference spectrophotometry, to give second derivative difference spectra, when enhanced discrimination against interfering substances and sharp fine structures are observed.

3.5.7.1 Advantages

- It can detect minute amount of sample such as microliters or micrograms.
- Quantitation of sample can be done precisely and reproducibly by this technique.

3.5.7.2 Limitations

- Extensive sample preparation is required.
- The sample should be purified prior to analysis.
- In this technique broad bands are obtained, so it is not a definite identification technique.

3.5.8 Microspectrophotometer

In Microspectrophotometer a microscope is linked with the spectrophotometer. When a beam of light directed on to the sample or particle under investigation then an absorption spectra is obtained depending upon the type of light radiation (i.e. either UV, Visible or IR). This spectra pattern viewed under the microscope linked through it and is used for studying biological material such as blood, pigments, fibre etc. It is also quite useful for the analysis of various physical evidences such as soil, paint, glass etc.

3.6 Atomic Absorption Spectroscopy

This technique was given by **Alan Walsh in 1955**. Atomic Absorption Spectroscopy is most useful technique for providing an accurate determination of an element's concentration in a sample. This technique is very sensitive for detection and quantitation of elements that are present at trace level.

3.6.1 Basic Principle

When a light radiation is pass through the gaseous state (atomic state) of an element, radiation of a particular wavelength is absorbed which is characteristic of that element. This absorption is proportional to the amount of atoms present in the element. The net energy of this state is equal to the energy of absorbed photon of light radiation.

It can be expressed as:-

$$E = h\nu = hc/\lambda$$

Where h	is plank's constant
λ	is the wavelength
c	is the velocity of light
E	is energy absorbed by the molecule

The only photon of a particular wavelength that is absorbed by the particular element may be analyzed.

3.6.2 Instrumentation

The Atomic Absorption Spectrophotometer consist of a source of light (hollow cathode lamp), an atom cell, a monochromator and a read out device. Which provides proper analysis of the element by measuring the absorption of constant intensity of electromagnetic radiation, passed through the sample (Fig. 3.9).

3.6.2.1 Light source

The most widely used light source is the hollow cathode lamp. It is made up of a glass envelope with a cathode of analyzing element and a suitable anode (tungsten). The closed glass envelope contains an inert gas, typically Neon or Argon at a pressure of 1 -5 Torr. When an electric potential is applied between cathode and anode, the metal atoms are excited and sputter (displace) out from the cathode. Now the collision takes place between gas ion and vaporized metal atoms from cathode resulting in the formation of characteristic spectrum of the metal that is used for making cathode.

Hollow Cathode Lamp is made up of pure element or alloy of several metals which is known as multielement cathode and used for the determination of more than one element at a time. Sometimes gas

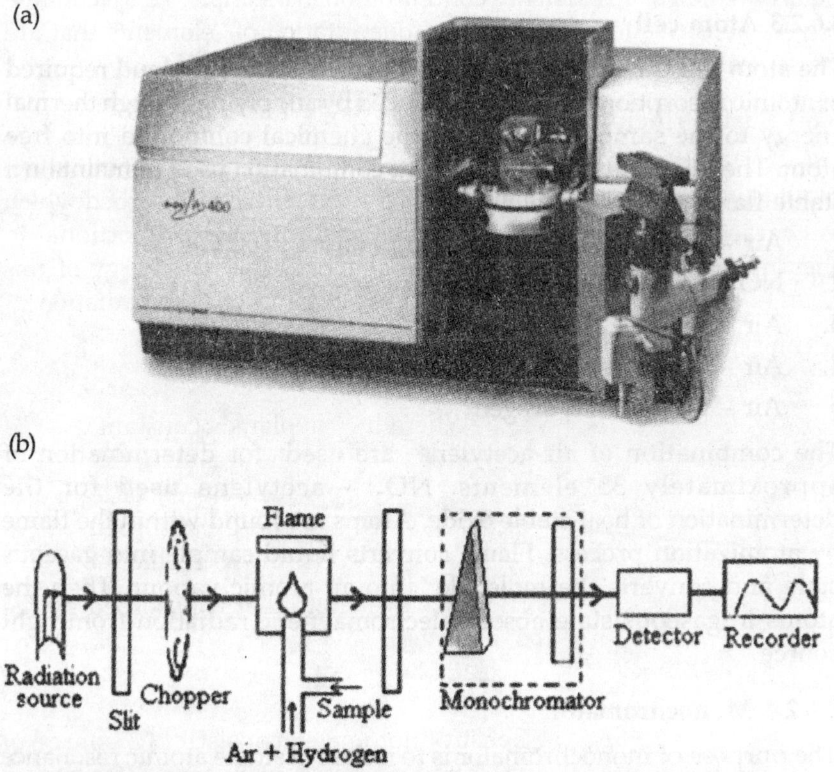

Fig. 3.9 (a) Atomic Absorption Spectroscopy, (b) Diagrammatic representation

discharge lamp (arc lamp) is also used in place of HCL for the estimation of alkali metals such as Cd, Hg, Zn etc. The advantage of HCL is that it generates very narrow spectral line, which is completely absorbed by the atom and is detected.

They are economical, simple to operate, produce stable and intense light and can be made for all chemical elements that can be analyzed by AAS.

3.6.2.2 Chopper

It is a wheel-like structure placed between HCL and flame. The main function of this is to break the steady light into pulsating light hence provide pulsating current to the detector. Light emitted by flame also produces a steady rate current but for preventing interference only pulsating current is amplified and recorded.

3.6.2.3 Atom cell

The atom cell is characterized by a flame. The atomic cloud required or atomic absorption element is produced by supplying enough thermal energy to the sample to dissolve the chemical compound into free atom. The most common fuel oxidant combination used to maintain a stable flame are given below:

1. Air - acetylene (operating temperature 2300°C)
2. NO_2 - acetylene (3000°C)
3. Air - Propane (1800°C)
4. Air - Hydrogen
5. Air - Argon - Hydrogen

The combination of air-acetylene are used for determination of approximately 35 elements. NO_2 - acetylene used for the determination of heat stable oxide. Atoms are found within the flame by atomization process. Flame converts liquid sample into gaseous state and converts the molecule into an atomic vapour. Then the atoms in gaseous state absorb electromagnetic radiation from light source.

3.6.2.4 Monochromator

The purpose of monochromator is to isolate a single atomic resonance line from the spectrum of lines emitted from the light source. Most of the Atomic absorption spectrophotometer use dispersive grating (prism) that have resolution in the range of 0.2 – 0.02 nm to separate light into different wavelengths.

3.6.2.5 Detection and Read-out Device

The most common type of detector is photomultiplier tube, which produces an electric signal, proportional to the intensity of electromagnetic radiation of the wavelength separated by the light dispersing monochromator. It detects the pulsating current only which is obtained by the sample, not by the flame. Hence characteristics band of sample is obtained.

The signal from the detector is amplified through amplifier device and transferred to the read-out system and the analytical result (output) is seen on the computer screen.

3.6.3 Application

- Atomic absorption spectroscopy is a very useful technique in the field of ceramics, mineralogy and biochemistry.

- It is used for the determination of various trace materials present in the soil and cement.
- It is best quantitative method for the analysis of metals.
- It is used in the analysis of gunshot residue.
- It is also useful in the analysis of plant and animal materials, food, beverages, chemical products and environmental studies.
- Some other informations like densities, temperature, abundance of elements may be obtained by studying the intensities of spectral lines.
- It is a useful technique for the determination of metallic poison in soft tissues of the body.
- This technique is very helpful in checking the adulteration of different materials.

3.6.4 Advantages

- It provides very high sensitivity, many elements can be detected at levels that approach one trillion of a gram.
- Hollow cathode lamp is used.
- It gives accurate results in the analysis of trace quality of elements.
- Technology is inexpensive.
- Technique is widely used for the measurement of gold, gold pathfinders and base metals.

3.6.5 Limitations

- In this technique chemical dissolution of the element is required.
- It is a sequential technique in which one element can be analyzed at a time.
- It shows reduction in sensitivity due to interference of other elements.
- For the analysis of a particular element proper lamp should be selected.

3.7 Flameless Atomic Absorption Spectroscopy

In Flameless Atomic Absorption Spectrophotometer in place of flame, a graphite burner is used for the analysis of solid samples. The use of graphite furnace is ideal for trace elemental analysis. Graphite furnace requires only a few microliters of sample. This technique can be used in solution where sample is in least quantity. The atomization process require a very high electric current passed through graphite tube on which sample is placed.

A comparative account of detection limit for metals in flame and graphite furnace is given as follows:-

Table 3.4

Element	Furnace (ppm)	Flame (ppm)
Ba	0.04	1.0
Cu	0.02	10.0
Pb	0.05	30.0
Sb	0.10	50.0
Ti	0.50	1.0
Zn	0.001	2.0

3.8 Atomic Emission Spectroscopy

Atomic Emission Spectrophotometer uses quantitative measurement of the optical emission from excited atoms to determine analyte concentration.

3.8.1 Basis Principle

Atomic Spectroscopy is based upon the ability of atoms to absorb or emit light. In AES the high temperature atomization source provides sufficient energy to promote the atom into excited high-energy electronic levels. As these electrons fall back to lower energy levels they emit light of specific wavelength, and produce characteristic spectral lines where the wavelength and relative intensity of these spectral lines are characteristic of the element and provide a means of identification. The intensity of emitted radiation is directly proportional to the concentration. A transition occurs between distinct atomic energy levels. The emission line in the spectra are narrow. The spectra of multielemental samples can be very congested, hence require a high-resolution spectrophotometer.

3.8.2 Instrumentation

In Atomic emission spectrophotometer the sample must be converted into free atoms, usually in a high temperature excitation source. The following components must be present in the AES (Fig. 3.10 & 3.11).

1. Excitation Source

2. Electric arc
3. Sample holder
4. Dispersive media
5. Detector
6. Recorder

3.8.2.1 Excitation Source and Electric arc

The excitation source must dissolve, atomize and excite the analyte atoms. Spark or arc excitation source use a spark (current pulse) or continuous electric discharge (arc) between two electrode to vaporize and excite analyte atoms. The electrodes are either metal or graphite. In case of metal sample it can be used as one electrode. Non-conducting samples are ground with graphite powder and placed into an electrode. The electric arc used at 220 volts and their temperature is about (5000° C to 8000° C).

3.8.2.2 Sample Holder

The radiation obtained from sources struck between two graphite electrodes which are a few mm apart. The sample is kept in lower electrode, the top of which is a cup-shaped structure.

There may be different types of electrodes configuration.

1. Point to point
2. Point to plane
3. Porous cup

The metal sample is analyzed directly because they conduct electricity easily whereas non-metallic samples are usually treated by wet or dry ashing to eliminate any organic material present. Nonconducting sample is mixed with graphite powder and put into cup-shaped lower electrode.

3.8.2.3 Dispersive Medium or Monochromator

The light produced by excitation is first passed through a narrow slit and collimated to form a parallel beam. It is then allowed to pass through a dispersing medium to separate the different wavelengths. The dispersing medium is either a quartz prism or diffraction grating.

3.8.2.4 Detector and Recorder

The spectrum which is in the series of line is commonly recorded on

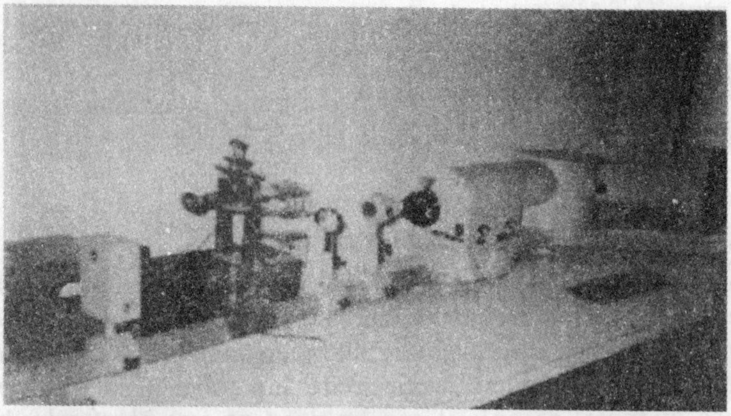

Fig. 3.10. Atomic Emission Spectrophotometer

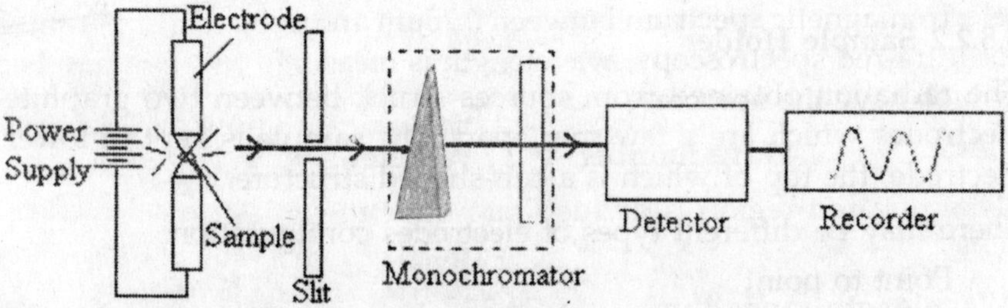

Fig. 3.11. Diagrammatic Representation of Atomic Emission Spectrophotometer

photographic film. Several spectra can be recorded on a single film by moving it after each exposure. Some modern spectrographs have photo multiplier tube to detect and record the spectrum.

3.8.3 Application of AES

- It is useful for qualitative and quantitative determination of sample.
- It is a destructive technique and very sensitive to detect the metallic element in various types of samples.
- It is useful for the detection of trace elements present in animal tissue and plant material.
- It is helpful in the field of archeology and restoration artifacts for the analysis of alloys, jewellery, coins, glasses, antique pieces, painting and ceramics.

- It is also helpful in the field of mineralogy and geology.
- Analysis of Ni and Cu in tea leaves.
- Antimony and silver in bullet lead.
- Quantitation of Fe in few green vegetables.
- Determination of Zn, K and Na in urine.
- Analysis of lead and other constituents in paint
- Water hardness
- Elemental composition of stature in Forensic anthropology.
- Determination of Ca and Mg in coal and coal ash.
- It is also used in other areas like biological, agriculture, industrial, food technology, forensic science and environmental analysis.

3.9 Infra-Red Spectroscopy

The Infra-red spectroscopy is the study of reflected, absorbed or transmitted radiant energy which covers the range of the electromagnetic spectrum between 0.78μm and 500μm. In the context of infra-red spectroscopy, wavelength is measured in wave numbers which have the unit cm^{-1}.

Wave number = 1 / Wavelength in cm

The infra-red region is divided into three regions:

	Near IR	Middle IR	Far IR
Wavelength range (μm)	0.78-25	2.5 – 25	25 - 500
Wave number (cm^{-1})	12800 – 4000	4000 – 400	400 - 20

Only the mid-infra-red region is considered here because it is the region which is widely used in the analysis of drugs and pesticides.

3.9.1 Basic Principle

Photon energy associated with this part of infra-red (from 1 to 15 kcal/mol) are not large enough to excite electron, but may induce vibrational excitation of covalently bonded atoms or group. The covalent bonds in molecule are like stiff springs that can be stretched and bent. IR Spectroscopy deals with the interaction of IR light with matter. The energy of an IR photon can be calculated by using the Plank energy relation.

$$E = h\nu = hc/\lambda$$

Where
- h is plank's constant
- λ is the wavelength
- c is the velocity of light
- E is energy absorbed by the molecule

When a molecule is subjected to IR radiation, transition takes place between rotational and vibrational energy level in the ground electronic state. These transition give rise to an absorption spectrum characteristic to the compound. In IR Spectroscopy the transition occurs at higher energy states and the absorption takes place only where the dipole movement of the molecule changes.

The particular bands or functional groups in a molecule have specific absorption band at given wave numbers. If the structure or physical state of molecule changes the wavelength of a band also changes.

Fingerprint region

A band formed in IR region is specific for a particular molecule and its identity is equal to fingerprints which are never duplicate. So it is known as fingerprint region. It includes wavelength from 1600 - 400 Cm^{-1}.

3.9.2 Theory of IR

In IR region the absorption takes place due to the changes in vibrational and rotational energy level. When radiation of less frequency pass through the sample molecule rotation takes place and when radiation of high frequency is passed, molecular vibration take place. Here the absorption by molecule is quantized, hence the band formed in discrete lines and appear as vibrational – rotational band due to energy changes.

When Infra-red light passes through the sample the vibrational and rotational energy of the molecule are increased. There are two types of variation of fundamental nature.

1. Stretching
2. Bending

3.9.2.1 Stretching: The position of atoms in the molecule are not fixed. In this mode the distance between the two atoms increases or decreases but the atoms remains in the same bond axis. There are two types of stretching vibration (Fig. 3.13).

(i) *Symmetric Stretching:-* The measurement of atom with respect to a particular atom occur in the same direction.

(ii) *Asymmetric Stretching:-* In this one atom approaches the central atom while the other depart from it.

3.9.2.2 Bending: In this there is change in bond angle with respect to original bond axis. It is of four types (Fig. 3.14).

(i) *Scissoring:-* In this type two atoms approach each other.

(ii) *Rocking:-* The movement of atom takes place in the same direction.

(iii) *Wagging :-* Two atoms move up and below the plane with respect to central atom.

(iv) *Twisting:-* In this type one of the atoms move up the plane while the other moves down the plane with respect to the central atom.

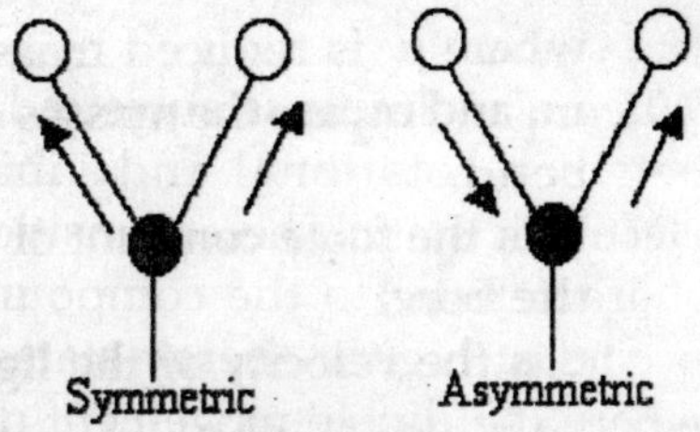

Fig. 3.13. Stretching Vibration in Molecules

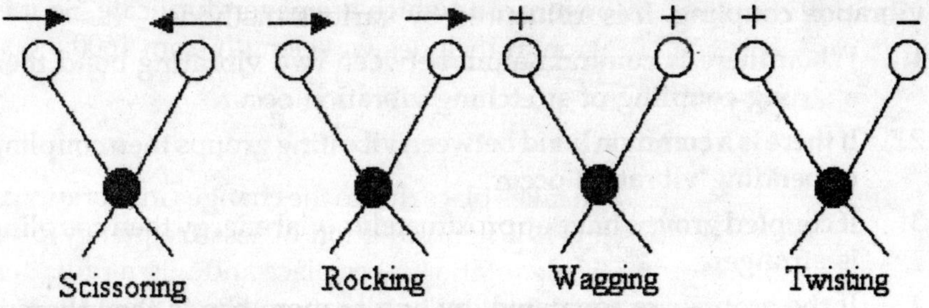

Fig. 3.14. Bending Vibration in Molecules

Bending vibration require lesser energy and hence occur at higher wavelength or lower numbers than stretching vibrations.

3.9.2.3 Vibrational Frequency

The value of the stretching vibrational frequency of a bond can be calculated accurately by the application of Hooke's Law.

It may be represented as–

$$V = \frac{1}{2\pi c}\left[\frac{k}{\frac{m_1 m_2}{m_1 + m_2}}\right]^{1/2}$$

$$= \frac{1}{2\pi c}\sqrt{\frac{k}{\mu}}$$

where μ is reduced mass

m_1 and m_2 are the masses of atom concerned in gms in a particular bond.

K is the force constant of the bond and relates to the strength of the bond

c is the velocity of the light radiation

Thus the value of vibrational frequency or wav umber depends upon bond strength and reduced mass. If the bonc strength increases or decreases, mass reduces and the value of the vibrational frequency increases.

3.9.2.4 Vibration Coupling

The interaction between vibration of molecular bond is known as vibration coupling. It is influenced by various methods.

1. When there is common atom between two vibrating bond then a strong coupling of stretching vibration occur.
2. If there is a common bond between vibrating groups then coupling of bending vibration occur.
3. If coupled groups have approximately equal energy then coupling is stronger.
4. If the groups are separated by two or more bonds then there is no coupling is seen.

3.9.3 Instrumentation

The IR Spectrophotometer comprises radiation source, monochromator, sample cell, detector and data output recorder. The

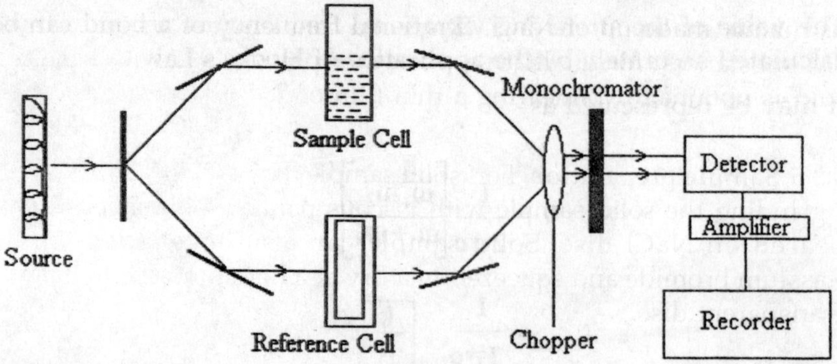

Fig. 3.12. Digrammatic Representation of Infra-red Spectrophotometer

optical components of IR Spectrophotometer cannot be made with glass or quartz material since they absorb IR radiation. For this purpose NaCl or other metal halides are commonly used (Fig. 3.12).

3.9.3.1 Radiation Source

An IR source should emit a continuous and high energy radiation. The most common radiation sources are–

(i) **Nernst Glower**: It consists of a rod of sintered mixture of the oxides of zirconium, Ytterbium and Erbium. The rod is electrically heated to 1500°C to produce Infra-red radiation.

(ii) **Nichrome Wire:** This source is simply a nichrome wire which emits IR radiation when heated by an electric current.

(iii **Glober**: It consists of rod of silicon carbide, produce IR radiation when electrically heated at 1100°C.

The light from radiation source split into two beams with the help of semi-reflecting mirror or prism, one is known as reference beam while another is sample beam.

3.9.3.2 Chopper: It is a circular device which rotates at a definite speed and reflect the sample and reference beam to a monochromator.

3.9.3.3 Monochromator

It is an optical prism or diffraction grating made up of sodium chloride. Because it is hygroscopic so protected from the condensation of moisture by working at suitable temperature. Diffraction grating gives better resolution at high temperature.

3.9.3.4 Sample Cell

It is mainly made up of NaCl. IR spectra runs on gaseous, liquid or solid substances; for qualitative work the spectrum of pure organic liquid is obtained by smearing a thin film of sample over the NaCl disc.

3.9.3.5 Sample preparation: For solid sample they are often prepared by grinding the solid sample with viscous paraffin oil and paste is smeared on NaCl disc. Solid sample can also be grinded with potassium bromide and squeezed in a dry at a high pressure to make a transparent disc.

3.9.3.6 Detector

It detects the absorption band formed in IR spectrum. There are many types of detectors used in IR spectrophotometer.

(i) **Semiconductor Type:** Semiconductor material such as indium, is used in this type of detector. When IR radiation falls on semiconductor material they are capable of exciting an electron to upper energy level. Thus creating a sufficient amount of electric current, measured by the detector in the form of electric signal.

(ii) **Thermocouple Type:** In this the radiation energy of detector element is being used, the temperature of which is measured to give output signals

(iii) **Bolometer:** It usually consists of a thin metal conductor. When IR radiation falls on this conductor its temperature and resistance changes. Thus the changes in temperature is regarded as a measure of the amount of radiation observed.

3.9.3.7 Data output Recorder: It is a device which facilitates the output of the printed absorption spectrum for recording purposes. This

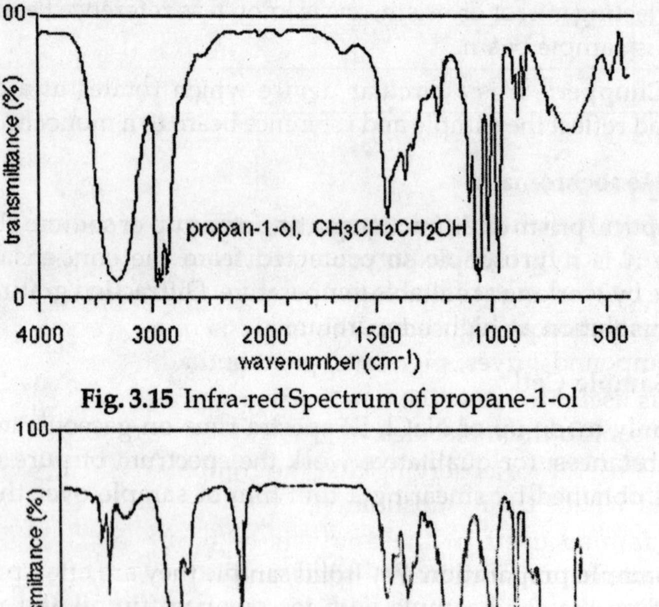

Fig. 3.15 Infra-red Spectrum of propane-1-ol

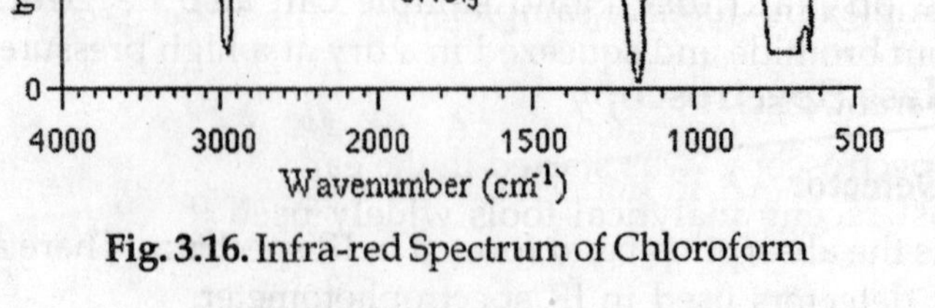

Fig. 3.16. Infra-red Spectrum of Chloroform

spectrum is in the form of graph and is known as IR - Spectrum. It consists of a PC and integrator or printer device.

Specific spectrum of propanol and chloroform obtained from IR spectrophotometer are as follows:-

Table 3.5. Some of the functional groups and their absorption frequencies are given for standard observation in the laboratory

S.N.	Functional group	Absorption Frequency
1.	- OH	3600 Cm^{-1}
2.	- NH	3500 Cm^{-1}
3.	- CH	3000 Cm^{-1}
4.	- C ≡ N	2250 Cm^{-1}
5.	-C ≡ C	2150 Cm^{-1}
6.	- C = O	1715 Cm^{-1}
7.	- C = C -	1650 Cm^{-1}
8.	- C – O -	1100 Cm^{-1}

3.9.4 Application

It is a non destructive technique and the sample as such can be preserved for further requirement. It includes many application in various field of scientific research.

- This technique is used in the analysis of explosives, polymeric compounds, dyes, pigments, paint and additives.
- It is useful to know the functional group such as C-H, O-H, N-H present in the molecules.
- It is useful for observing that the compound is aromatic or not and what's their substitution.
- It is also used in the analysis of biological materials for identification of proteins, lipids, and nucleic acids.
- Library search facilities are also available for identification of complex mixtures of sample.

3.10 Mass Spectroscopy

Mass Spectroscopy was started in the early 20th Century. It is one of the most recent analytical tools widely used to identify unknown compounds by determining their molecular weight at the expense of negligible amount of sample.

In this technique molecules are ionized and broken up into many fragments, where each kind of ion has its particular mass to charge ratio (m/e) known as mass number. For most ions the charge is 1 and m/e ratio is simply the molecular mass of the ion, where these different molecular masses are separated by means of electric and magnetic fields. The ions are thus reflected and the intensity of the output signal is a measure of amount of various ions produced. The output signal is called mass spectrum which provide a detailed picture of the elemental composition of parent ion and hence called fingerprint of the compound.

3.10.1 Theory and Principle

The basic principle of mass spectrometer is that the organic molecules are vaporized and bombarded with a beam of high energy electrons. The resulting collisons impart considerable energy to the molecule, which in turn emits electrons to produce positively charged ions.

$$ABC + 2e \rightarrow ABC^{+} + 2e$$

$$AB^{+} + C$$

$$A^{+} + BC$$

(Molecular ions)

The positively charged ions are accelerated towards a negatively charged plate by passing them through a magnetic field, which deflects the ions. The ions of lighter mass are deflected more than heavier ions. Each kind of ion has a particular mass to charge (m/e) ratio. It is therefore useful for quantitation of atoms or molecule and also for determining chemical and structural information about molecule. The ion separation power of a mass spectrometer is described by the resolution, which may be defined as:–

$$R = m / \delta m$$

Where m is the mass of ion

δ m is the difference in mass between two resolvable peaks in a mass spectrum

3.10.2 Base Peak

The largest peak found in a mass spectrum (highest intensity) is called the base peak, and is given the numerical value of 100. The intensities of all other peaks are expressed relative to the height of the base peak. A mass spectrum is highly characteristic of a particular compound (Fig. 3.17).

3.10.3 Molecular Ion

The ion formed by removing one electron from the parent molecule called molecular ion peak is usually represented as M^+. It may or may not be the peak, of highest intensity. The molecular ion is the most important ion, since its mass is the molecular weight of the parent molecule.

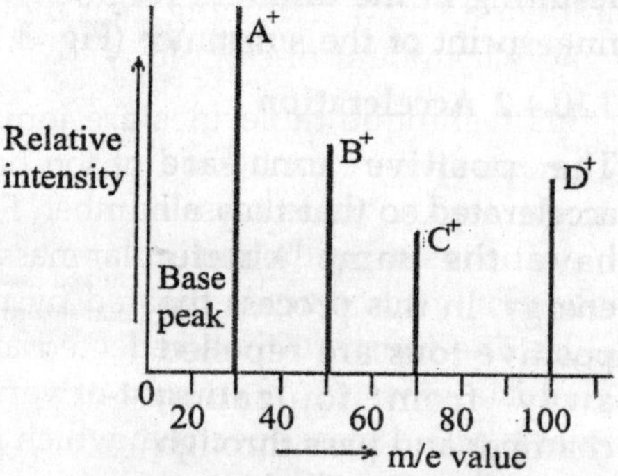

Fig. 3.17. Base Peak in Mass Spectrophotometer

3.10.4 Instrumentation

The Mass spectrophotometer consists of ion source, mass selective analyzer and detector. The general process of mass spectrometer include:

3.10.4.1 Ionization: It is done by means of electron impact ionization method. The sample vapour passes into the ionization chamber. The electrically-heated metal coil (70ev energy) gives off electrons which are attracted to the electron trap (positively charged plate). The particles in the sample bombarded with stream of electrons and make positive ions. During the electron impact process the charge acquired by the molecules is predominantly one and therefore their m/e ratio is one important parameter in separating them. The mass spectrum produced by electron impact shows a number of peaks

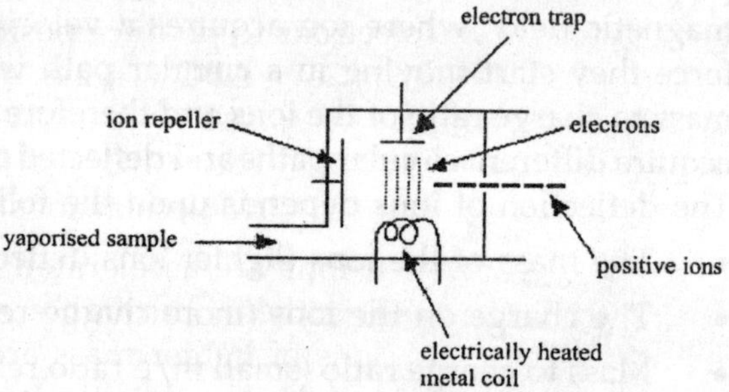

Fig. 3.18. Ionisation of Sample

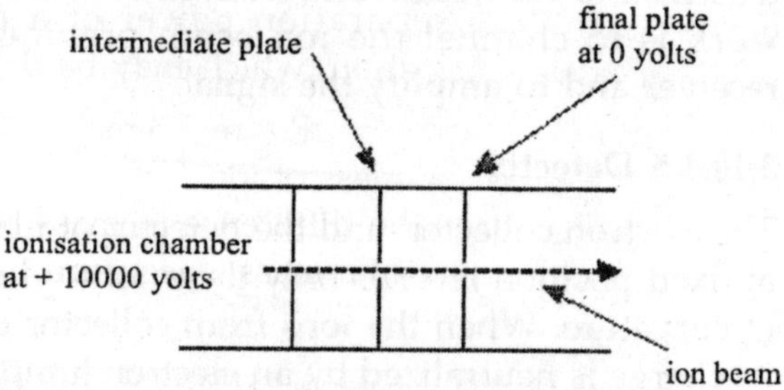

Fig. 3.19. Ionised Sample

resulting in the different fragments and has been considered as the fingerprint of the substance (Fig. 3.18).

3.10.4.2 Acceleration

The positive ions are accelerated so that they all have the same kinetic energy. In this process the positive ions are repelled away from ionization chamber and pass through three slits. The final slit is at 0 volts (Fig. 3.20).

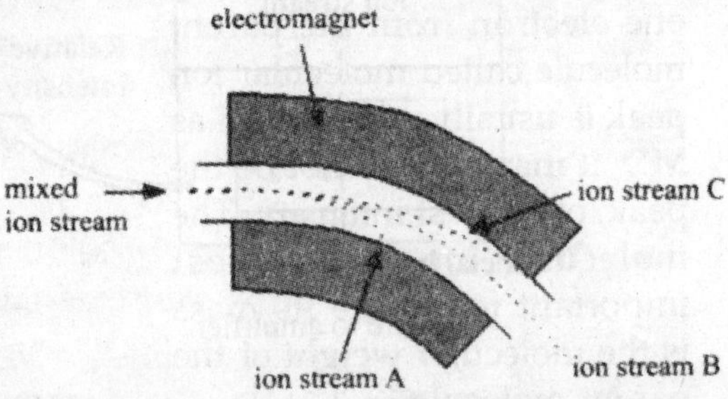

Fig. 3.20. Acceleration of Sample

3.10.4.3 Mass Analyzer

The beam of positive ions are drawn into an evacuated chamber by an electric potential difference and a magnetic field is applied in perpendicular direction. The moving ion beam leads through this magnetic field where ion acquires a velocity and due to magnetic force they start moving in a circular path which depends upon the mass to charge ratio of the ions and therefore the ion from the sample acquire different circular paths and deflected through a magnetic field. The deflection of ions depends upon the following factors :-

- The mass of the ions (lighter ions deflected more than heavier).
- The charge on the ions (more charge results more deflection).
- Mass to charge ratio (small m/e ratio results in more deflection).

3.10.4.4 Collector Device

It consists of electrodes technically known as **Faraday's cylinder** whose work is to channel the ion beam previously dispersed towards receiver and to amplify the signal.

3.10.4.5 Detector

The electron collector and the detector of mass spectrometer situated at fixed position records only those ions which have a correct radius of curvature. When the ions from collector device hit the metal box, its charge is neutralized by an electron jumping from the metal on to the ion that leaves a space among the electrons in the metal and the electrons on the wire move to fill the space. Now the flow of electrons in the wire is detected as an electric current that can be amplified and recorded. The current is proportional to the number of positive ions.

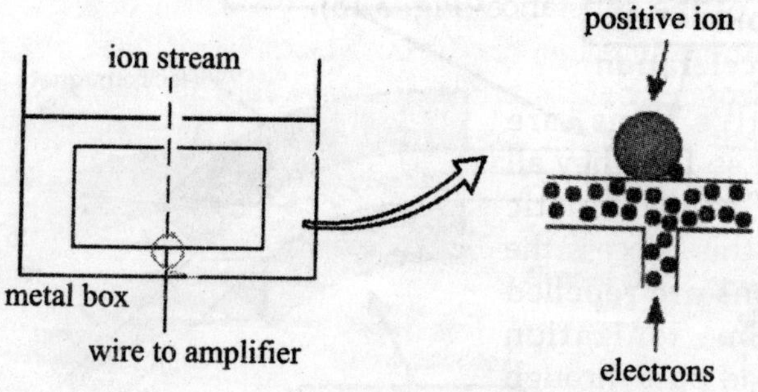

Fig. 3.21. Detection of Ions from Sample

There are two types of detector basically used in Mass Spectrometer.

(i) Photographic Films

(ii) Electron Multiplier

(i) Photographic Films: The Photographic film has been used for the detection of the ions which gives a latent image developed by the conventional methods. The position of the line on the plate indicates the mass of ions and its intensity is a measure of its quantity. The plate is calibrated with standard available.

(ii) Electron Multiplier: Another type of detector used nowadays are electron multiplier. They have a high detection sensitivity and high speed of recording. For this purpose mainly photo multiplier tube is used.

3.10.4.6 Resolution and Scanning

The two important considerations in mass spectrometer are resolution and scan speed, where the resolution is the ability to separate two adjacent masses and scan speed is the time taken to scan the entire mass.

3.10.5 Application

The most important application of mass spectrometry is the unequal identification of unknown compounds from their mass spectra.

- It has become the powerful analytical tool for monitoring environmental pollutants.
- Pesticides and insecticides residues in food, water and soil can be easily analyzed by mass spectrometry at part per billion and trillions levels.

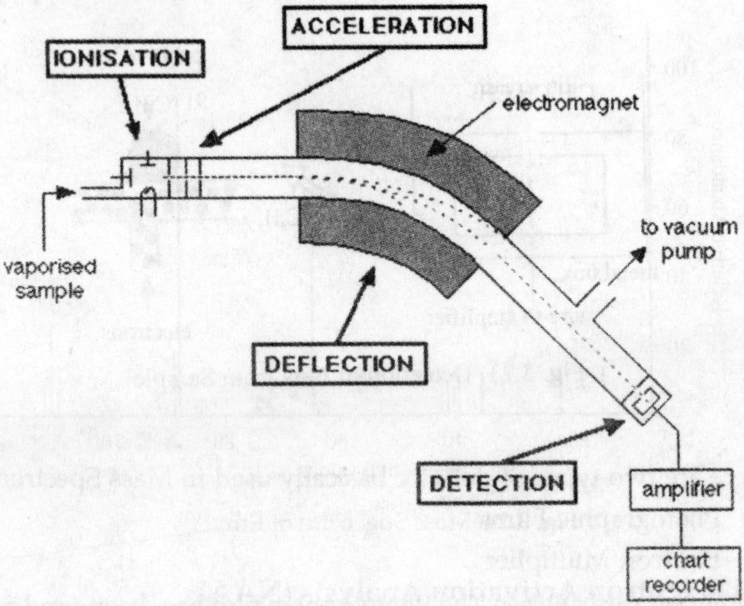

Fig. 3.22. Schematic Representation of Mass Spectrophotometer

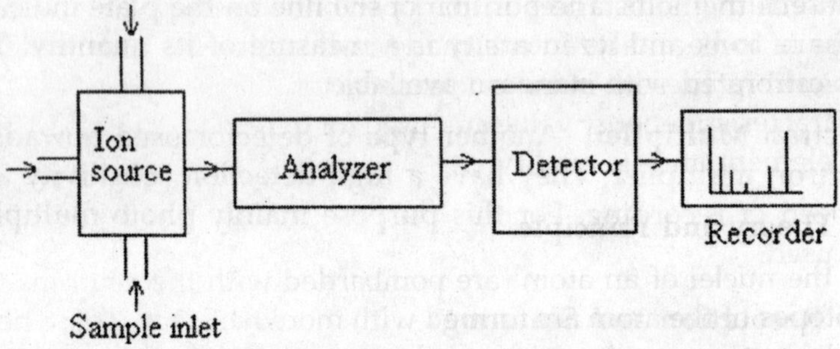

Fig. 3.23. Digrammatic Representation of Mass Spectrophotometer

- Identification of explosive residues recovered from the crime scene is often analyzed by Mass spectrometer.
- It is used in the analysis of synthetic polymers.
- It is used for all kinds of chemical analysis, ranging from environmental analysis (e.g.. Detection of poison such as dioxin) to the analysis of petroleum products, trace metals and biological materials (including products of genetic engineering).
- Tiny amount of proteins can be identified by mass spectrometer.

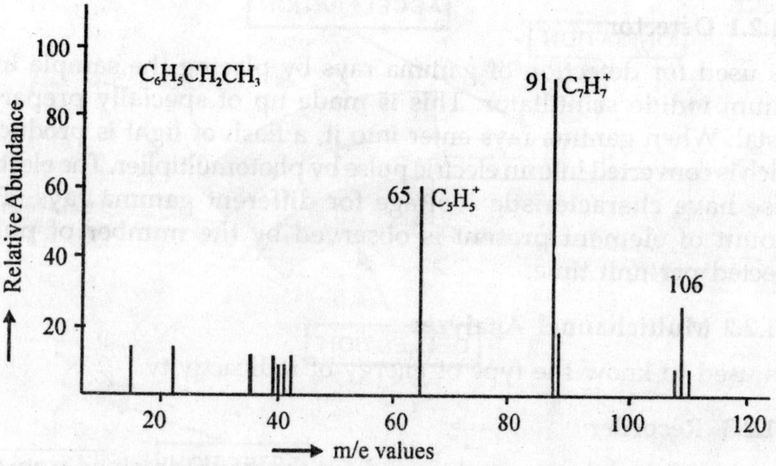

Fig. 3.24. Mass Spectrum of Ethyl Benzene

3.11 Neutron Activation Analysis (NAA)

Neutron activation analysis is a technique for detecting and analyzing highly sensitive substances in part per billion range. The elements which are to be analyzed are made radioactive by bombarding it with neutrons present in the nuclear reactor. Hence the radioactivity has characteristic energy value and used for detection, characterization of the element and its quality.

3.11.1 Theory and Principle

When the nuclei of an atom are bombarded with the neutrons then the isotopes of the atom are formed with more neutrons. These newly formed isotopes are decomposed due to radioactive decay with the liberation of α, β and γ rays. Alfa rays are positively-charged particle, beta rays are electron and gamma rays are electromagnetic radiation.

In a nuclear reactor when neutron enters into the nucleus of an atom then gamma rays are produced due to disintegration. These gamma rays have characteristic energy value which is used to know the type of atom or element and its intensity tells about the concentration of the element present in a substance.

3.11.2 Measurements of Radioactivity

The measurement of gamma rays energy includes the following equipments:-

3.11.2.1 Detector

It is used for detection of gamma rays by placing the sample into sodium iodide scintillator. This is made up of specially prepared crystal. When gamma rays enter into it, a flash of light is produced which is converted into an electric pulse by photomultiplier. The electric pulse have characteristic voltage for different gamma rays. The amount of element present is observed by the number of pulse detected per unit time.

3.11.2.2 Multichannel Analyzer

It is used to know the type of energy of radioactivity.

3.11.2.3 Recorder

It is an electrical device used to read out the signal obtained from the detector on a computer screen.

3.11.3 Application

- It is used to analyze many complex organic substances at a time in one billionth of a gram.
- It is used to detect trace element in hair, gunpowder deposits around a firearm wound, gunshot residue particles on the hand of user of a gun etc.

3.12 Nuclear Magnetic Resonance (NMR)

Nuclear magnetic resonance is related with the magnetic properties of certain nuclei. The nuclei of Hydrogen atom behave as a magnet and generate a magnetic field. NMR may be defined as the interaction between oscillating field of electromagnetic radiation and the magnetic energy of nucleus of H or other atom, placed in an external magnetic field. When an electromagnetic radiation passes through the sample, it absorbs radiation of radio wave region at different frequencies and absorption depends upon the type of nuclei (proton) in the sample.

3.12.1 Basic Principle

Radio waves are formed as the lowest form of the electromagnetic radiation. Their energy is too small to vibrate, rotate and excite an atom or molecule but this energy is sufficient to effect the nuclear spin of the atom of a molecule. Therefore the nucleus of the atom in a molecule on absorbing radio frequency may change their direction of spin. Now if a proton is placed in a magnetic field, it starts resonance at a certain frequency in radio wave region. The energy required to bring about the transition ($\Delta E = h\nu$) or to resonate the proton depends upon the external magnetic field (Fig. 3.25).

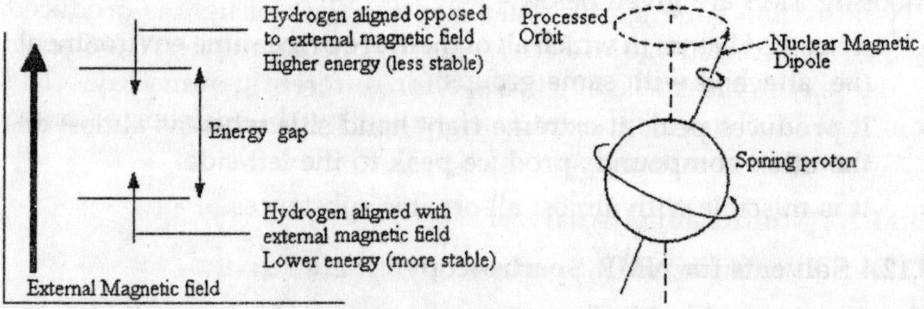

Fig. 3.25. (a) Resonance of proton in magnetic field **(b)** Spining of proton

Hydrogen nuclei can also be aligned or opposed to external magnetic field, where it is opposed to the field, is less stable (at a higher energy). It can bring from more stable state to less stable state by supplying it exact amount of energy.

3.12.2 Number of Signal or Peaks

In the NMR spectrum the number of signal or peaks depends upon the number of H-atom present in different environments.

$^{a}CH_3CO^{a}CH_3$ $\qquad$ $^{a}CH_3 - COOH^{b}$

In Acetone, only one signal is obtained because H-atom is attached with two same groups (i.e. in same environment) whereas in acetic acid two signals are obtained because H-atom is attached with two different groups (i.e. in different environment). The proton attached in the same environment are called **equivalent protons** while the protons attached with different environment (groups) are known as **non equivalent protons**. The size of the peaks give information about the number of H-atom (proton) present in each environment (groups). It can be observed by measuring the area below the peaks (not by the height of the peaks). NMR spectrometer has a device which draws another line on the spectrum called as integrator trace by which relative area below the peak can be measured.

3.12.3 Standard for Comparison

The horizontal scale of NMR spectrum has a zero point at right hand end of the scale. At this point a peak is formed by tetramethylsilane

(TMS). It is standard for all the compounds and everything can be compared with this compound. If in a NMR spectrum there is a peak at zero point, ignore it because it is TMS peak. The advantage of choosing TMS are given below:-

- It has 12-H atom in which all of them are in the same environment (i.e. attached with same groups)
- It produces peak at extreme right hand side whereas almost all the other compounds produce peak to the left side.
- It is miscible with almost all organic substances.

3.12.4 Solvents for NMR Spectroscopy

The solvent used in NMR spectroscopy never contain any hydrogen atom because it generates confusing peaks in the spectrum. So tetrachloromethane (CCL_4) or Carbon disulphide (CS_2) may be used. We can also use a solvent in which the ordinary H-atom is replaced by its isotope (i.e. deuterium) such as $CDCl_3$ in place of $CHCl_3$.

3.12.5 Low Resolution NMR Spectra

A low resolution NMR spectra is much simple than high resolution NMR spectra because it does not distinguish between the individual peaks in the various groups of peaks (Fig. 3.26).

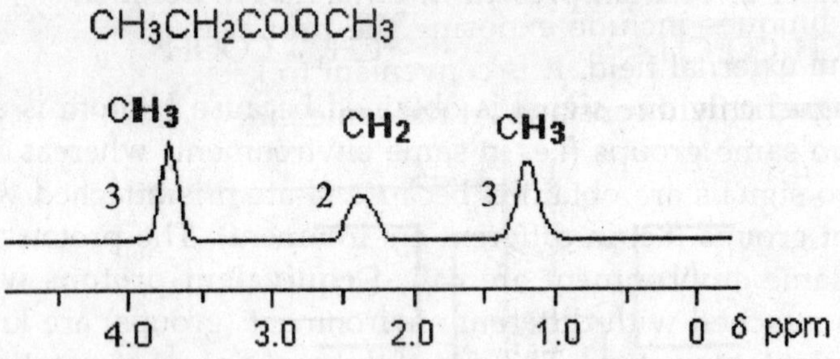

Fig. 3.26. Low Resolution NMR Spectrum of Methyl Propane

3.12.6 High Resolution NMR Spectra

The high resolution NMR spectra shows that a single peak in low resolution spectra split into cluster of peaks (Fig. 3.27).

3.12.7 Chemical Shift

The position of the peaks in spectrum indicates the type of group present (i.e. aliphatic, aromatic or acetylenic) while the number of

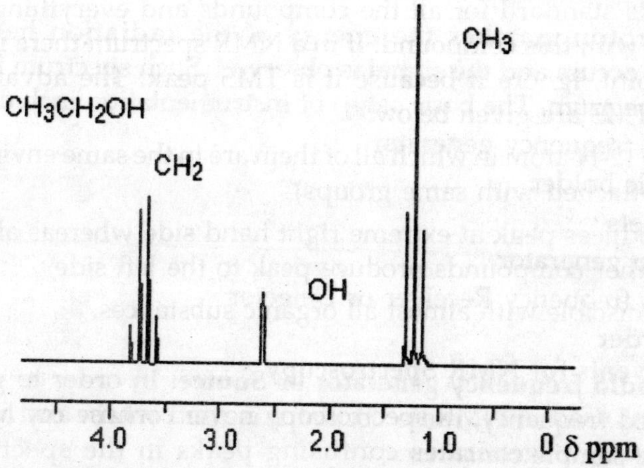

Fig. 3.27. High Resolution NMR Spectrum of Ethanol

peaks tell the number of sets of H-atom (proton) present in the molecule. Each type of proton has different electronic environment hence they absorb specific amount of energy. This difference in the absorption position (energy) of the H-atom with respect to standard TMS peak is known as chemical shift. It is expressed as δ value.

3.12.8 Instrumentation and Technique

The techniques include exposing the proton on the sample to the powerful external field. It is convenient to keep the radio frequency and magnetic field constant. At the same time the energy required to

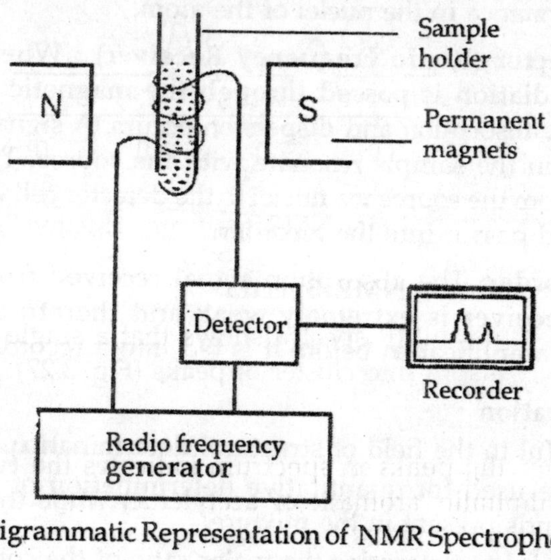

Fig. 3.28 Digrammatic Representation of NMR Spectrophotometer

flip the proton matches the energy of the radiation hence the absorption occurs and the signal is observed. Such spectrum is called as NMR spectrum. The basic setup of instrumentation includes

- Radio frequency generator
- Sample holder
- Magnets
- Sweep generator
- Radio frequency Receiver or Detector
- Recorder

3.12.8.1 Radio frequency generator or Source: In order to generate the required frequency, radio oscillator is used whose coil is bound around the sample container.

3.12.8.2 Sample Holder: 7.5 cm long and approximately 3.0 cm in diameter glass tube is taken which should be chemically inert and transparent.

3.12.8.3 Magnets: Permanent magnets or electromagnets can be used. The magnet should give homogenous magnetic field that is the strength and direction of the magnetic field should not change from point to point.

3.12.8.4 Sweep generator: The variation in current can be done by fixing a pair of "Helmoltz coil" in the pole faces of main magnets. The magnetic field induced by these coils can be varied by varying the current flowing through them. Thus radio frequency radiation brings about the resonance in the nuclei of the atom.

3.12.8.5 Detector (Radio Frequency Receiver) : When the Radio frequency radiation is passed through the magnetic sample two phenomenon, absorption and dispersion occurs. A signal is detected if the nuclei in the sample resonate with the source. The energy is transferred from the source via nuclei to the detector cell which absorb the signal and pass it into the recorder.

3.12.8.6 Recorder: The absorption signal received from the radio frequency receiver is extremely weak and therefore it requires considerable amplification before it is fed into a recorder.

3.12.9 Application

- It is useful in the field of structural determination.
- It can be used for quantitative determination of one or more compounds present in the mixture.
- It is helpful to determine the molar ratio of the component in a

mixture.

- It can be used for studying the hydrogen bonding in the metal chelates.

3.13 X- Ray Spectroscopy

3.13.1 Introduction

X- rays was discovered by **Rontgen in 1895**. These rays are generally invisible and travel in straight lines at the speed of light. Although they cannot be deflected by means of a lens and prism. The beam can be diffracted or bent by a crystalline grid. When passing through a material X- rays are partialy absorbed in the transmission direction. The relation between absorption and penetration depends on the kind of material (its atomic number) and on the energy of the X- rays. The energy itself is a function of the acceleration of the emitted electrons (the high voltage connected between anode and cathode) and the electrical current passing the filament wire. Another important property of X- rays is that they can destroy or impair living cells.

3.13.2 X- Ray Diffraction

X- ray diffraction is a versatile, non-destructive analytical technique for identification and quantitative determination of the various crystalline forms, known as 'phases' of compounds present in powdered and solid samples.

Identification is achieved by comparing the X- ray diffraction pattern or 'diffractogram' obtained from an unknown sample with an internationally recognized database containing reference pattern for more than 70,000 phases.

3.13.3 Basic Principle

When X- rays pass through the crystalline surface they are reflected or scattered by these planes. Most of the reflected X- rays interfere with each other in a destructive manner. Some rays however depend upon the angle of incidence i.e. interfere in constructive manner resulting is the reinforcement of the X- rays. Such reinforcement is given by Bragg's equation

$$N\lambda = 2d \sin\theta$$

Where λ is wavelength

d is spacing between crystal

$\sin\theta$ is the angle between incident ray and reflecting ray

3.13.4 Properties of X-Rays

- They travel in vacuum with the speed of light (3×10^8m/sec).
- They are not deviated by electric or magnetic field.
- They affect photographic plate very intensly.
- They ionize the gas through which they pass.
- They cause fluorescence in substance such as Zinc sulphate, Barium platino, calcium tungustate.
- They produce photoelectric effect
- These rays cannot penetrate bone and heavy metals but penetrates paper, thin sheet of metal, wood, flesh etc.

3.13.5 Diffraction

When a monochromatic X- ray beam with wavelength λ is incident on a lattice plane in a crystal at an angle θ, diffraction occurs only when the distance travelled by the rays reflected from successive plains differ by a complete number of wavelength.

By varying the angle θ, the Bragg's law conditions are satisfied by different d- spacing in polycrystalline materials. Plotting the angular positions and intensities of the resultant diffraction peaks produce a pattern which is characteristics of the sample. Where a mixture of different phases are present, the diffractogram is formed by addition of the individual pattern (Fig. 3.29).

A crystal may be defined as a piece of solid matter in which the atoms are regularly arranged in space. An example is aluminum, in which the arrangement is described as **"Face-Centered Cubic"** or "FCC".

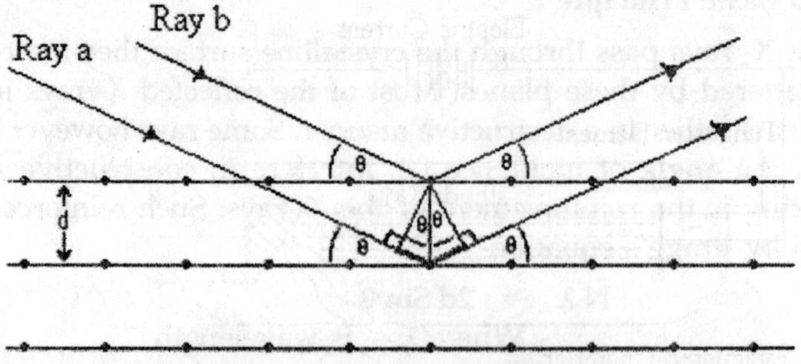

Fig. 3.29. Diffraction of X-ray Beam

In crystals, atoms are arranged in a definite and synthetic pattern. This technique is used to determine the crystal structure of chemical compounds. (Fig 3.30)

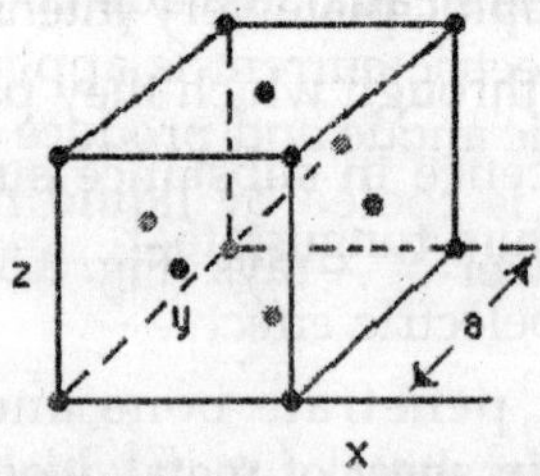

Fig. 3.30. Structure of a Crystal

3.13.6 Size of Crystallites

The size of crystals can be determined by identifying the structure of peaks from X-ray diffractogram. The widths of the peak in a particular phase pattern provide an indication of the average crystal size. Large crystallites give rise to sharp peaks while the peak width increases as crystallites size reduces.

3.13.7 Instrumentation

X-rays diffraction have the following components:-

1. X-rays source
2. Sample holder
3. Collimator
4. Detector and Recorder

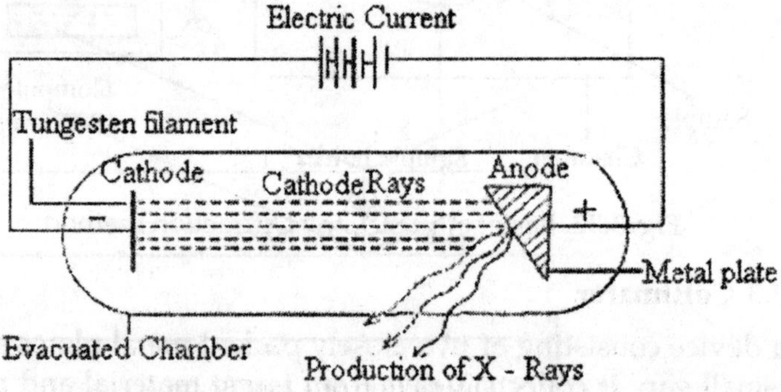

Fig. 3.31 Production of X-rays by Coolidge Tube

3.13.7.1 X-Rays Source

The main component of X-rays source is a X-ray tube or **Coolidge tube.** It consists of a glass bulb or metal envelope under vacuum. In the evacuated area there is a cathode made up of tungsten and anode of metal plate. When electric current is applied, the electrons from cathode strike on metallic anode and produce X-rays. To prevent the anode from damage, it is cooled by liquid material (water) or air depending upon the power of X-rays (Fig. 3.31).

3.13.7.2 Sample holder

Sample holder is a circular metal disc in which a space in the middle is provided for putting the sample. It should be clean with acetone after and before use. Sample should be in powder form, paste, fibrous or metallic. After putting the sample in the sample holder, its upper surface should be made plane with the help of glass slide and care should be taken that no trace or crystal of sample should remain left on sample holder other than the space provided for putting the sample. The sides of the sample holder must be clean with acetone and sample should be placed too tightly, that it should not fall out by moving it at 45° degree angle.

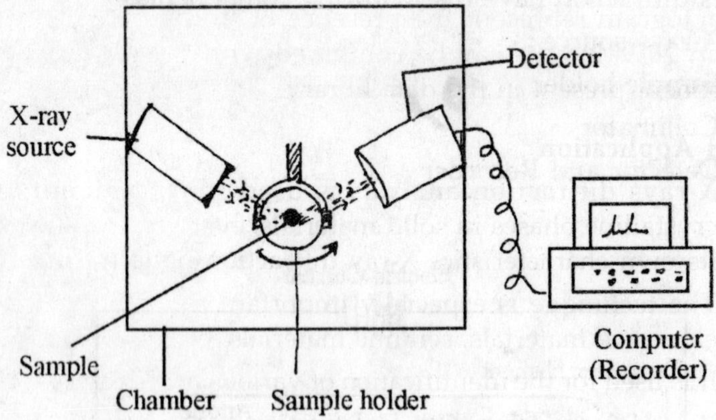

Fig. 3.32. Basic setup of X-ray Diffraction method

3.13.7.3 Collimator

It is a device consisting of two closely packed metal plates separated by a small gap. It collects X-rays from target material and provide a narrow beam of X-rays.

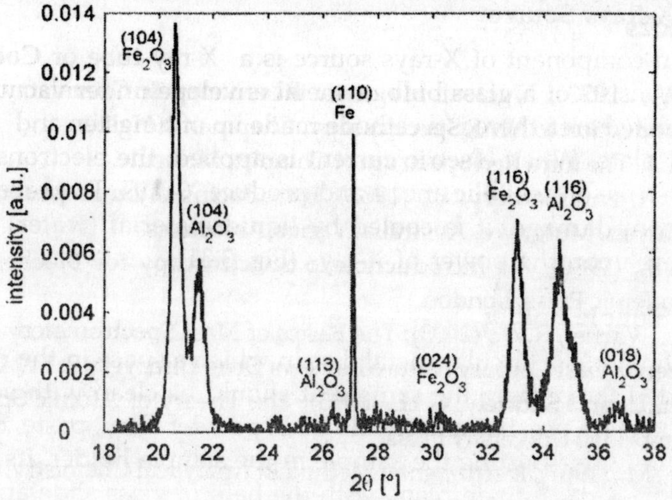

Fig. 3.33. X-ray Diffractogram

3.13.7.4 Detector and Recorder

The detector in X-rays diffraction is based on photoelectric effect. The diffracting X-rays give information about the sample molecule in the form of peaks on graph known as diffractogram. Each peak in diffractogram represent the presence of individual component at certain 2θ value. It may be compared with the standard peaks of component present in the data library.

3.13.8 Application

- X-rays diffraction analysis is used for the identification of crystalline phases in solid materials; every crystalline phase has its own characteristics X-ray diffraction pattern (fingerprint).
- The technique is especially important for the identification of explosive materials, ceramic materials, building materials etc.
- It is used for the identification of various metals and metal alloys.
- It is also used for the identification of soil, paint, cloth piece, fibres, lipstick, toothpaste or anything which may be held in sample holder.
- X-rays are also used for industrial applications such as X-rays inspection of casting products for the automobile industry or for analytical application.

References

Akitt, J.W., (1973); Nuclear Magnetic Resonance & Chemistry : An Introduction to NMR Spectroscopy, Chapman & Hall.

Bellamy, L.J. The Infra Red Spectrum of Complex Molecule.

Bennet, P.A. and Rothery, E., (1983); Introducing Atomic Absorption Analysis, Mulgrave, Australia: Varian Associates.

Brown, S.B., (1980); An Introduction to Spectroscopy for Biochemists. Academic Press, London.

Clish, G.L., Vachet, R.W., (2003); The Basics of Mass Spectrometery in the Twenty-First Century Nature Reviews Drug Discovery 2: 140:150.

Condon, E.U. and Shortely; G.H., (1963); The Theory of Atomic Spectra, Cambridge University Press.

Donbrow., M., (1967); Instrumental Method in Analytical Chemistry, Vol.@ Optical Methods, London, Pitman.

Dyer, J.R.,(1965); Application of Absorption Spectroscopy of Organic Compounds, Prentice Hall, Eaglewood Cliffs, N. J.

Ebdon, L., (1982); An Introduction to Atomic Absorption Analysis; A Self Teaching Approach, London: Heyden.

Flemming, I. and William, D.H.(1973); Spectroscopic Methods in Organic Chemistry, McGraw Hill.

Goldberg, Leo., (1988); Atomic Spectroscopy & Astrophysics. Physics Today 38-45, August.

Knowles, A. and Burgess, C., (1984); Practical Absorption Spectrometery, London, Chapman and Hall.

Rao,C.N.R.,(1975); Ultraviolet & Visible Spectroscopy, Chemical Applications. plenum Press.

Scheinmann, F, Ed. An Introduction of Spectroscopic Methods for the identification of organic compounds, Pergamon Press, New York.

Sharma, Y.R., (2006); Elementary Orgaic Spectroscopy S. Chand & Co. Ltd: New Delhi.

Shrader, S.R., (1971); Introduction to Mass Spectrometery, Boston, Allyn & Bacon.

Skoog, Holler and Nieman, Principles of Instrumental Analysis. Chapter 8 and 9, pages 192 - 227.

Tatum, R., (2002); Instrumental Analysis Notes. La Sierra Unioversity. Riverside CA. Winter.

Willard, H., Merritt, L., Dean, A., Settle, A., (1986); Instrumental Method of analysis, 7th edition.

CHAPTER 4

Chromatography

4.1 A Journey to Chromatography

The first chromatographic technique was invented by Russian botanist Mikhail Tsvet in 1901 during his research on chlorophyll.

Neubaur (1938) separated neutral amino acids and observed that the partition of acetylated amino acids between water and immiscible organic solvents differed for various amino acids.

Fritz Prior developed solid-state gas chromatography in 1947. Archer John Porter Martin, was awarded the Noble Prize for his work in developing liquid - liquid and paper chromatography in the year 1941-1944 respectively and he laid down the foundation for the development of gas chromatography and later produced liquid-gas chromatography in the year 1950.

In 1952 A.J. Porter Martin and Richard Laurence Millington Synge was awarded the Nobel Prize for their invention of partition chromatography.

Nowadays many advanced, high technical performance chromatographic techniques are developed by which we can resolve even similar molecules.

4.2 Introduction

A homogenous mixture or mass is divided into its component, individual unit or even into elements by using separation technique that are based on their physical or chemical properties. Some methods used for separation are distillation, crystallization and electrolytic precipitation. The commonly used separation technique is chromatography that finds application to all biological sciences.

The term "Chromatography" is derived from two Greek words *chroma-* "colour" and *graphein* - "to write". Russian botanist **Mikhail Tsvet** first used chromatography in 1906 to describe his work. He separated plant pigments(chlorophyll) into band by using a column of finely divided calcium carbonate (chalk). Chromatography is a flexible yet powerful analytical procedure but remains a separation technique. It may be considered as an analytical technique used for the purification and separation of organic and inorganic substance, closely related compounds such as isomer and in the isolation of unstable substances.

Recently the International Union of Pure and Applied Chemistry has defined chromatography as:

"A method used primarily for the separation of the components of a sample, in which the components are distributed between two phase. One of which is stationary while the other moves. The stationary phase may be solid, or a liquid supported on a solid or a gel. The stationary phase may be packed in the column spread as a layer, or distributed as a film etc. The mobile phase may be gaseous or liquid".

It may be used in different ways; some people use chromatography to find out component in a solid or liquid. It is also used to determine the presence of cocaine in urine, alcohol in blood, PCB's in fish, lead in water, explosives in debris, poison in viscera, alkaloids in plant extracts and different other components. The Police, F.B.I. and other Forensic Scientists use chromatography for the analysis of clue materials.

4.2.1 Basic Principle

Chromatography is based on the principle of selective distribution of the components of a mixture between two phases one of which is fixed (stationary) phase and the other is moving (mobile) phase. The stationary phase can be a solid or a liquid while the moving phase is a liquid or gas. When the stationary phase is a solid, the basis is adsorption and when it is a liquid the basis is partition.

4.2.2 Retention: The retention is the measure of speed at which substances move in chromatographic system. In continuous development system like HPLC and GC, where the compound are eluted with the eluent, the retention is usually measured as the retention time Rt (i.e. the time between injection and detection). But in TLC the Retention is measured as the Retention factor Rf. It can be denoted as:

$$Rf = \frac{\text{Distance moved by sample}}{\text{Distance moved by eluent (mobile phase)}}$$

This Retention factor depends upon stationary phase, temperature and setup of the instrument. It is therefore important to compare the retention of test compound with standard under absolute identical conditions.

4.2.3 Plate Theory

This theory was developed by **A.J. Porter Martin** and **Richard Laurence Millington Synge.** This theory describe the chromatographic system as being in equilibrium.

The partition coefficient K is based on this equation and is defined by following equation –

$$K = \frac{\text{Concentration of solute in stationary phase}}{\text{Concentration of sample in mobile phase}}$$

K is the partition coefficient and can be changed if experimental condition of chromatographic system is changed. For a column of fixed length and flow, the retention time (Rt) and retention volume (Vr) can be measured that is useful to calculate partition coefficient (K).

4.2.4 Basic Procedure

The mixture to be analyzed dissolved in a suitable solvent and passed through a column containing an adsorbing material. The component of the mixture would be held back by the material to different extant, the extant of such retention depends upon the "Partition Coefficient" i.e. the relative affinity of each compound to the solvent and adsorbing material as the solvent continuously flow through the column. The components are separated and appear in the effluent at different times. The components with the least affinity to the stationary phase appear first and one with stronger affinity appear at the last.

4.3 Classification of Chromatography

Chromatography is a technique that involves separation of solutes based on selective interaction between a stationary phase and a liquid (mobile phase).

(i) If the stationary phase is a solid support or a liquid coated solid support and the mobile phase is a liquid, the technique is known as liquid chromatography.

(ii) If the stationary phase is applied as a layer, the technique is referred to as thin layer and paper chromatography.

(iii) When the stationary phase is placed in a column it is said to be liquid column chromatography.

(iv) In gas chromatography the stationary phase is a solid support or a liquid coated solid support and the mobile phase is a gas.

Chromatography can be classified according to the nature of stationary or mobile phase. If the stationary phase is a solid the process is called **adsorption chromatography**. It can be understood by following table:

Table1.1

Stationary phase	Mobile Phase	Process	Technique
Solid	Liquid	Adsorption	LSC
Solid	Gas	Adsorption	GSC
Liquid	Liquid	Partition	LLC
Liquid	Gas	Partition	GLC

4.4 Paper Chromatography

Paper chromatography is frequently used by students in the research laboratory. It is an analytical technique for separating and identifying pigments and other molecules from complex mixture. In this sample is dissolved in a suitable solvent which run on the paper by capillary action and hence the sample become attracted towards the paper at different degrees and is separated.

4.4.1 Basic Principle

The basic principle of paper chromatography is that chemical interaction of compound with the paper makes it travel at different rates, mainly due to the hydrogen bonding. This is done by the differences in partition coefficient (K) (Fig. 4.1).

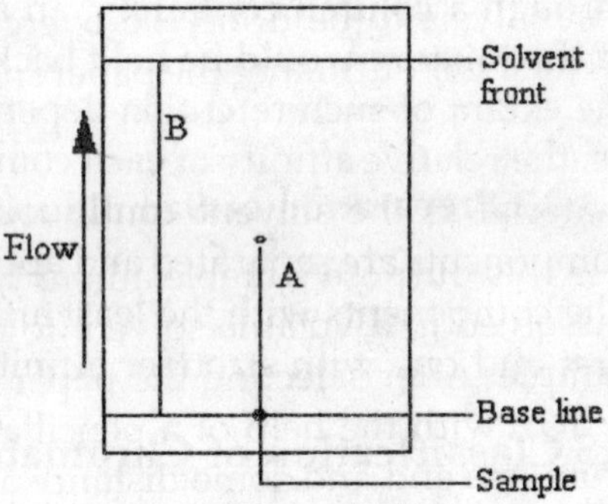

Fig. 4.1. Principle of Paper chromatography

$$Rf = \frac{\text{Distance moved by sample}}{\text{Distance moved by solvent}}$$

$$Rf = \frac{A}{B}$$

4.4.2 Types of Paper Chromatography

It is of the following two types:–

4.4.2.1 Paper Partition Chromatography

In this technique Whatman No. 1 filter paper is used as an inert support with the mobile and stationary phase respectively. The solvent used in mobile phase run on the paper and separates the mixture into its components.

4.4.2.2 Paper Adsorption Chromatography

In this technique paper is impregnated with an adsorbent like silica or alumina and single solvent is used to flow over the unknown sample.

4.4.3 Experimental Procedure

4.4.3.1 Materials Required

In this technique Whatman No. 1 filter paper is used, which is made up of cellulose and should possess the following characteristics.

- It should have maximum degree and clarity of separation.
- It should be devoid of diffusion of spot.
- It should inhibit the tailing of substance to be analyzed.
- It should have excellent movement of solvent front during analysis.
- It should also inhibit the vertical movement of sample.

The shape and size of the filter paper may vary according to the type of analysis to be done. To overcome the problem of diffusion and reducing of substance the paper should be washed with acetone before use.

4.4.3.2 Preparation of Sample and its Application on the Paper

For this purpose suitable amount of solid sample weighted and then dissolved in a volatile solvent to form a concentrated solution of the sample. After selecting the paper of specific shape and size, a line is drawn with the help of a pencil at a suitable distance (about 2.0 cm) from one end and some distance also left from two ends of the paper. This line works as a platform for the sample. Some points are marked on this line at equal distances, on which the sample is placed.

The minimum amount of concentrated solution is then applied on these points with the help of fine capillary tube achieving the diameter of 5 mm. Then each spot should be dried by a stream of hot air or N_2 for preventing the diffusion.

4.4.3.3 Selection of Solvent

The selection of proper solvent depends upon the type of sample to be separated. Since the polar solvent is adsorbed on paper, it is used more frequently. These polar solvents are known as mobile phase and move on the paper by means of capillary action (since paper is made up of many cellulose fiber and they occupy different fine capillaries between them by which solvent run over the paper). In various type of separation the solvent may consist of different proportion of components such as :-

- Water : n butanol : Acetic acid (5:4:1)
- Isopropanol : Ammonia : Water (7:1: 2)
- Phenol : Water (7:3)
- Benzene : Chloroform (7:3)

Some times alcohol, acids, ketones, esters, and phenols etc. can also be used.

4.4.3.4 Development of Chromatogram

Before developing the chromatogram the glass jar should be saturated with the solvent. It can be developed by one of the following methods:-

- Ascending method
- Descending method
- One dimensional method
- Two dimensional method
- Radial or Disc development

(i) Ascending Method

It is simple from all other methods. In this method the lower end of the paper containing sample is dipped into the solvent and allowed to run the solvent by capillary action in a glass jar. The solvent runs along the paper upwardly and separates the sample material into its components. The low Rf value substances are not completely separated by this technique; for such compound descending method is applied.

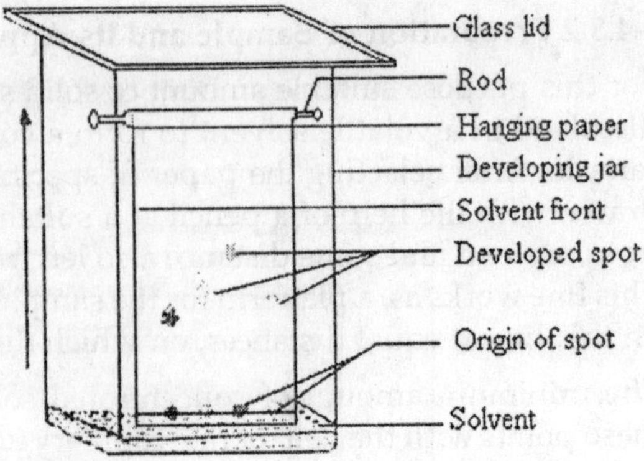

Fig. 4.2. Schemetic Representation of Paper Chromatography

Care should be taken that the sample spot does not dip in the solvent. If the paper is rolled into a cylinder its two ends can never be touched by using paper clips (Fig. 4.3).

(ii) Descending Method

In this method the paper has to be hanged with the help of a glass rod at the upper side of the glass jar. Here the solvent is placed at the upper side and spotted end of paper should be put towards the solvent. And then allow to run the solvent from top to bottom. The solvent front is the lower end of paper. This method is useful for the

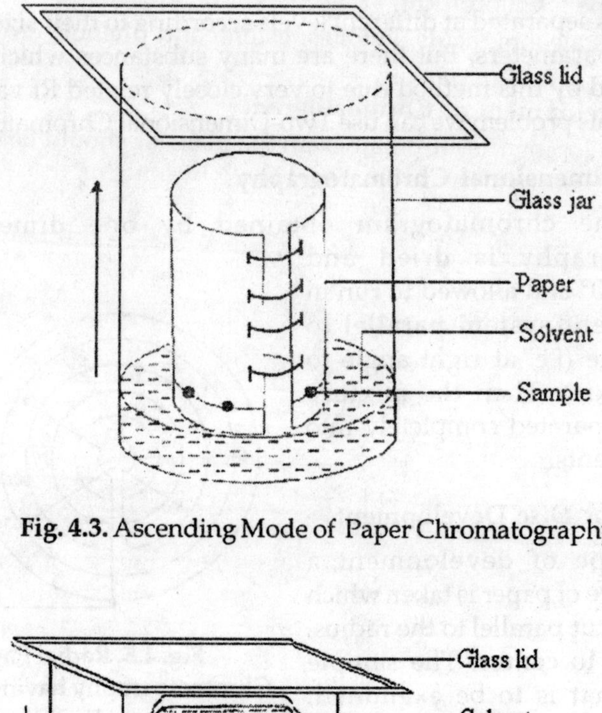

Fig. 4.3. Ascending Mode of Paper Chromatography

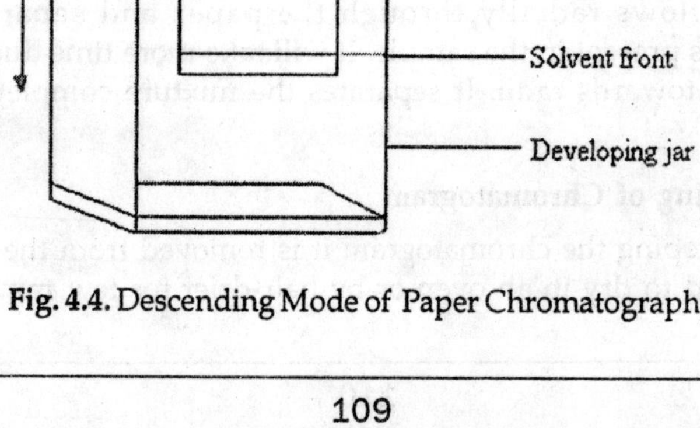

Fig. 4.4. Descending Mode of Paper Chromatography

components having closely related Rf values. The Rf value affected by gravity so that the substance is compared with suitable standard compound (Fig. 4.4).

(iii) One Dimensional Method

A complex mixture is generally separated by this method. In this the sample is placed at the corner of the paper instead of their margin. And then put into suitable solvent and allowed to run. The different components separated at different levels according to their size, nature and other parameters. But there are many substances which cannot be separated by this method due to very closely related Rf values. To overcome this problem we can use Two-Dimensional Chromatography.

(vi) Two-Dimensional Chromatography

In this the chromatogram obtained by one dimensional chromatography is dried and rotated at 90° and allowed to run in other solvent system parallel to second edge (i.e. at right angle to the first axis). Then the mixture becomes separated completely into its components.

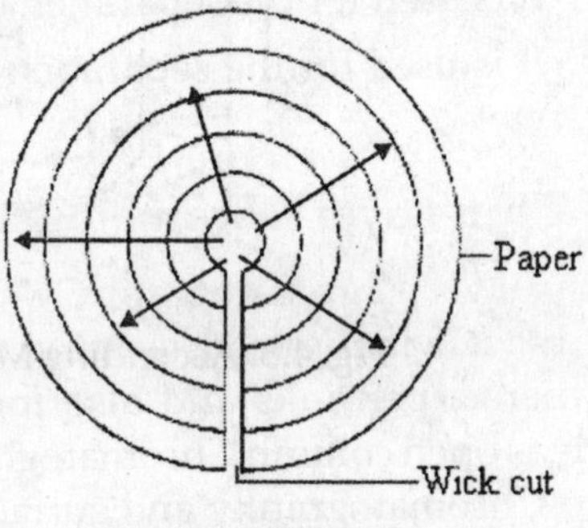

Fig. 4.5. Radial Paper Chromatography having Round Paper and Wick cut in it

(v) Radial or Disc Development

In this type of development a circular piece of paper is taken which has a wick cut parallel to the radius, from edge to center. The sample material that is to be examined, spotted to the center of the paper and upper end of the wick. This paper is laid on the edge of a circular disc and wick dipping in the solvent at the bottom of the dish. The liquid ascends through the wick and flows radially through the paper and separates the components present in the sample. It will take more time due to slow movement towards radii. It separates the mixture completely (Fig. 4.5).

4.4.3.5 Drying of Chromatogram

After developing the chromatogram it is removed from the glass jar and allowed to dry in an oven or by hair-drier for few minutes.

4.4.3.6 Location of Separated Components

The coloured components separated easily but colourless component can be located by means of physical or chemical treatment.

By UV rays : The sample can be located by examining under UV light.

Radioactive material can be located by various radiation methods.

The locating reagent like ninhydrin and diphenylamine spray on the sample spot and it becomes visible.

4.4.4 Application

- It is used to separate amino-acids and anions.
- It is used in RNA typing.
- Sometimes it may be useful for separating and testing histamines and antibiotics.
- It is used for the separation of various insecticides and pesticides.
- It is used for the separation of plant pigments, dyes and pen ink etc.

4.5 Thin Layer Chromatography

Thin Layer Chromatography was developed by **Stahl in 1958**. It is the most widely used technique for the separation of drugs, plant pigments, pen inks and also for explosive materials. Other names such as open column Chromatography, spread layer Chromatography, strip Chromatography and surface Chromatography are given to this technique.

4.5.1 Basic Principle

It is based on the principle that a mobile phase moves by capillary action across a uniform thin layer of finely divided stationary phase (adsorbent like silica gel) bonded on to a plate. When a mixture of sample is applied to the plate and developed with the mobile phase, the sample components move across the plate at different degrees depending on their solubility, i.e. pKa values and capability of hydrogen bonding and hence become separated.

$$Rf = \frac{\text{Distance moved by sample}}{\text{Distance moved by solvent}}$$

$$Rf = \frac{A}{B}$$

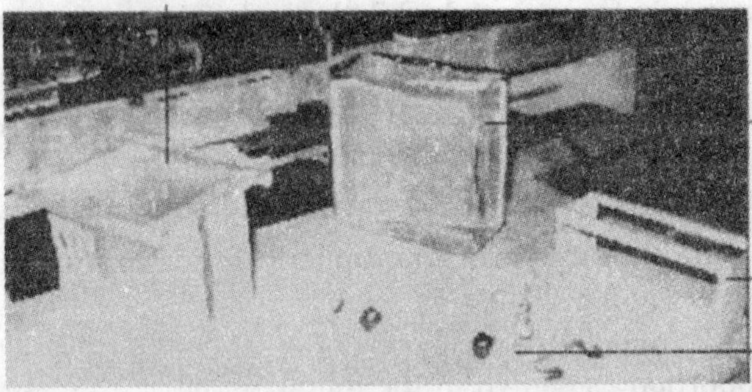

Fig. 4.6. Thin Layer Chromatography Kit having Developing Chamber, TLC Plates, Gel Applicator and Stand

4.5.2 Experimental Procedure

In Thin layer chromatography a number of steps like preparation of TLC plate, sample application, development of TLC plate and locating the spot have to be done. These steps are given as follows:-

4.5.2.1 Materials Required

Silica gel is used in making stationary phase while water and other organic solvents are used as mobile phase. Glass, plastic plate or aluminum foil are used for the binding up the stationary phase (Fig. 4.6).

(i) Stationary Phase

Stationary phase consist of a thin layer of adsorbent material like silica gel, alumina, Kieselghur, magnesium silicate or powdered cellulose, which is bonded on to a suitable plate. Due to flexibility of aluminum foil or plastic plate, it may be cut into small plates before use. On the basis of nature of stationary phase it may be divided into two categories.

(a) Normal Phase System

When the stationary phase is more polar than the mobile phase the system is known as normal phase system. In this the silica gel is mixed with water, acts as stationary phase and the mobile phase has a volatile non-polar organic solvent.

(b) Reversed Phase System

When the mobile phase is more polar than the stationary phase the system is termed as reversed phase system. In this the TLC plate impregnated with materials like heavy oil, liquid paraffin, silicon oil, fat etc. and the mobile phase containing water.

Methanol : Water or **Acetonitrile : Water** can also be used as mobile phase. These systems give good separation for different drugs but have the disadvantages of being slow running and having poor reproducibility.

(ii) Mobile Phase

The choice of mobile phase depends upon the compound to be separated and stationary phase to be used. It should not react with the substance to be separated. It either may be organic volatile polar solvent or water. It may be a single solvent or a mixture of solvents in different proportion as shown in the following table:

Table 1.2

S. No.	Solvent	Ratio
1.	Acetone: Chloroform	90 :10
2.	Toluene: Cyclohexane	70 :30
3.	Methanol: Toluene	80 :20
4.	Methanol: Formic Acid	80 :20
5.	Methanol: Acetonitrile	60 :40

These are the best known mobile phase used for various drugs and explosive analysis in controlled conditions.

When complex separation is required the size of TLC plate is 20 cm otherwise the plate size down to 7.5 x 2.5 cm may be used to save time and material. The TLC plate is used to be 2 mm thick for common analysis.

4.5.2.2 Preparation of TLC Plate

TLC plate may be prepared by using various methods like spreading, pouring, dipping, etc. but the spreading is reliable and the most commonly used method. For this purpose 6 gm of silica gel G (having grain size 2 - 25 m) is mixed with 12 ml of water and stirred gently to remove all air bubbles then simply poured on to the glass plates which is manipulated to obtain a thin layer. It can also be prepared with the help of an applicator known as Stahl applicator. The prepared slurry of material is put inside the applicator and kept on to the glass plate and the knob is allowed to move in the opposite direction. The slurry pours on the glass plate with a uniform layer of 250 μm thickness. Nowadays the prepared TLC plates are also available in the market. These are aluminum plates coated with silica gel G and suitable for handling. (Fig 4.7)

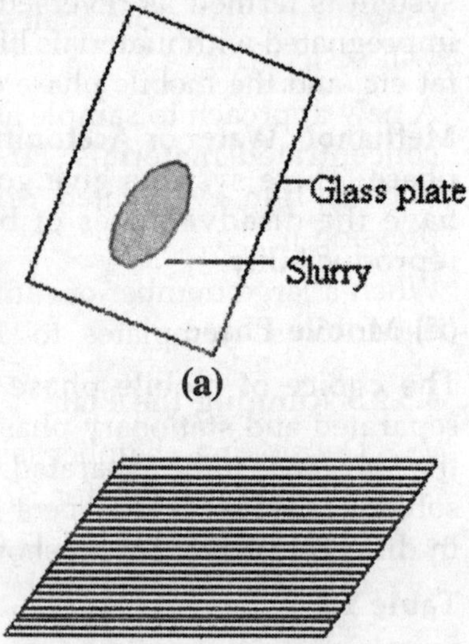

Fig. 4.7. (a) and (b) Preparation of TLC plate

4.5.2.3 Activation of TLC Plate

Prepared TLC plate is kept in the oven at 110°C for 1 hour for activation. It increases its absorptive effect and so increase retention. Now the plate is ready for use.

4.5.2.4 Sample Application on Plate

When the plate is activated it is removed from oven. Then a parallel line is drawn with the help of a pencil from 2 cm bottom of the plate. Now some points are also marked on this line 2 cm from the side and at least 1 cm from each other. Sample is spotted on these points and is known as origin of the sample. Another line also drawn at about 10 cm from origin known as solvent front. The sample is applied in its minimum volume (about 1 – 10 μg) with the help of a fine capillary or micropipette. The spot

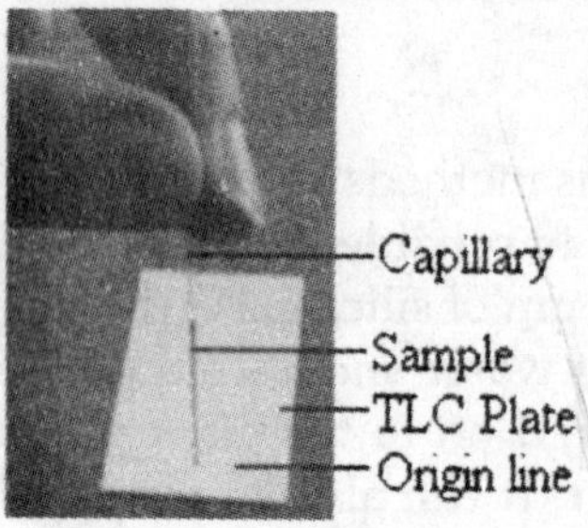

Fig. 4.8. Loading of Sample on TLC Plate

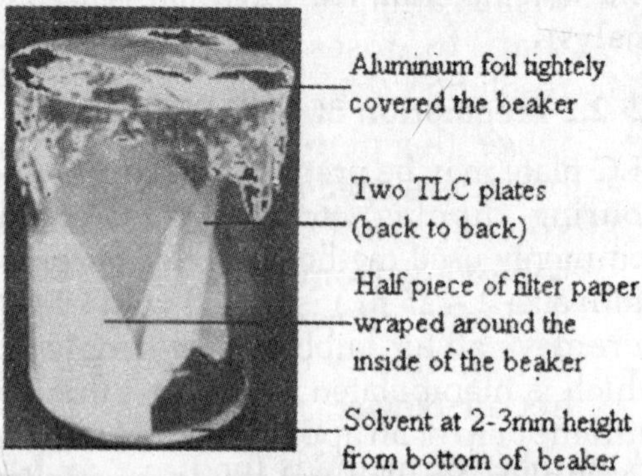

Fig. 4.9. Development of TLC Plate

should not be more than 4mm in diameter, otherwise resolution will be lost (Fig. 4.8).

A new approach to sample application is used for more viscous and concentrated materials. First sample is loaded on non wettable Polymer film, evaporated, dried and then transferred to the plate by pressing it.

When a large number of samples are loaded on to a glass plate, it is better to use templates to know the position of the spot accurately.

4.5.2.5 Running the Plate

- Developing chamber (size 5″x 9″) should be saturated first by allowing it stable for 30 minutes.
- Now sample loaded TLC plate (20 x 20 cm) is placed vertically into developing chamber filled with suitable mobile phase (100 ml).
- Special racks are also available that allow up to 5 plates placed vertically may be developed simultaneously.
- The care should be taken that the origin line is above the level of mobile phase. Then the level opening tank is covered with a glass lid. The mobile phase move ascending by capillary action on to the glass plate and separate the mixture into its components.
- The mobile phase take time about few minutes to 1 hour to develop the plate at solvent front of about 10 cm. It may take about 2 hours in case of viscous mobile phase. This time can be reduced when the plate is run only for 5 cm. This gives advantage of increasing sensitivity and saving of materials, but the disadvantages are that it loses the resolution (Fig. 4.10).
- Once the plate has been developed to the solvent front, it is removed from the tank and allowed to dry naturally or by hot air blower.

A number of methods for development have been reported in thin layer

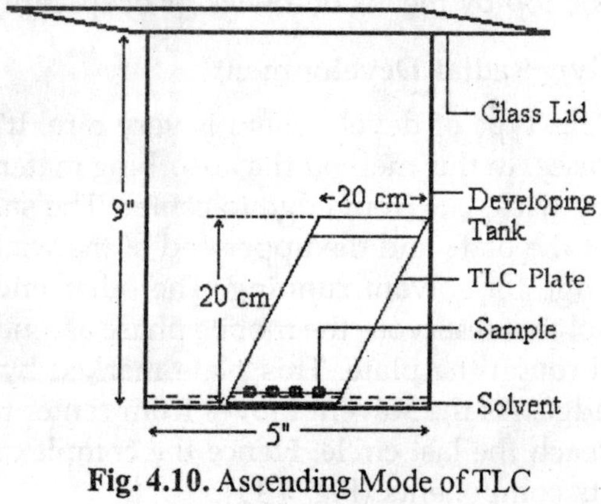

Fig. 4.10. Ascending Mode of TLC Development

chromatography.

(i) Ascending

(ii) Descending

(iii) Continuous

(iv) Radial development

(v) Multiple development

(vi) Two dimensional

(vii) Gradient elution

(i) Ascending Development

In this method the TLC plate is kept vertically into the developing tank and allowed to run the mobile phase. The solvent run upwardly due to capillary action and separates the component of the mixture known as ascending development method.

(ii) Descending Method

In this method the TLC plate is kept opposite the developing tank i.e. the spotted line towards upper side and solvent front from the base of the tank. Then solvent is allowed to run from upper to lower side with the help of a reservoir containing solvent. It runs more frequently due to gravitational force. This method is used for the component having low Rf value.

(iii) Continuous Development Method

A single development will not separate all the components in a mixture. It may be possible by using continuous development. In this method the mobile phase running up the plate and removing it from the top by means of a wick or evaporating by means of IR lamp.

(iv) Radial Development

This type of development is very rare. It is used only in very special cases. In this method the adsorbing material on to the plate is scraped by wick, cut from edge to center. The sample is placed at the center of the plate and the upper end of the wick, which is placed in cutting edge for solvent running. The other end of the wick is kept in the solvent reservoir, the mobile phase ascends the wick and flow radially through the plate. This plate marked by few circles from center to edge. As the solvent moves from center to radius, takes more time to reach the last circle. Hence the complex mixture is also separated in its components (Fig. 4.11).

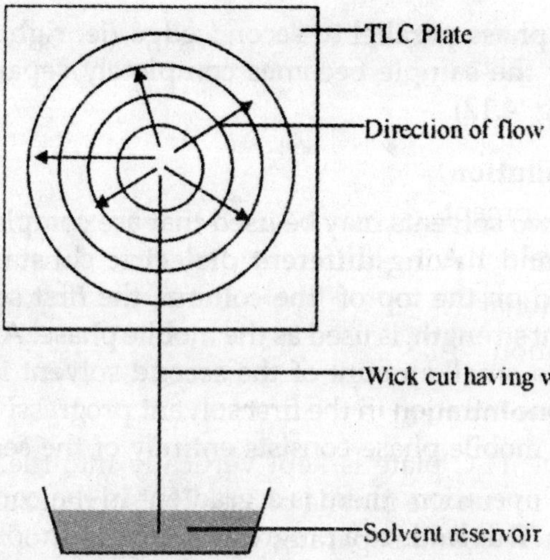

Fig. 4.11. Radial Development Method

(v) Multiple Development

In this type of development the plate is run in one mobile phase and allowed to dry. After that it is again run in the same direction by using the same or other more polar mobile phase. This procedure may be repeated a number of times to obtain the required separation. It is useful to analyze the components having different polarities.

(vi) Two-Dimensional Development

In this method the TLC plate of separated chromatogram is obtained from one dimensional method (Ascending Method). After that the plate is dried and rotated at 90° and then allowed to run by using

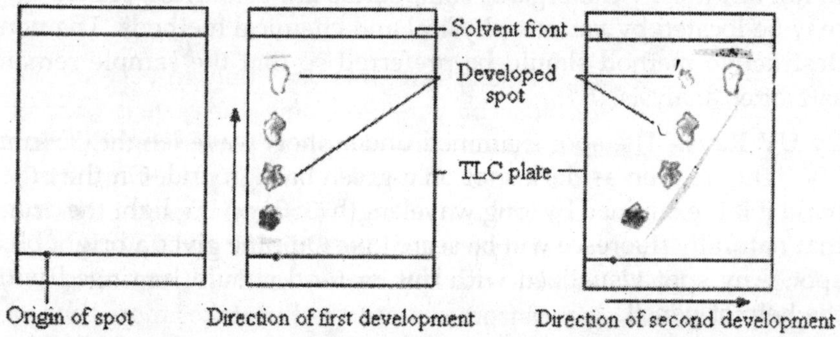

Fig. 4.12. Two-dimensional Method of Development

another mobile phase parallel to second edge (ie. right angle to the first axis). Now the sample becomes completely separated into its components (Fig. 4.12).

(vii) Gradient Elution

In this system two solvents may be used that are completely miscible in each other, and having different dielectric constant. After the sample is loaded on the top of the column, the first solvent, which has lower solvent strength, is used as the mobile phase. After a suitable period of time a small amount of the second solvent is introduced. With time, its concentration in the first solvent progressively increases until the finally mobile phase consists entirely of the second solvent.

Throughout the operation there is a gradient in the concentration of the two solvents. This leads to a progressive change in solvent strength and in the solubility of some of the components of the sample. Solvents that are somewhat different in their properties are selected in order to separate a greater range of components. Commonly used solvents are :-

Water : Acetonitrile
Water : Methanol
Dioxane : Tetrahydrofuron

An unknown compound can be identified according to their retention time or factor that can be confirmed by comparison with a known standard.

4.5.2.6 Location of Separated Components

After the plate is developed it is taken out from the glass jar and the solvent front is noted. The solvent evaporates naturally or by exposing to hot air. Mostly the organic compounds are colourless. Hence they may be located by various physical and chemical methods. The non-destructive method should be preferred so that the sample remain safe after analysis.

By UV Rays:- The spot examined under short wave lenght (254nm) UV light are seen as dark spot on a green background. On the other hand if it is examined by long wavelength (350nm) UV light the drugs that naturally fluoresce will be seen. Like Quinine gives a bright blue spot. Any spot visualized with this method should be ringed with the help of pencil.

Further nondestructive chemical methods can be performed, such as putting the plate in a tank of iodine vapour to see the brown spot. Photographic plate can also be used to determine radioactive drugs.

Another very useful but destructive test is to spray H_2SO_4 (sulphuric acid) on the plate and gently warm it, the organic material of the spot char and give brown or black colour.

Dragendorff reagent may be sprayed for the detection of alkaloids, besides that Morquis reagent and Mandelin's reagent are also helpful in the identification procedure.

4.5.2.7 Storage of Chromatogram

Aluminium and plastic TLC plates are flexible and stored as it is. But TLC glass plate can be photographed or photocopied. The colour reproduction than black and white picture are more useful. The actual layer on a glass plate can be preserved and removed by spraying with a solution of polymer.

Example : Polyvinyl propionate, which sets a clear pliable plastic film.

4.5.3 Rf Value

The Rf value of TLC is defined as:-

$$Rf = \frac{\text{Distance travelled by the Substance from the origin}}{\text{Distance travelled by the Solvent from the origin}}$$

Table1.3. Rf value of different Pesticides using a single solvent system of different chemicals

Substance (Pesticides)	Rf value with Solvent System Cyclohexane:Acetone: Chloroform (70 : 25 :05)	Locating reagent (for all groups)
Diazinone	82	Spray with Molybdate-antimony Reagent and then Lightly overspray with ascorbic acid reagent
Dimethoate	19	
Disulfoton	100	
Malathion	74	
Parathion	81	
Phorate	100	
Trichlorphon	09	

This Rf value have no unit and never exceed from 1. It is more useful to repeat Rf x 100 value to avoid decimal. This may also be referred to as hRf value. The distance traveled by the sample is measured from the center of spot.

Table1.4. Some Imporatnt Standard Rf value of common drugs and alkaloids by using different solvents:

Substances	Rf value with different solvent systems				Colour with locating reagent		
(Drugs and alkaloids)	Cyclohexane : Toluene : Diethylamine (75:15:10)	Chloroform : Methanol (90 : 10)	Chloroform : Acetone (4:1)	Ethyl Acetate	Ninhydrin Reagent	Dragondorff Spray	Van Urk Reagent / Chromic Acid
Amphetamine	15	09	– –	– –	Violet/Pink	Orange/Red	– –
Asprin	– –	– –	18	30	– –	– –	Pink
Barbitone	– –	– –	41	– –	Violet	Violet/Pink	Pink
Caffine	03	58	– –	– –	Yellow	Red/Brown	Pink
Diclofenac	– –	– –	25	40	– –	– –	Red
Dipteromine	24	04	– –	– –	Violet/Pink	Violet	Pink
Doxepin	52	37	– –	– –	Violet/Pink	Orange	– –
Ephedrine	05	05	– –	– –	Pink	Orange	Blue
Nicotine	39	35	– –	– –	Violet	Brown	– –
Paracetamol	– –	– –	15	34	– –	Violet	Pink
Trazadone	09	58	– –	– –	Violet	Red	– –
Zimeldine	27	25	– –	– –	Violet	Red/Orange	Violet

Rf values are affected by a number of external factors which enhance separation and change the Rf value. These are given below:-

- The type of adsorbent and binder, presence of impurities and uniform thickness must be checked carefully. The TLC plate should be stored at room temperature and the solvent used for applying the sample completely removed before running the plate.
- The solvent used for mobile phase should be prepared accurately and fresh for each analysis. It may be highly volatile or hygroscopic.
- The developing tank should be properly saturated before running the plate. It can be done by using a small tank with filter paper liners and sufficient solvent. The covered glass lid must be well fitted
- As the temperature increases the volatile solvents evaporate more quickly and run faster. It may cause slight decrease in Rf value. So the tank should be kept away from source of heat and direct sunlight etc.
- If the solvent front is increased the Rf value may also increase due to increased running distance and evaporation of the solvent from the upper part of the plate.
- If the mass of sample is increased on to the plate, it will cause tailing of the spot and change the Rf value of the sample and it will not be distinguished easily.

Test sample of known Rf value should be run to compare the results simultaneously.

4.5.4 Application of TLC

- It is used in the detection of various plant pigments and alkaloids.
- It is useful technique to analyze the poison from viscera.
- By TLC we can also do preliminary test for high explosive materials.
- It is quite useful in examination of various drugs like benzodiazepines, aspirin, amphetamines, barbiturates etc.
- We can also analyze sulphonamide and different pesticides by this methods.

4.5.5 Advantage of TLC over Paper Chromatography

It is superior than paper chromatography due to the following reasons:

- In TLC the separation is sharper.
- The separation requires less time (15 – 50 minutes) and less substance (micrograms).
- The individual spot is less diffused hence the sensitivity of detection is increased.
- We can provide higher temperature to TLC plates without damaging it.

4.5.6 Precautions

- Apply sufficient amount of concentrated sample on to the TLC plate (do not overload).
- Do not drop any other organic compound on to the TLC Plate.
- Origin of sample should always be marked with the help of pencil (not with pen).
- Do not disturb the developing chamber at the time of running of plate.

4.6 Column Chromatography

Column chromatography is defined as uniform movement of liquid (mobile phase) through a column of finely divided adsorbing material (stationary phase).

4.6.1 Basic Principle

The chromatographic column is being composed of a series of separate but adjoining, narrow, horizontal layers called theoretical plates. The running of sample between two phases is assumed to occur at each plate and the movement of solute and solvent is then viewed as a series of stepwise movement from one plate to another.

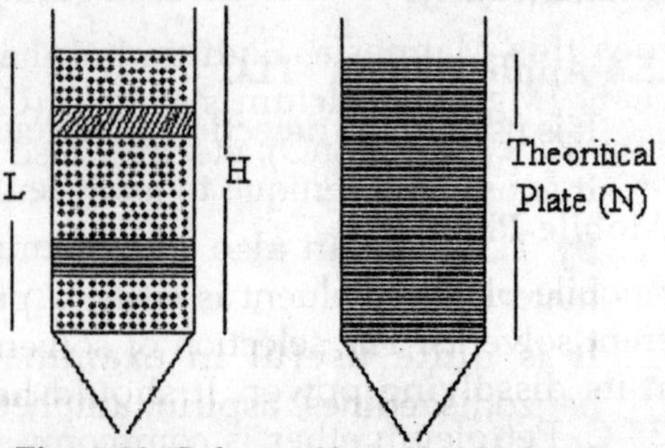

Fig. 4.13. Column Showing Separation Band and Theoritical Plates

The efficiency of the chromatographic column improves as the number of theoretical plate increases. Thus the number of theoretical plate (N) is used as a measure of column efficiency. The height of the column (H) also serve for this purpose. The relationship between these two parameters is –

$$N = \frac{L}{H}$$

Where L is length of column packing. It may be noted that H decreases as the efficiency of column become greater. That is as H becomes smaller, the number of equilibrium that occur in a given length of column becomes larger (Fig. 4.13).

Adsorbents like silica gel and alumina are the same ones used in TLC. The sample is dissolved in a small quantity of solvent (the eluent) and applied to the top of the column. The eluent, flows down through the column filled with the adsorbent. But in TLC it runs via a capillary action.

4.6.2 Experimental Procedure

4.6.2.1 Materials Required

The material required for column chromatography is same as for TLC, instead of TLC plates column is used for the analysis.

(i) Stationary Phase

In column chromatography the stationary phase or adsorbent is a solid. The most common stationary phase for column chromatography is silica gel. Alumina and cellulose powder were often used in the past. The stationary phase are usually finely ground powders or gel and micro porous, for an increased surface.

Besides this Magnesia, Sodium sulphate(Na_2SO_4), Magnesium sulphate ($MgSO_4$),Calcium sulphate ($Ca_3(PO_4)_2$),Barium sulphate ($BaSO_4$), Zinc oxide (ZnO), etc. may also be used as adsorbent.

(ii) Mobile Phase

The mobile phase or eluent is either a pure solvent or a mixture of different solvents. The selection of solvent or mobile phase depends upon its dissolving power. It should have boiling point between 60-85° C. Petroleum ether is commonly used for this purpose. The other solvents are Benzene (C_6H_6), Cyclohexane, Chloroform, (CCl_4) Carbon disulphide (CS_2), Ethyl alcohal (C_2H_5OH), Acetic acid (CH_3COOH), and Ethyl acetate ($CH_3COOC_2H_5$) also used.The solvent used in chromatography occupy following function:

- The solvent dissolves the mixture of various constituents and introduce it into column. The solvents are generally non-polar. (like Benzene, Petroleum, Ether etc.) so that the adsorption takes place more rapidly from such solvents.
- After passing through the column, chromatogram is developed and each chromatogram gets separated sharply from one another.
- Solvents are used for removing the various constituents of a mixture from the chromatogram; they are known as eluents. A good eluent should be a liquid which is capable of dissolving the various components of the given mixture. Its boiling point should be low so that it can easily be removed from the recovered component.

(iii) Developers

Developers are chemicals like H_2S, $(NH_4)_2S$ etc. used to produce colour with colourless solution.

4.6.2.2 Packing of Column

The packing of column is done by two methods.

In wet packing method the adsorbent is mixed with solvent and then poured this slurry into the prepared column. Before pouring the slurry the column is clamped in vertical position and its lower end is covered with glass wool plug. If there is some air bubble in the plug or at the bottom of the column, it should be removed by pushing it with a glass rod; the pouring of slurry should be continued to a desired height (Fig. 4.14, 4.15).

The excess of solvent may be removed by the lower end of the column. The common material used for column packing is Al_2O_3. MgO etc.

The dry pack method for packing the column is easier, but can lead to bubbles in the column. In this method first of all take an empty column, plug it with a small piece of glass wool, and affix a pinch clamp to the bottom of the column. Then clamp the column in a vertical position, close the pinch clamp and fill the column with solvent. By using a dry funnel, 8 g of alumina sprinkle into the solvent and allow to drain from the column to prevent overflowing. Now the alumina settles and gently tap the column with a pencil or glass rod so that the alumina will pack tightly into the column. Drain the solvent until the solvent level is just even with the surface of the alumina.

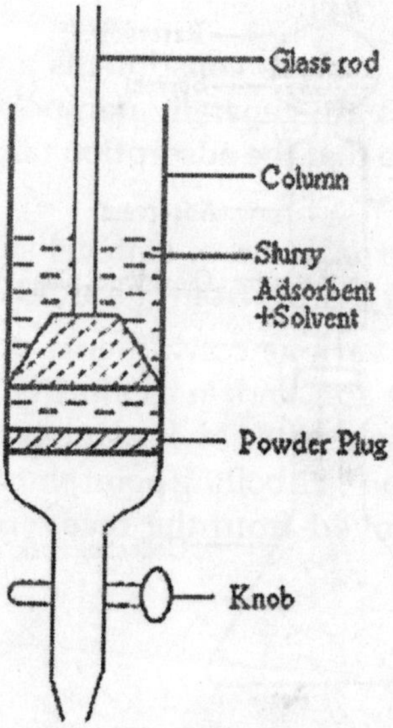

Fig. 4.14. Packing of Column with the help of Glass Rod and Silica Gel

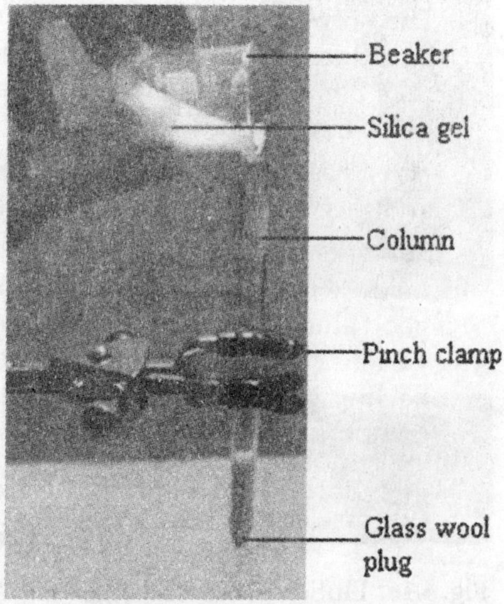

Fig. 4.15. Packing of Column with Silica

4.6.2.3 Procedure of Column Chromatography

The sample to be analyzed is dissolved in a very small amount of solvent to make a concentrated solution. This solution is then added to the top of column with the help of a pipette. The pinch clamp is opened and the solvent is allowed to run down. Then the eluting solvent is added into the column at the top and allow to flow through the medium. The solvent may be changed to more polar during the eluting processes. The flow of solvent continues until the sample mixture is completely separated into its components in the form of band or different zones (Fig. 4.16, 4.17).

After separation the adsorbent with the zone is taken out and each zone is separated with the help of a knife, and each zone may be dissolved in suitable solvents for further identification of the components. Such a set-up of separation is based on the polarity of the substances. The silica and associated solvents forms an extremely polar matrix. Thus more polar substances in the sample will adsorb more strongly to the stationary phase and elute slowlv from the column.

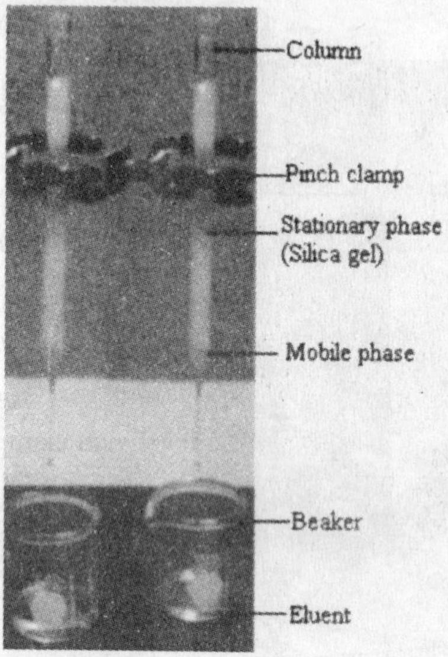

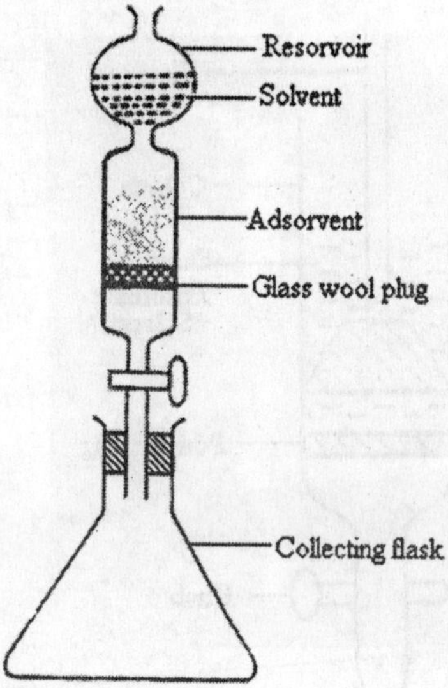

Fig. 4.16. Elution of Solvent with Separation of Sample Mixture

Fig. 4.17. Schematic Representation of Column Chromatography

On the other hand less polar substances in the sample adsorb weakly to the stationary phase and are quickly pushed through the column by the mobile phase.

4.6.3 Flash Column Chromatography

In column chromatography the silica or alumina gel makes the stationary phase quite dense. Hence mobile phase is moved very slowly through the column only due to gravitational force. This process can be speeded up by using a syringe attached to the bottom of the column for providing vacuum suction that fascilates quicker elution. It may also done by using high gas pressure at the top of the column to push the mobile phase more quickly. This method is called flash column chromatography (Fig. 4.18, 4.19).

4.6.4 Advantages of Column Chromatography

- It can be used in both analytical and preparative application.
- By this method we cannot only determine the number of components present in the mixture but also separate and purify substantial quantity of the component.
- This is in contrast to paper chromatography which is an analytical method.

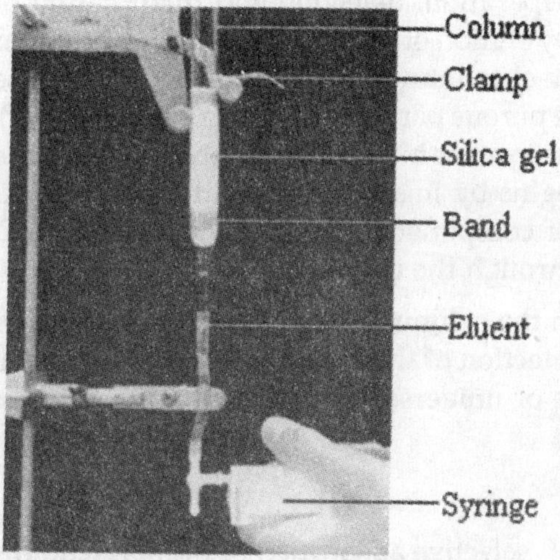

Fig. 4.18. Method of Flash column Chromatography showing Syringe attached to the Bottom of the Column

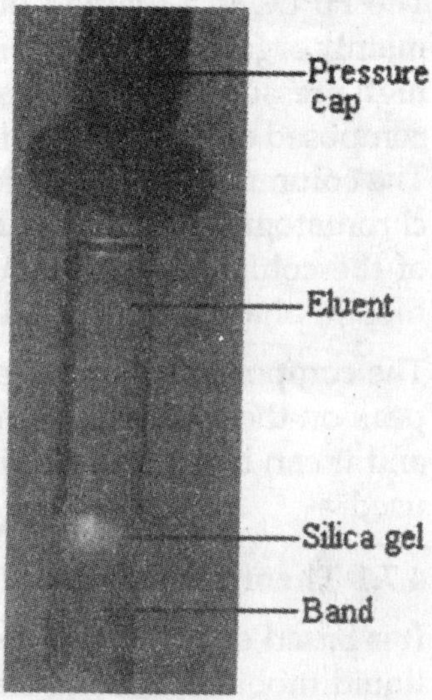

Fig. 4.19. Method of Flash Column Chromatography showing Air Pressure at the Top of the Column

4.6.5 Disadvantages

- For proper setting of the column it requires some manual skill and time.
- It is less foolproof than paper chromatography and requires constant attention while the experiment is being done.
- It is a time-consuming method, especially for large samples.
- It is not easy to perform like paper chromatography.

4.6.6 Application of Column Chromatography

- It is used for quantitative separation of two or more component in the mixture.
- It purifies the substance from its contaminants.
- It is helpful to concentrate the solute from its dilute solution.
- It is also used for identification of technical products.

4.7 High Pressure Liquid Chromatography (HPLC)

The modern form of column liquid chromatography is known as High Performance, High Pressure, High Resolution and High Speed liquid chromatography.

The HPLC is a method of separation, detection and quantitation of mainly organic compounds by elution of a liquid (mobile phase) under high pressure in a stainless steel column packed with stationary phase composed of micrometer size porous particles (10 µm or less diameter). The column is the heart of the system in which separation occurs. The chromatographic process begins by injecting the solute onto the top of the column. Separation of components occur as the analytes and mobile phase are pumped through the column.

The components eluted from the column appear as a narrow band or peak on the recorder. The detection of these components is important and it can be either selective or universal, depending on the detector used.

4.7.1 Theory and Principle

It is based on the principle of selective adsorption of the solute to the liquid mobile and solid stationary phase. A sample to be analyzed is injected into the column which carries through mobile phase. The different components in the sample are retarded at different degrees depending on their interaction with stationary phase.

Retention is a necessary factor for achieving good and contrast separation in chromatography. It is a measure of the speed at which a substance moves in chromatographic system and is expressed as Rt or t_R.

The fundamental relation between retention volume (Vr), the quantity of stationary phase (Vs) and the partition cofficient (K) is expressed as follows:-

$$Vr = Vm + KVs$$

Where Vm is the volume of mobile phase within the column, it may be determined by the chromatogram.

$$Vr = f \times Rt$$

Where f = flow rate of solvent

Rt = retention time of component

Similarly

$$Vm = f \times t_m$$

Where t_m = time taken by a unretained compound to traverse the column.

For evaluating the value of partition coefficient (K) the value of Vr must be known.

$$\text{Partition coefficient (K)} = \frac{\text{Concentration of sample in stationary phase}}{\text{Concentration of sample in mobile phase}}$$

The capacity factor K′ is related to K by following equation :

$$K' = K\frac{Vs}{Vm} = \frac{ns}{nm} = \frac{\text{number of moles of solute in stationary phase}}{\text{number of moles of solute in mobile phase}}$$

The capacity factor can be expressed as:-

$$Vr = Vm\ (1 + K')$$

The empirical expression derived are generally applicable to all types of column chromatography and are used universally.

First of all we measure the column efficiency, which is expressed in terms of number of theoretical plates (N) and height equivalent of theoretical plate denoted by (H) and after that we measure the resolution (Rs) which is attained in chromatogram.

A measure of column efficiency can be done by a number of theoretical plates that is expressed in terms of Retention time (Rt) and Base width (w).

$$N = 16\left(\frac{Rt}{w}\right)^2$$

$$N = a\frac{Rt^2}{w^2}$$

a is constant dependent on height where peak width is measured.

The efficiency of any column is best measured by the height equivalent to a theoretical plate which is expressed as :-

$$H = \frac{L}{N}$$

Where L is the length of the column

H is the height of the column

N is the number of theoretical plates.

Separation is the fundamental importance of any chromatographic method. The quantitative description of the separation is known as resolution which can be obtained between two peaks.

It is expressed as follows –

$$R = \frac{t_2 - t_1}{\frac{1}{2}w_1 - w_2} = \frac{2\Delta t}{w_1 - w_2}$$

The separation between two peaks is taken as the distance between the band centers divided by the average peak widths.

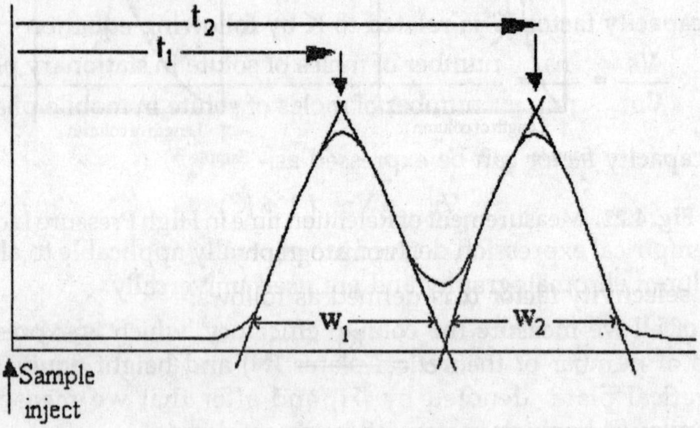

Fig. 4.20. Measurement of Resolution in High Pressure Liquid Chromatography

Thus greater the separation in retention times, narrower the peaks which influences higher resolution.

For quantitative work the aim to be minimum resolution is of 1, while for qualitative work a smaller resolution may be tolerated.

An unretained peak can be defined as :-

$$t_m = \frac{L}{u}$$

$$\text{but } Rt = t_m (1+K')$$

$$\text{So that } Rt = \frac{L}{u(1+K')}$$

where L is the length of column in cm

and u is the linear velocity of the mobile phase in cm / sec.

Thus the longer the column, the greater the retention time and smaller the linear velocity of the mobile phase and longer the retention of a component (Fig. 4.21).

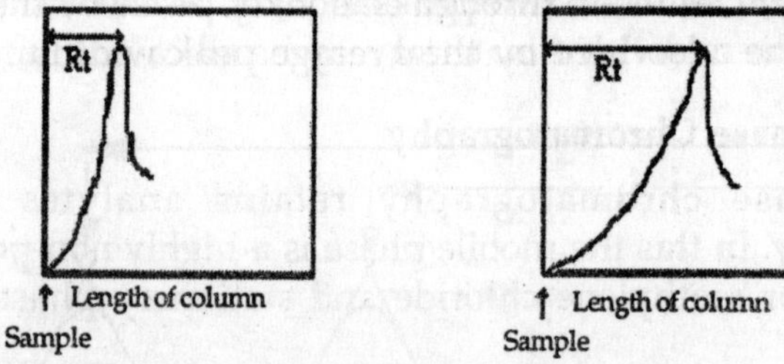

Fig. 4.21. Measurement of Retention time in High Pressure Liquid Chromatography

The selectivity factor α is defined as follows:-

$$\alpha = \frac{K'_2}{K'_1}$$

The relation between selectivity factor, resolution, capacity factor and column efficiency are expressed as :-

$$R = \frac{1}{4}\left[\frac{K'}{K'+1}\left(\alpha - 1\right)\right]N^{1/2}$$

where N, α and K′ are the fundamental parameters of chromatography.

A small increase in α will affect resolution significantly. If $\alpha = 1$, $K' = 2$ and $n = 1600$ then $R = 0$, which means no separation

Hence

$$K'_1 = K'_2$$

If we now increase α to 1.1 and keep the other conditions constant resolution will be approximately 0.7

If we now increase α to 1.2 while K′ and N are kept constant, resolution will be doubled.

4.7.2 Modes of Chromatography

HPLC carried out in various modes in which adsorption, partition, ion exchange, size exclusion and affinity are possible with great success.

4.7.2.1. Liquid Solid Chromatography (Adsorption)

In this separation mode the stationary phase is a solid and the mobile phase is a non-polar solvent such as hexane or methylene chloride.

The solute particles retain through stationary phase by the process of adsorption. The adsorbent material may be silica or alumina.

(i) Normal Phase Chromatography

Normal phase chromatography retains analytes based on hydrophilicity. In this the mobile phase is a highly non-polar solvent like hexane or methylene chloride and stationary phase is a polar solvent.

(ii) Reversed Phase Chromatography

In this type of chromatography the non-polar polymer beads can be used as a stationary phase with relatively polar solvents such as water, acetonitrile or methanol as the mobile phase. This type of separation mode is referred to as reversed phase adsorption.

4.7.2.2. Partition

In partition chromatography the separation is based on partition coefficient of sample between the stationary phase and mobile phase.

(i) Liquid – Liquid Partition

In this chromatographic mode the stationary phase is a liquid (i.e. tightly bound water act as stationary phase) and the separation occurs as a result of partitioning between two liquid – liquid phase.

If the stationary phase is polar and the mobile phase is non-polar, the chromatographic mode is known as Normal Phase Partition Chromatography. But in the opposite case it refers to as Reversed Phase Partition Chromatography. It suffers from the disadvantages of that stationary phase always, has some solubility in the mobile phase; thus precaution must be taken.

(ii) Chemically Bonded Partition

To overcome the disadvantage of liquid-liquid partition chromatography the stationary phase is developed with chemically bonded or organo bonded soluble matrix. The most common one is Octadecylsilane (ODS), which is bonded to a silica support via a silylether linkage (Siloxane). Such a packing material is used with a polar eluent like methanol or water – methanol. Thus the stationary phase is stable and chromatographic mode does not suffer any disadvantages. If the bonded phase is polar then non-polar mobile phase is employed, and technique is known as normal phase chromatography.

Table 1.5

Phase	Type of Solvent	Mode of Chromatography
Mobile Phase	Polar	Reversed Phase Chromatography
Stationary Phase	Non Polar	
Mobile Phase	Non Polar	Normal Phase Chromatography
Stationary Phase	Polar	

4.7.2.3 Size Exclusion Chromatography

In this mode the molecules are separated on the basis of their size. This method is employed basically for the analysis of polymer molecule weight or molar mass. At the time of separation the smaller molecules of the sample enters into porous medium and take more time to exit the column whereas larger particles leave the column first.

4.7.2.4 Ion Exchange Chromatography

In Ion exchange Chromatography it uses a charged stationary phase, which is usually a ion exchange resin (like zeolite) that carries charged functional groups which interact with the oppositively charged groups of the sample which is to be analyzed and run through the column with mobile phase. The positively charged ion exchanger interact with anion while negatively charged ion exchanger interact with cations.

4.7.2.5 Affinity Chromatography

Affinity Chromatography is based on selective non-covalent interaction between an analyte and specific molecule. It is very specific and often used in biochemistry for the purification of proteins.

4.7.3 Instrumentation

It includes various parts which are described below :-

4.7.3.1. Stationary Phase

The Stationary phase in HPLC refers to the solid support through which mobile phase flows. The sample is injected into the mobile phase of the assay through the injecting port. As the sample solution flows with the mobile phase through the stationary phase, the components of that sample solution will migrate according to the interaction of the compound with stationary phase.

The chemical interaction of the stationary phase and the sample with the mobile phase, determines the degree of migration and separation of the components contained in the sample.

Those samples which have stronger interaction with the stationary phase than with the mobile phase will elute from the column less quickly, and thus have a longer retention time, while the reverse also as such. Column may contain any mode of stationary phase as described before such as adsorption, partition, Ion exchange, Size exclusion or Affinity chromatographic mode.

4.7.3.2. Mobile Phase

The mobile phase in HPLC refers to the solvent being continuously flowing to the column. The mobile phase acts as carrier for the sample solution, which flows through a column with the mobile phase, the component of that solution migrate according to the interaction of the compound with the column.

Ex: Those samples which have stronger interaction with the mobile phase than with the stationary phase will elute from the column faster, and thus have a shorter retention time, while the reverse is also as such.

A good quality solvent should be used because soluble impurities may give noisy baseline and spurious peak and also change the retention time. It can also alter the column resolution. Generally the mixture of methanol with aqueous solution or buffers are suitable eluents for many separations, water should be distilled from glass and never stored in plastic container. Acetonitrile is a particularly difficult solvent used for separation. If air is dissolved in mobile phase it must be removed because it can lead to problems. The air bubble in a pump head usually reduces or stops eluent flow while the bubble formed in detector can affect the detection response, the solvent are easily degassed by warming the solvent or by applying weak vacuum to the solvent reservoir for 1 -2 minutes.

The pH of mobile phase is also adjusted (i.e. 2 to 8) because high pH may dissolve the silica support of stationary phase. It can be minimized or adjusted by using correct choice of solvent and base.

Mobile phase should have the following properties:-

1. It should have low viscosity
2. It should have compatibility with detector (e.g. for UV detector, solvent should not absorb UV light).

3. It should have high purity and stability.
4. It should be volatile.

Commonly used mobile phase are given below:-

- Methanol
- Acetonitrile
- Ethanol isooctane
- Water

These may be used in their mixture of different proportions depending on the type of analysis.

1. Acetonitrile : Water (70 : 30)
2. Isooctane : Dichloromethane : Methanol (165: 35 : 100)
3. Acetonitrile : Methanol (50 : 50)

While preparing an eluent it is usually best to dissolve the required buffer salt in water at the appropriate concentration. Adjust the pH, then mix this solution (v/v) with the organic solvent.

The choice of mobile phase to be used in any separation will depend on the type of separation to be achieved.

4.7.3.3. Solvent Supply System or Pumping System

HPLC is equipped with one or more glass or stainless steel reservoirs each of which contains 1-2 liters of a solvent. These reservoirs are equipped with degasser system for removing the air bubble from the solvent. Degassers may consist of a vacuum pumping system, a distillation system, or a device for heating and stirring the solvent.

Modern HPLC is generally equipped with devices that introduce solvent from two or more reservoirs into a mixing chamber at rates that vary continuously, the volume ratio of the solvent may then be altered linearly with time. Thus solvent is supplied into the column with the pressure of 5×10^7 pascal. It should never flow in the form of pulses (i.e. variation in the pressure) because it may affect the detection response. Various pumping systems are available for supply of the solvent at a constant pressure.

4.7.3.4. Pumps

The pumps are the specific device to flow the solvent into the column with pressure and constant flow rate. The flow rate through the column is generally between 1-3 ml/min. and pressure ranging from 3.4 - 27.6 Mpa or 5×10^7 pascal. The pumps show minimum fluctuation within these ranges to achieve maximum stability of the detector response.

(i) Reciprocal Piston Pump

It is widely used and some time also used for column packing. It consists of a small motor-driven piston which moves rapidly back and forth in a hydraulic chamber that may vary from 35 – 400 µl in volume. On the back stroke, the separation column valve is closed and the piston pulls in solvents from the mobile phase reservoir. On the forward stroke, the pump pushes solvent out to the column from the reservoir. They give a constant solvent flow which can be regulated but it does not eliminate pulsation due to reciprocating action of piston pump.

(ii) Syringe Type Pump

It is most suitable for small bore column because this pump delivers only a limited volume of mobile phase before it has to be refilled. These pumps have a volume between 250 – 500 ml. The pump operates by a motorized lead screw that delivers the mobile phase to the column at a constant rate. The rate of solvent delivery is controlled by changing the voltage on the motor.

It provides pulseless solvent flow and requires to refill after each interval due to limited capacity of solvent.

(iii) Constant Pressure Pump

In this pump gas pressure is used to regulate the flow of eluents. A low pressure gas source can generate high liquid pressure. The valving arrangement allows the rapid refill of the solvent chamber whose capacity is about 70 ml. This provides continuous mobile phase and flow rates of about 1 – 2 ml / min.

4.7.3.5. Sample Injecting System

The sample is injected in the HPLC via an injecting port. It mainly consists of an injection valve and the sample loop. In liquid chromatography, liquid sample may be injected directly and solid sample needs to be dissolved in an appropriate solvent (prefer mobile phase).

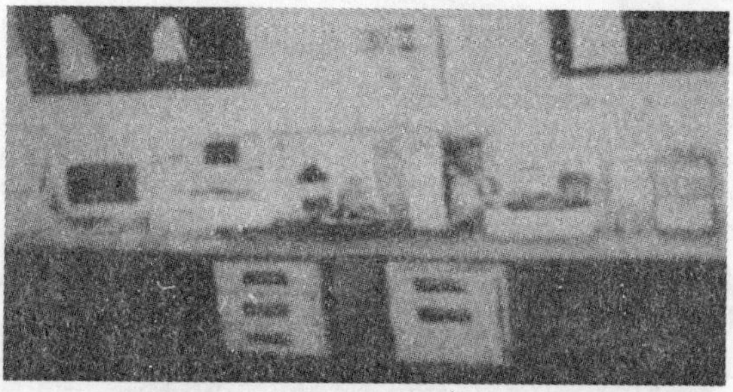

Fig. 4.22 High pressure liquid chromatography

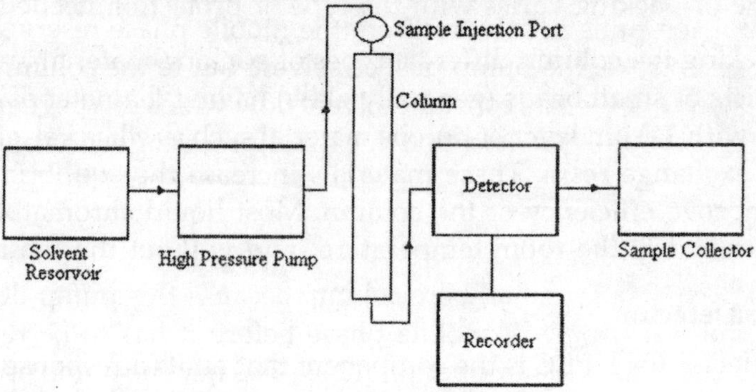

Fig. 4.23. Digrammatic Representation of High Pressure Liquid Chromatography

The sample is then drawn into a syringe and injected into the loop via the injecting valve placed onto the head of the column. A rotation of the valve rotor closes the valve and opens the loop in order to inject the sample into the stream of the mobile phase. Loop volume can range between 10 µl - 500 µl sample. In modern HPLC systems, the sample injection is typically automated.

4.7.3.6.Column

In HPLC there are various type of column used depending on the type of analysis, but basically two types of columns are adopted.

1. Analytical column
2. Guard column

(i) Analytical Column

The column is made of glass tubing or stainless steel tubing having a polished inner surface. The typical column is 10 - 30 cm in length and

4.0 – 5.0 mm internal diameter are normally used.

(ii) Guard Column

It is a short column which is placed between the injector and the HPLC column. This serves as a protective factor that prolongs the life and usefulness of the column. It also protects the column from damage or loss of efficiency caused by particulate matter or strongly absorbed substances in sample or solvents. These column must be changed on a regular interval to optimize their protective function. It may be packed with microparticulate stationary phase or layer beads. The size of packing varies with the type of protection needed.

For packing the column different types of packing material are used. It consists of small beads (generally glass) having diameter of 40 μm, coated with 1-3 μm layer of porous material such as silica gel, alumina or ion exchange resin. These materials increase the equlibrium rate and improve efficiency of the column. Most liquid chromatography is performed at the room temperature and without thermostating.

4.7.3.7. Detector

The detector for HPLC is the component that emits a response due to the eluting sample compound and subsequently signals a peak on the chromatogram. It is situated immediately posterior to the stationary phase in order to detect the compounds as they elute from the column.

The bandwidth and height of the peaks may usually be adjusted using the coarse and fine tunning controls.There are many types of detector that can be used with HPLC. Some most common detectors include:

(i) UV - Detector

The most commonly detector in liquid chromatography is the UV-absorption detector. It is based on the principle of absorption of UV light. The main source of UV light is mercury lamp which emits intense radiation at 254 nm. Some compounds do not absorb light at the above wavelength hence, the sensitivity is very poor. To increase the sensitivity and specificity the Hg lamp has been replaced by the deuterium (190 – 400 nm) and the tungsten (400 – 700 nm) lamps.

(ii) Refractive Index Detector

The refractive index detector can be considered as a universal detector because all compounds cause a change in refractive index when dissolved in eluent. The eluent emerges from the column and passes into the absorption or refractive index cell. If a solute is present, its absorption or refractive index changes and is plotted on a recorder to provide the chromatogram. For better detection system a double beam principle is used. Hence the Refractive Index of the sample cell is measured and compared with the reference cell.

(iii) Photodiode Array Detector

It is another type of UV detector in which polychromatic light is passed through the flow cell. The emerging radiation is diffracted by a grating and then allowed to fall on to an array of photodiodes, each photodiode receiving a different narrow wavelength band. The photodiode array is a row of detector (up to 400) mounted on a 1cm silicon chip, each diode receiving a different wavelength.

When transmitted radiation falls on the photodiode, photocurrents are generated. The electronic signals from each photodiode detector is processed to give absorbance data, which is then displayed as a spectrum. The absorption data can be displayed as a function of wavelength and time.

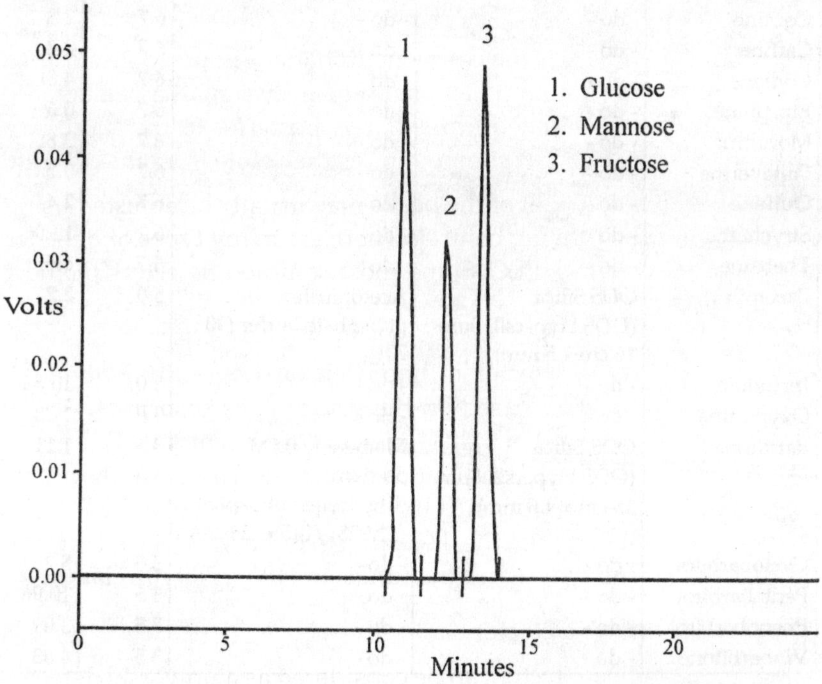

Fig. 4.24. Separated Chromatogram of Carbohydrates by HPLC

Table 1.6. Different types of drugs and narcotic substances with K' value

Substance	Column	Eluent	pH Value	K' Value
Aderanaline	Silica (Spherisorb, 5μm, 25cm x 5mm)	Methanol: Ammonium nitrate buffer solution (90 : 10)	10	0.63
Amphetamine	- do -	- do -	10	0.98
Bezephetamine	- do -	- do -	10	0.15
Caffiene	- do -	- do -	10	0.26
Ephedrine	- do -	- do -	10	1.79
Pipradrol	- do -	- do -	10	0.69
Amitriptyline	Silica (Spherisorb, S5W, 5 μm 12.5 cm x 4.9 mm)	1.175 g (0.01 M) of Ammonium perchlorate 1000 ml of methanol	6.7	1.8
Antazoline	- do -	- do -	6.7	1.8
Deptropine	- do -	- do -	6.7	5.0t
Ergosine	- do -	- do -	6.7	0.3
Lysergic acid	- do -	- do -	6.7	0.8t
Cocaine	- do -	- do -	6.7	2.8
Caffine	- do -	- do -	6.7	0.2
Codiene	- do -	- do -	6.7	4.8t
Etorphine	- do -	- do -	6.7	0.6
Morphine	- do -	- do -	6.7	3.8t
Papaverine	- do -	- do -	6.7	0.3
Quinine	- do -	- do -	6.7	2.4
Strychnine	- do -	- do -	6.7	13.0t
Thebaine	- do -	- do -	6.7	4.6t
Doxepin	ODS Silica (ODS Hypersil, 5μm 16 cm x 5 mm)	Acetonitrile : phosphate buffer (30 : 70)	3.0	2.27
Iprindole	- do -	- do -	3.0	10.83
Oxypertine	- do -	- do -	3.0	1.33
Barbitone	ODS Silica (ODS Hypersil, 5μm 15 cm x 4.6 mm)	Methanol : 0.1M Sodium dihydrogen phosphate (11.998g/l)(55 : 25 :20)	3.5	1.11
Cyclobarbitol	- do -	- do -	3.5	5.25
Pentabarbitol	- do -	- do -	3.5	10.96
Phenobarbitol	- do -	- do -	3.5	3.09
Vinbarbitone	- do -	- do -	3.5	4.83

t - tailing peak
Flow rate: 1.5 - 2 ml / min.

4.7.4. Application

HPLC has been applied to a great varieties of areas such as, pharmaceutical analysis, clinical chemistry, environmental monitoring, forensic science and toxicology. This chromatography finds utility in crime and research laboratories in the last few decades.

- It is used for the separation of anion and cation in Inorganic Chemistry
- It is used in the detection of a large number of toxicants and poisons.
- It is also used in the detection of additive drugs.
- It may be used in the separation of Steroids, lipids, carbohydrates, vitamins and preservatives.
- It is used in the separation and purification of Nucleic acid.
- It is used for the separation and identification of Psycotropic drugs in body fluids.
- HPLC is mainly used for the analysis of drugs which are polar (e.g. asprin) and thermally unstable (Benzodiazepines)
- It can also be applied to natural products such as coal, oil, cannabis, resin and alkaloids that contains numerous component.

Table 1.7. Retention time of High explosive materials analysed by HPLC

Explosives	Column	Flow rate	Solvent used	Rt value
RDX	μ Bondapok·	1.5 ml/min.	Isooctane :	1.436
PETN	CN column		Dichloromethane	2.203
TNT	10 μm particle		: Methanol	2.799
HMX	size		(165 : 35 : 100)	3.064

4.7.5. Advantages over Gas Chromatography

It has advantage to analyze the non-volatile substances and thermally unstable materials because it works on room temperature while in Gas Chromatography it is not possible to analyze these materials due to operating at high temperature.

4.8. Size Exclusion Chromatography

This chromatography is also known as Gel permeation or Sephadex gel chromatography. It separates the molecule on the basis of their size. The stationary phase consists of polymer or silica-based support material of controlled pore sizes. This method is most widely used in the analysis of polymer molecular weight (or molar mass). In the starting of this technique people use simple glass column filled with silica gel and perform Gel permeation chromatography, but nowadays HPLC columns are used.

4.8.1. Theory and Principle

In Size exclusion chromatography the column is made up of stainless steel having 500 - 1000 mm length and typically 10 mm in diameter. The column is packed with a porous material, it may be micro porous silica and solvent is forced through the column with flow rate of 1ml/min. and pressure of 50 - 200 bar.

A sample is dissolved in the same solvent that is running through the column and is then introduced into solvent stream going through the column. Inside the column, molecules are separated based on their hydrodynamic volume (volume occupied by molecule in dilute solution). By studying the polymers in particular solvent and by calibrating each column set up with sample of known molecular weight, it is possible to get a relative distribution of molecular weights for a given polymer sample.

4.8.2. Separation Procedure

When a molecule flows through the column it passes by a number of porous beads. If the molecule can fit inside the pore then it is drawn in by the force of diffusion. There it stays a short while and then moves on. If a molecule cannot fit into a pore then it continues following the solvent flow. Due to this the molecule of large size will elute first than the molecule of smaller size. The effective range of the column is determined by the pore size of the packing.

SEC is a useful tool for determining molecular weight in polymers but it is essential that the column and instrument operate carefully and properly calibrated for good results. The resolution of SEC is relatively low and careful column selection is important for each application. The column of SEC has a limited size for achieving good separation.

4.8.3. Application

This chromatography is widely used in the separation of sugars, polypeptides, proteins, lipids, polyethylenes, polystyrene, silicons and many other biological materials.

4.9. Affinity Chromatography

Affinity chromatography is a biochemical separation method which is the combination of size exclusion chromatography (SEC) and a specifically designed stationary phase that has the ability to reversibly bind to a known sample molecules. In this method a specific buffer solution is also used which elutes the sample molecules from the stationary phase.

4.9.1. Basic Principle

Affinity chromoatogrphy involves solid phase (column) and binding molecules of the sample mixture. It is based on the principal of binding of sample molecules with the solid medium packed into the column. The initial sample mixture is passed through the column and wash buffer is allowed to pass through it which eluted the sample. This elutes sample is collected in a vessel.

4.9.2. General Procedure

- Pack the column with solid packing material (Silica, alumina or polymer beads). Thus solid stationary phase is ready.
- Now allow to flow the sample mixture through the column.
- Molecules of sample mixture will be trapped on the solid stationary phase, while the other molecules of heterogenous mixture become free.
- Now allow to run the wash buffer through the solid stationary phase in order to elute the molecules of sample mixture (entrapped molecules).
- The solid support medium may again be used for binding of another molecules.
- The elution mixture may be used for further analytical purpose.

4.9.3 Application

Affinity chromatography is used for the purification of Nucleic acid, blood serum, cell extract etc.

4.10. Ion Exchange Chromatography

It is a column chromatography that uses a charged stationary phase that is usually an ion exchange resin which carries charged functional groups that interact with opposite charged groups of the sample compound.

4.10.1 Theory and Principle

Ion exchange chromatography involves charged stationary phase which is usually ion exchange resin (beeds of polymerized organic materials with acidic or basic groups) carrying charged functioal groups. These groups interact with opposite charged groups of sample compound to be separated or retained.

The cation exchangers exchange cation (e.g. Na^{+2} ion in Zeolite) while the anion exchagers exchange with anion. Polystyrene divenyl benzene a co-polymer structure is the most common component of widely used resins.

Although the resins are insoluble in water, yet their active functional groups are hydrophylic (water loving) having varying degree of affinity for ionic species.

Table1.6. Commonly used cation and anion exchanger.

Type	Cation exchanger	Anion exchanger
Natural	Zeolite, clays,	Dolomite
Inorganic	MgO , SiO_2, Al_2O_3	Heavy metal silicates
Organic	Liginite, sulphonated coal	

The ion exchange chromatograply should have the following qualities for proper selectivity and good retention.

- The size and charge on sample ion should be uniform.
- The pH of the mobile phase should be properly adjusted.
- The mobile phase should have the proper concentration (total concentration) of ion species.
- The addition of the organic solvent to the eluent should be properly caliberated (i.e. volume should be considered).
- Temperature of the column should be adjusted according to the sample mixture (optimum temperature).

4.10.2. Qualitative and Quantitative Analysis

The chromatography is a method of closely related chemical compounds. It is also used for qualitative identification and quantitative determination of separated components in the mixture.

4.10.2.1. Qualitative Analysis

The qualitative identification of a compound may be got by the chromatogram of separated species. This chromatogram provides retention time and its position on the stationary phase after a elution time. Other factors like temperature variation and quality of mobile and stationary phase can also be derived from the chromatogram.

4.10.2.2. Quantitative Analysis

This technique provide useful quantitative information about the separated species. It may be done by the analysis of peak area or peak height derived by the chromatogram of a separated component.

4.10.3. Calibration with Standard

For calibration with standard sample, it is necessary to prepare a standard solution that approximate the composition of unknown. Then the chromatogram of standard solution is obtained and peak height and peak area are plotted as a function of the concentration present in the standard.

The analysis are based on this plot. Differences in peak height and peak area may indicate the concentration of component in the analyzing sample mixture. The concentration of the analyte is found from the ratio of a peak area to the total area of all peaks.

4.10.4. Application

- It is most widely used in the identification of 30 or more amino acids in a protein.
- It is used for the separation of anions and cations.
- It is also used to separate charged molecules in biological samples.

4.11 Gas Chromatography

Gas Chromatography is one of the most versatile of all the chromatographic techniques. It was first described by James and Martin in 1952.

Gas Chromatography is a special form of the general chromatography used for separating and identifying chemicals in a sample. It involves the separation of volatile material in the vapour state i.e. the boiling point of the sample is the main criteria of their separation. It is most widely used for the qualitative and quantitative analysis of a large number of compounds because it has high sensitivity, reproducibility and speed of resolution. In this chromatography both absorption and partition phenomenon are possible. If absorption process takes place, the technique is known as Gas solid chromatography (GSC) whereas when partition process takes place it is known as Gas liquid chromatography (GLC).

4.11.1 Basic Principle

Gas Chromatography separates the mixture on the basis of difference in the partition coefficient of the volatilized compounds between the stationary liquid or solid phase and moving gas phase. As the compounds are carried through the column by the carrier gas and after leaving the column it passes through a detector that is linked via an amplifier to a chart recorder, which in turn records a peak as each analyte passes through the detector.

4.11.2 Instrumentation

The Gas Chromatography basically consists of the following equipments (Fig. 4.25 & 4.26).

4.11.2.1. Carrier gas

The most commonly used carrier gases in Gas Chromatography are Helium, Nitrogen, Hydrogen and a mixture of 95 % Argon and 5 % Methane. The selection of the carrier gas depends on the type of detector used. Hydrogen and Helium gas are the most suitable used carrier gas with thermal conductivity detector (TCD) because of their thermal conductivity. Nitrogen and Helium are good carrier gas with Flame Ionisation Detector (FID). Argon - Methane combination is also used for the Electron Capture Detector.

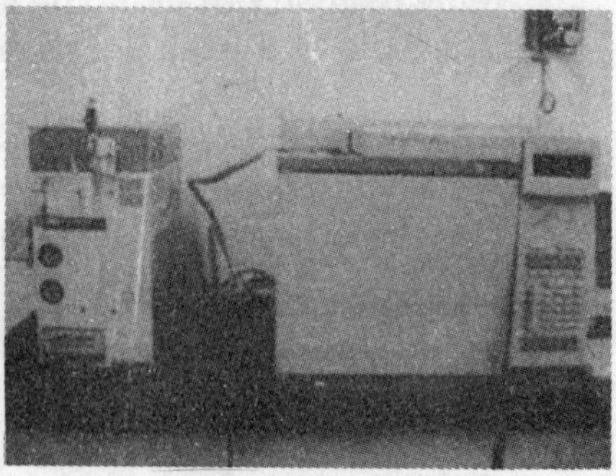

Fig : 4.25 Gas Chromatography instrument

4.11.2.2. Flow Control: It is used to regulate flow of carrier gas.

4.11.2.3. Injecting Port or Sample Inlet System

The sample for chromatographic analysis is dissolved in a suitable solvent such as acetone, heptane or methanol. Chlorinated organic solvents are generally avoided as they contaminate the detector. The sample inlet system called the injector port is generally heated to high temperature (about 50°C) for vaporizing the sample quickly which is to be analyzed. After diluting the sample in a suitable solvent it is

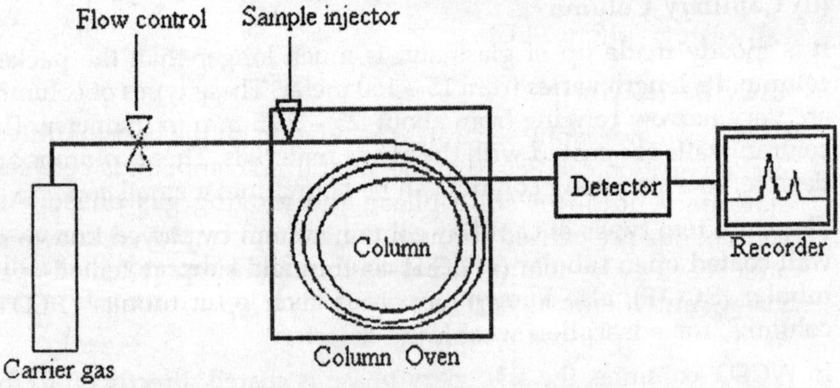

Fig. 4.26. Schematic Representation of Gas Chromatography

introduced into the injecting port with the help of a micro-syringe. The sample should not be too large. The slow injection of the large samples may cause band broadening and loss of resolution. Various modes are available to introduce the sample into the system such as direct injection, split, splitless etc.

4.11.2.4. Stationary Phase

It is thin film of liquid contained within the column categorised as gas liquid chromatography, whereas in gas solid chromatography the fixed phase consists of solid material such as granular silica, alumina and porous polymers. In gas liquid chromatography stationary phase is non-volatile liquid eg: Polyethylene glycol squalene or polymethyl siloxane liquids are held as thin layer on solid support such as silica or Keiselgurh.

4.11.2.5. Column

Generally the column is made of copper, aluminium, stainless steel and glass. Glass is mostly preferred due to its inert nature. There are two types of column commonly employed in GLC (Fig. 4.27).

(i) Packed Column

In packed column the stationary phase is thin film of liquid that is fixed on to the small granular particles (commonly based on diatomaceous earth) packed into column. This column is usually made up of stainless steel or glass. These are 1.5 to 10 m in length and have an internal diameter of 2- 4 mm. For packed columns, the sample size ranges from tenths of a microlitre up to 20 μl.

(ii) Capillary Column

It is mostly made up of glass and is much longer than the packed column. Its length varies from 15 - 160 meter. These types of columns are very narrow ranging from about .25 - 2.75 mm in diameter. The column walls are coated with the active materials. These columns are flexible, so a very long column can be bound into a small coil.

There are two types of capillary column system employed known as wall coated open tubular (**WCOT**) column and support coated open tubular (**SCOT**), also known as porous layer open tubular (**PLOT**) columns, for adsorption work.

In **WCOT** columns, the stationary phase is coated directly on to the walls of the capillary tubing. As due to the presence of very small amount of stationary phase only small amount of samples may be chromatographed. For this purpose a splitter system has to be used at the sample injection port so that only a small fraction of the injected sample reaches the column.

In **SCOT** columns a support material is bonded to the walls of the capillary column and the stationary phase is coated on to the support. The capacity of **SCOT** columns is considerably higher than that of **WCOT** columns and consequently small samples can be injected directly on to such columns without the need for a splitter system. **SCOT** system are therefore much simpler to use of quantitative analysis than for **WCOT** systems.

These columns have much thinner walls than the glass capillary columns, and are given strength by the polyamide coating. These are flexible and can be wound into coils.

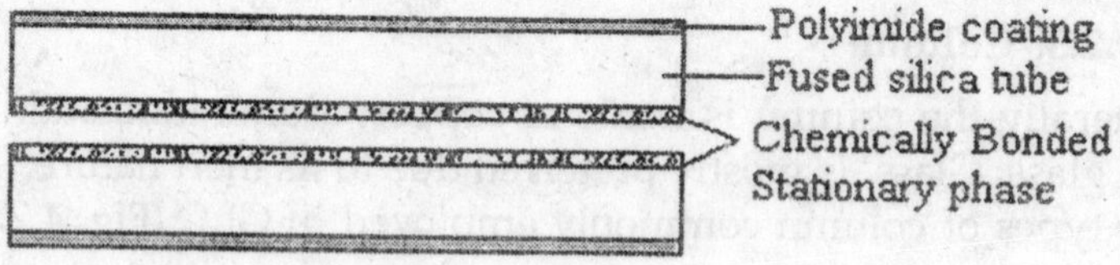

Fig. 4.27. Column of Gas Chromatography

(iii) Column Temperature

The column temperature depends upon the boiling point of the sample. Minimal temperature gives good resolution, but increase elution times. If a sample has a wide boiling range then temperature programming can be useful. The column temperature increases as separation proceeds.

4.11.2.6. Detector

Several detectors have been developed for the analysis of the GLC effluents. The function of the detector is to detect and measure the different components of the sample as they emerge out of the column. The performance of the detector can be judged from its noise, sensitivity, linearity, specificity and response time.

The choice of the detectors depends on the type of the analysis being performed. The most widely used detectors are :

(i) Thermal Conductivity Detector

In TCD there is a heated filament over which the carrier gas flows at a steady speed. The heat loss is constant and the filament remains at a constant temperature. When a carrier gas flows through it the component in the carrier gas change the rate of heat loss. Therefore the temperature of tungsten filament is altered which further changes the filament resistance and then converted into an electric signal with the help of appropriate circuit. It works on **Wheatstone Bridge principle.** This electric signal is amplified and recorded since the thermal conductivity of gases are different. Therefore a change in the composition of the gases causes the changes in thermal conductivity and become detected. It is a universally used detector. It has detectivity of 1 ng.

(ii) Flame Ionization Detector

FID has become the most commonly used detector in Gas Chromatography. In the FID a flame is maintained by an independent stream of air and hydrogen near which a metal loop electrode is positioned and kept at a constant electric potential.

When carrier gas passes through this flame along with the analytical components it decomposes the analytical components producing positive and negative ions that changes the electrode potential. These

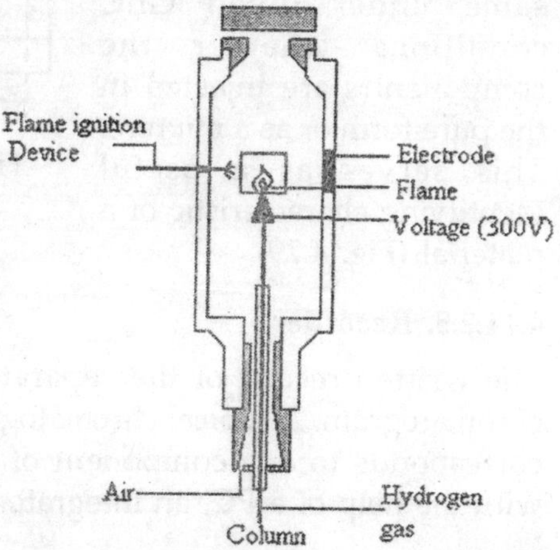

Fig. 4.28. Flame Ionisation Detector

changes are recorded as a signal on a chart, indicating the arrival of the sample components. It is used for the detection of most organic compounds. It has detectivity of 100 pg (Fig. 4.28).

(iii) Electron Capture Detector

This detector is mostly used for electronegative species e.g. halogenated compounds having chlorine, bromine, fluorine and also pesticides. In this type of detector when an electronegative species passes through the detector it captures low energy electrons, so that current is changed and thus sensed by the detector. It has selectivity of halides, nitrates, nitriles and anhydrous organometallic compounds. It has detectivity of 50 fg.

Numerous selective detectors other than the detector described above are also used in Gas Chromatography depending upon the nature of analytes. Some of them are flame photometric detector, microwave plasma detector and the ultrasonic detector etc.

4.11.2.7. Retention Time

It may be defined as the interval of time between the introduction of the sample mixture into the column and elution of a component from it. Retention time or volume of a component remains the same under given GLC conditions whether the componentrs are injected in the pure form or as a mixture. This serves as a useful identifying characteristic of a material (Fig. 4.29).

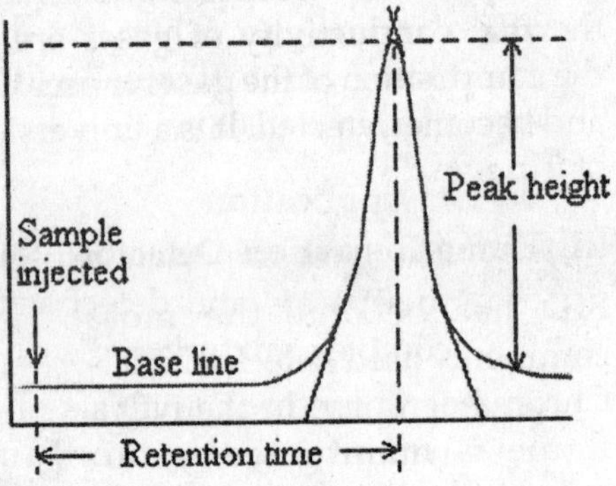

Fig : 4.29 Measurement of Retention Time

4.11.2.8. Recorder

The written record of the separation of the component is called chromatogram. A typical chromatogram will show a number of peaks corresponds to one component of the mixture. It can be obtained with the help of a PC, an integrator or Printer (Fig. 4.30).

4.11.3. Basic Theory of Instrument

In Gas Chromatography the carrier gases like N_2, H_2, He, Ar or mixture of any two is used, which is obtained from a cylinder and passed through pressure adjusting valve, drying tube, flow regulator to get an even flow of the carrier gas.

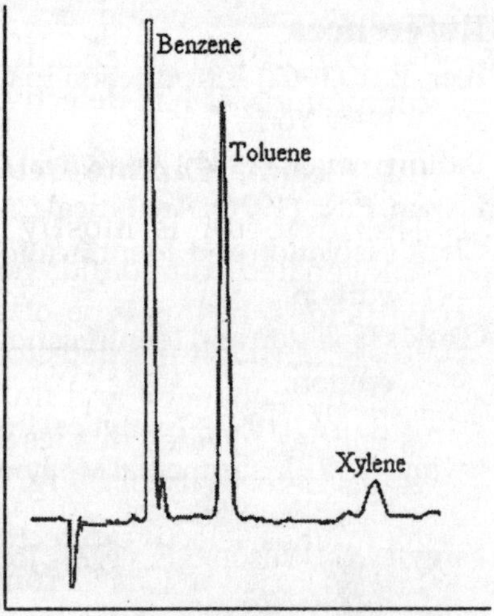

Fig. 4.30. Gas Chromatogram of Different Organic Compounds

The gas is then passed through the sample injecting port where it picks up the sample mixture for analysis. The carrier gas containing sample mixture enters into the column where the mixture get separated. The carrier gas containing the separated vapours of the compounds of the sample emerge from the column and pass through the detector. The detector measures the concentration of the vapours in the carrier gas. Then finally a chromatogram is obtained with the help of recorder and electronic signal from detector.

4.11.4. Application

- The most important aspect of Gas Chromatography is its ability to separate and detect small amount of a variety of drugs in a complex mixture.
- It is used for analysis of gases such as carbon monoxide or natural gases by directly injecting it into the column.
- It is used in blood alcohol analysis. The blood is usually diluted approximately in the ratio of 1:1 with distilled water and injected into Gas Chromatography column.
- It is also used for the analysis of paints, fibers, polymers. These samples are heated upto 1000°C in an external chamber called pyrolyzer, connected to Gas Chromatography. The long chain molecules are broken into simple volatile product and get detected.
- It finds diverse application in toxicological analysis viz. alcohol, volatile poison, drugs, plant poisons etc.
- The petroleum product like kerosene, petrol, diesel, turpentine oil etc. are detected by this method successfully.

References

Bair, E.J., (1962) Introduction to Chemical Instrumentation. McGraw Hill, New York.

Bidlingmeyer, (1984); Analytical Chemistry, Vol 56, Pg. No. 1583 – 1596.

Brown, P.R., (1990); Analytical Chemistry, Vol. 62, Pg No. 995.

Clark's Isolation and Identification of Drugs, The Pharmaceutical Press 2nd edition.

Clark's Isolation and Identification of Drugs, the Pharmaceutical Press, 2nd edition.

Edwin, G.W., (1997); Analytical Instrumentation Handbook, Marcel Dekker.

Ewing, G.W., Instrumental Method of Chemical Analysis, McGraw Hill Book Co., New York.

Farey, M.G., Wilson, S.E., (1975); Journal of Chromatographic Science, Vol.114, Pg No. 261.

Grob, R.L., (1977); Modern Practice of Gas Chromatography. John Wiley, New York.

Jinno, K., (1996); Chromatographic Separation based on Molecular Recognition. Wiley VCH, New York.

Lurie, L.S. and Walker, J.D.,(1983); High Performance Liquid Chromatography in Forensic Chemistry, New York, Marcel Dekker.

Phama. Acta Helv., (1986); Vol. 61, Pg. No. 167 - 176.

Plummer, D.T., (1987); An Introduction to Practical Biochemistry. McGraw Hill.Co. (UK)

Pryde, A. and Gilbert, M.T., (1979); Application of High Performance Liquid Chromatography, London, Chapman and Hall.

Shellard, E.J., (1975); Quantitative Paper and Thin layer Chromatography, London, Academic Press.

Strobel, H. A., (1973); Chemical Instrumentation 2nd ed. Addision - Wesley, Reading, Mass.

Touchstone, J.C., and Dobbins, M.F., (1983); Practice of Thin layer Chromatography.

Vinson, J.A., Hooyman, A.A.S., Ward, C.E., (1974); Identification of Street Drugs by TLC and a single Visualization reagent. Journal of Forensic Science, Pg.No. 552.

Willard, H., Merritt, L., Dean, A., Settle, A., (1986); Instrumental method of Analysis 7th edition, Wadswaeth Publishing Co.

Zweig, G., and Sherma, J., (1972); Handbook of Chromatography, vol I and II, Boca Raton, Florida, CRC Press.

CHAPTER 5

Electrophoresis

5.1 A Journey to Electrophoresis

The term electrophoresis refers to the separation technique involving the movement of charged particles through a matrix under the influence of an applied electric field.

Tiselius in 1937 designed an apparatus to separate serum proteins. His method was known as Tiselius moving boundary method or zone electrophoresis. He separated α, β and γ fractions of the serum protein.

In 1940's Swensson and Longsworth developed more advanced optical system for the quantitative estimation of serum proteins (α_1, β_1, β_2, γ_1 and γ_2) by this technique and it was useful for clinical investigations.

Further developments between 1940-1950 in electrophoretic techniques resulted in two more advanced techniques known as Isoelectrofocussing and Isotachophoresis. These techniques were very useful in separation of a mixture of proteins. The technique involved the use of different matrices such as paper, gel-like agrose or starch for different protein samples.

Smithies in 1955 used starch gel as a medium for electrophoresis while Kohn in 1957 used cellulose acetate as the support medium for electrophoresis.

In 1959 Raymond and Weintraub used polyacrylamide gel for the first time in disc gel electrophoresis. Lammli in 1970 used acrylamide gel for protein separation in SDS polyacrylamide gel electrophoresis. Two Dimensional gel electrophoresis was used by Klose (1974) and O' Farrell. Jorgenson and Lukacs in 1981-1983 introduced capillary as matrices for the first time.

5.2. Introduction

The term electrophoresis describe the migration of charged particles under the influence of an electric field. "Electro" refers to the energy of electricity and "Phoresis", from the Greek word "Phoros", means "to carry across."

In electrophoretic technique an electric current is applied across a chromatographic medium so that one end has a positive charge and the other a negative charge. The individual molecule in the mixture move towards the positive or negative end depending upon their relative mass and charge. The molecule can be characterized by their rate of movement in an electric field. The electrophoretic technique is mainly applied for the separation and identification of ionisable groups of compounds like nucleic acids, amino acids, proteins, nucleotides etc.

5.2.1. Basic Principle

The principle of electrophoresis states that a charged ion or group will migrate towards one end of the electrode after placing it in an electric field at a given pH.

If a particle having charge q placed in an insulating medium of an electric field E, then the particle will move at a constant velocity (V) towards one end of the electrode. It is determined by the balance between the electric force Eq, and the viscous drag, fv, whereas f is the frictional coefficient.

It can be expressed as :-

$$Eq = fv$$

$$V = Eq / f$$

Where E = electric field
q = net charge on particle
f = frictional coefficient
V = velocity

5.2.2. Electrophoretic Mobility

The movement of particles is due to the electric field and potential differences which is known as its electrophoretic mobility. It can be expressed as :-

$$V = Eq / f$$

$$V = \mu E \quad (\mu = q / f \text{ and } f = 6\pi\eta r)$$

$$\text{So} \quad \mu = q / 6\pi\eta r$$

$$(6\pi = \text{constant})$$

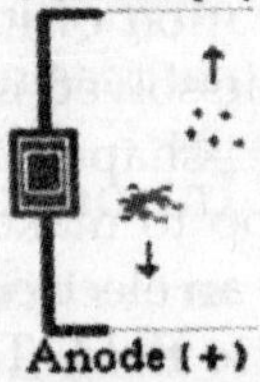

Fig. 5.1 Movement of Charged Particles

μ depends on the following factors:-

1. Frictional coefficient (f)
2. Viscosity of the medium (η)

3. Size, shape and radius (r) of the molecule.
4. Charge (q) on the molecule.

Thus molecule separated on the basis of differences in charge to mass ratio. The separation of the molecule can be achieved by using appropriate medium and suitable pH.

5.3.Types of Electrophoresis

There are following types of electrophoretic techniques:-

1. Moving Boundary method
2. Zone Electrophoresis
   a. Paper electrophoresis
   b. Cellular acetate strip electrophoresis
   c. Gel electrophoresis
3. Agrose gel Electrophoresis
4. Polyacrylamide Gel Electrophoresis (PAGE – SDS)
5. Rotating Gel Electrophoresis
6. Gradient Electrophoresis
7. Two Dimensional Electrophoresis (Combined Electrophoresis)
8. Capillary Electrophoresis
9. Immunoelectrophoresis
10. Isoelectric Focusing
11. Isotachophoresis

5.4. Moving Boundary Method

Historically this was the first form of electrophoresis that found application on a large scale. This type of electrophoresis demands relatively sophisticated equipment and does not result in an efficient separation of ion. It consists of mixture of sample to be separated and dissolved in a buffer of known pH being placed at the bottom of the U-shaped tube. More pure buffer is carefully added further on the top to make a clear boundary between pure buffer and mixture. Then an electrode is placed at both ends of the U tube and applied an electric field. The positively charged molecules move towards the cathode, while the negatively charged molecules move towards anode (i.e. towards the region of pure buffer). As well as the charged ions moves towards electrodes changing refractive indices indicating the electrophoretic band pattern (Fig. 5.2).

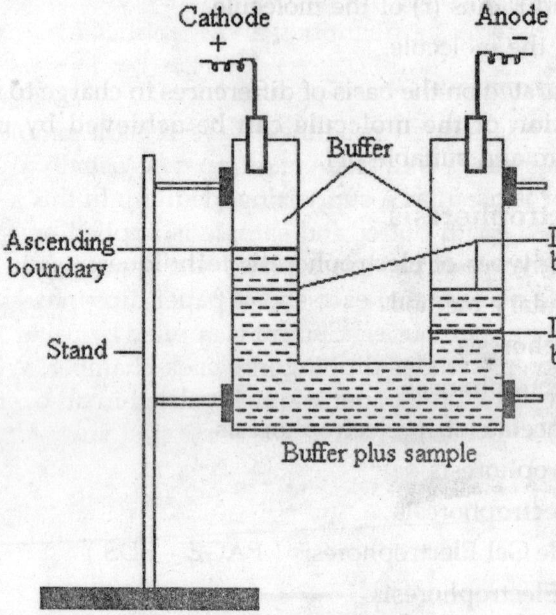

Fig. 5.2. Moving Boundary Method of Separation

5.4.1. Disadvantages

This form of electrophoresis suffers a drawback of diffusion of separated components, because it is carried out in free solution. To overcome the problem of mixing solution, the solution to be separated held in a stable medium such as paper or gel (Agrose, Polyacrylamide, Starch etc.)

5.5. Zone Electrophoresis

Zone electrophoresis was discovered by **Koenig at Brazil in 1837.** When we use paper or gel as a stabilizing medium for separating the mixture of samples, then the separation is achieved in different zones so that this technique is known as zone electrophoresis. The molecules are separated on the basis of their mass to charge ratio. It is the most common method because very small amount of sample is required for separation. There are various supporting materials used depending upon the analysis and compatibility. It posseses higher resolution than moving boundary method because paper or gel provide three dimensional network of pores which inhibit mixture particles according to their molecular size. The quantitative value of electrophoretic mobility can never be determined because value obtained are always relative to the supporting medium. The separated zones (bands) are stable for quantition and identification.

5.5.1. Paper Electrophoresis

Paper electrophoresis is rarely used these days. It is the simplest form of zone electrophoresis. It is carried out on a paper (usually Whatman No. 1 filter paper is used) as a supporting medium. In this a strip of paper is moistened with buffer and sample is applied on that and then it is placed between two glass plates like a sandwich. This is arranged in such a manner that each end of paper dips into a separate chamber, containing pure buffer. Current is applied by using 120 volt battery and carbon electrodes dipping into each chamber. When the separation is completed, the paper is quickly dried in an oven and a locating reagent is sprayed to locate the separated substances (Fig. 5.3).

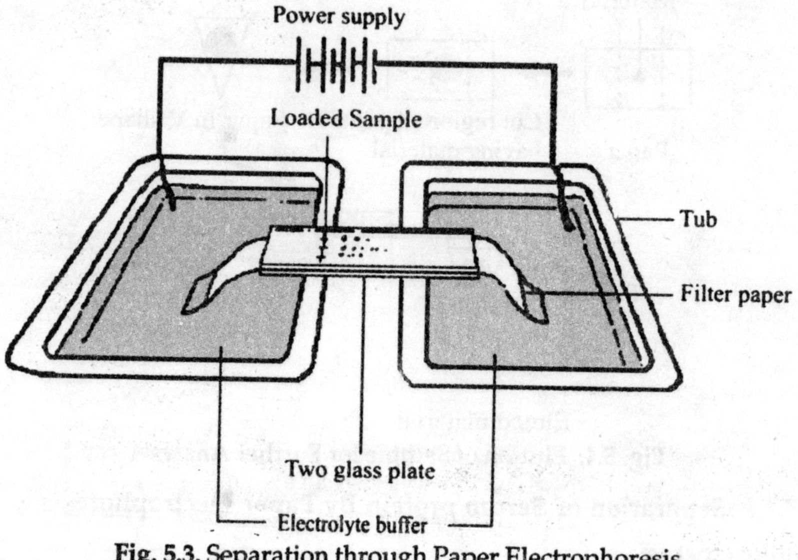

Fig. 5.3. Separation through Paper Electrophoresis

There are two types of system that works :

(i) **Continuous Buffer System:** When the buffer used on the paper and the chamber are the same then it is referred to as continuous buffer system.

(ii) **Discontinuous Buffer System:** In this system the buffer contained in chamber is chemically different and also has a different pH to that of supporting medium (i.e. Paper). This results in faster movement and sharper resolution of zones and separated component located by its colour, fluorescence or by staining with various dyes. If the sample is radioactive, spots can be located by counting radioactivity or autoradiography of the whole sheet using X-ray film.

The sample material required to be elute from the paper for further analysis may be accomplished by the following ways:-

- Cutting the region of the paper, having material to be eluted.
- The paper is soaked into small volume of eluting buffer.
- The spot is cut out as a V-shaped piece of paper.
- Now the eluting buffer is poured from the base of triangle of paper and drops containing the substance, to be eluted are collected from lower vertex of triangle opposite to base (Fig. 5.4).

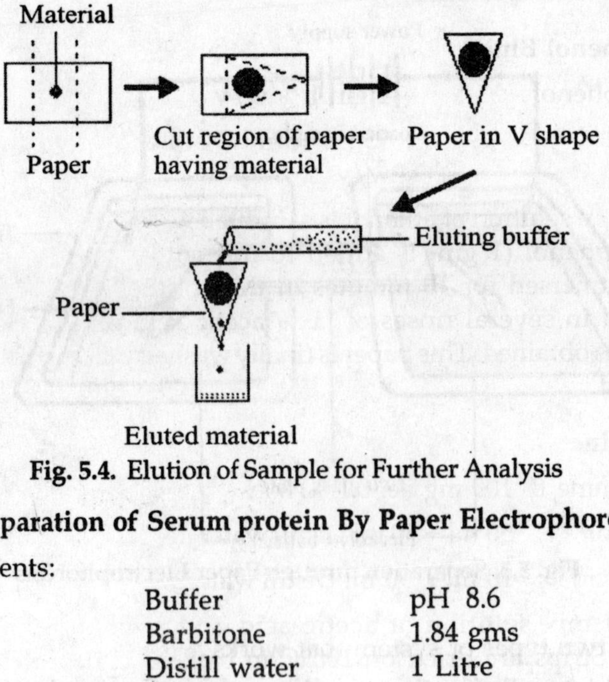

Fig. 5.4. Elution of Sample for Further Analysis

5.5.1.1. Separation of Serum protein By Paper Electrophoresis

Requirements:

Buffer	pH 8.6
Barbitone	1.84 gms
Distill water	1 Litre
Voltage	Constant 250 volts
Time	4 hrs
Current	22.5 mA
Distance travelled	10 cm
Dye	Bromophenol

In this method Whatman No. 3 paper strips were cut into 5 x 30 cm sizes. About four strips may be put at a time. Then a pencil line is drawn across the paper about one-third of the distance from one end after which the papers are dipped in the buffer. The strips are then placed on the electrophoretic tank in such a way so that the pencil line is nearest the cathode end. It is preferable to pass current for about 30 minutes through strips for ionic equilibrium.

Now the serum sample is allowed along the pencil line to widthen or spread about 0.5 cm of each end of paper. About 4 µl of undiluted serum sample is applied per cm width of paper. The path of electrophoresis is best followed by addition of a drop of bromophenol blue dye (in distill water). This dye is fairly tightly bound to serum albumin during the coarse of electrophoresis and does not alter the mobility of albumen.

5.5.1.2. Stains and Destains

(a) Bromophenol Blue

Bromophenol	1 gm 1 % w/v
Ethanol	95 ml +5 ml Distilled water i.e. 95 % w/v

This 95 % w/v solution of ethanol is saturated with mercuric chloride then Bromophenol (1 gm) is added to this solution. The strips of paper are immersed for 10 minutes in this solution. The strips are then washed in several rinses of 1 % acetic acid until a cleansed background is obtained. This paper is finally washed twice in methanol and air dried.

(b) Azocarmine

Azocarmine B	100 mg i.e. 0.1 % w/v
Methanol	50 ml + 50 ml Distill water i.e. 50% w/v methanol
Acetic acid	10 ml + 90 ml Distill water i.e. 10 % w/v

Take 100 ml mix solution of acetic acid and Methanol and add azocarmine. Strips are dried on 100°C in bath so that proteins are denatured and fixed. Now immerse these strips for 10 minutes in the stain. Excess dye is removed by rinsing in 10 % v/v. acetic acid and finally by methanol.

5.5.1.3. Comments

Normal sera yields five protein components on paper electrophoresis, all of which (except γ globulin) move towards the anode in alkaline buffers. The γ globulin fraction appear to move towards the cathod due to electroendosmosis, since the fraction is electrically neutral albumin moves furthest towards the anode in alkaline buffer being followed by α_1 globulin, α_2 globulin, β globulin, and finally the γ globulin fractions. The zone are not very sharp in paper electrophoresis.

5.5.1.4.Disadvantages

- Supporting medium is not a homogenous medium.
- Medium is not inert.
- Electroendosmosis affects the ionic strength of buffer.
- There is much adsorption of serum protein in supporting media.
- Protein molecules adsorbed by cellulose (i.e. cellulose hydroxyl groups) and it results in low resolution and tailing of the spot or band.
- Supporting medium (paper) increased resistance due to which current is increased as a result heat is generated which sometimes destroys the protein and band cannot be identified.

5.5.1.5. High and Low Voltage Electrophoresis

It works on low and high voltage. In low voltage paper electrophoresis (LVPE) voltage does not exceed 400 volts and is used for the separation of proteins and enzymes. Whereas the high voltage paper electrophoresis (HVPE) is used for the separation of small molecules like amino acids, peptides, indoles, phenols, purine and pyrimidines. It has the advantage of high speed and sharp resolution.

5.5.2. Cellulose Acetate Membrane Electrophoresis (CAM)

In Cellulose Acetate Strip Electrophoresis instead of paper a cellulose acetate membrane is used which shows the following advantages:-

- Hydrxyl group is converted into acetate group which do not show adsorption.
- It results in the reduction of background staining and improves the sensitivity of detection.
- The separated material is transparent which facilitates spectrometric analysis.
- In this the separated spot is smaller having a high concentration of material so that it is easily detected.

- Simultaneous staining for protein, lipids and carbohydrates.

Cellulose Acetate Membrane is easily available in variety of sizes e.g.. 2.5 x 12 cm, 2.5 x 16 cm etc. The strips are insoluble in water, alcohol, ether and most of the hydrocarbons but are soluble in phenol and acetone. The following solvents are of particular value in dissolving cellulose acetate membrane.

- Dichloromethane : ethanol (9:1)
- Chloroform : ethanol (9:1)
- Dichloromethane : Acetone (1:1)

5.5.2.1 Buffers Used

Any of the following buffers are suitable for performing CAM Electrophoresis.

(i) Barbitone Acetate Buffer: pH 8.6

Sodium Acetate	6.5 gm
Barbitone sodium	8.87 gm
Barbitone	1.13 gm
Distill water	1 litre

(ii) Barbitone buffer pH 8.6

Barbitone sodium	10.3 gm
Barbitone	1.84 gm
Distill water	1 litre

This buffer is used in Electrode and buffer compartments and also for soaking strips.

(iii) Tris EDTA borate buffer pH 9.0

Tris (2-amino-2 hydroxy-methyl- propane - 1, 3 di al)	78.65 gm
EDTA	7.8 gm
Boric acid	5.98 gm
Distill water	1 litre

5.5.2.2. Basic Procedure

Cellulose acetate membrane such as Celagram (Supplied by Shandon) are good to handle. First strips should be soaked in buffer. Strips are dropped into a shallow tray containing buffer so that only the lower surface is in contact with the buffer. This is best done by holding the strips at both ends by means of curved forceps, bringing the strips as closely over the surface of the buffer as possible and releasing both ends of the strips at the same time. The strips will then float on the surface of the buffer and will soak almost immediately. If buffer is allowed to flow on the top surface of the strips, before the under surface is wetted then opaque areas are apparent on the surface and the strips will be useless for electrophoresis. The strips can not be simply immersed in the buffer as this results in air bubbles being entrapped in the strip and these may take several hours to disappear. Badly soaked strips show opaque areas. After soaking the strips are blotted between filter paper.

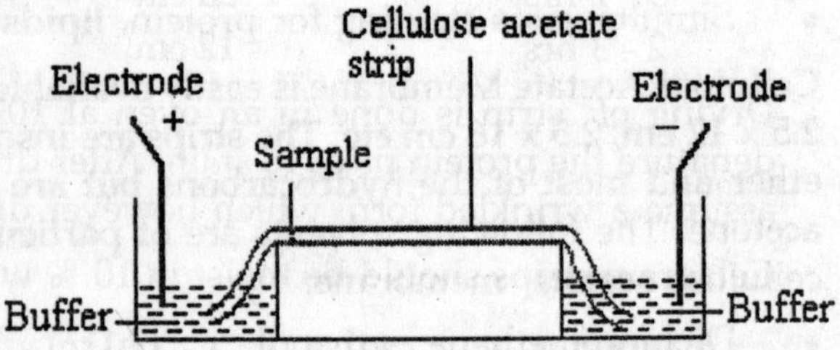

Fig. 5.5. Cellulose Acetate Strip Electrophoresis

The strips are then immediately placed in the tank and current switched on. If there is drying during this process again reimpregnation with buffer is done. About 15 minutes are allowed between switching of current and application of sample, in order to allow equilibrium condition. The sample is applied in a straight continous line about one-third of the cathod end of the strip for alkaline buffer.

Strip width	Sample applied in µg
2.5 cm	350 µg
5 cm	700 µg

About 10 and 20 µl of sample can be adsorbed by strips of 2.0 cm wide 5.0 cm wide. Sample may be applied with the help of micropipette. About 0.5 cm should be left clear at either end of the strip. After applying the sample, the origin is marked by a few crystal of bromophenol blue.

5.5.2.3. Current and Voltage

mA	=	0.4 mA per cm width of paper
V	=	6 - 8 mA per cm width of paper
Time		according to strip Length

5 - 7 hrs	20 cm
2 - 3 hrs	12 cm

Drying of strip is done in an oven at 100ºC for 10 minutes. This denature the protein prior to stain. After drying the strips frequently assume a wrinkled form which however disappear after staining.

Celagram strips should be moist in 10 % w/v Trichloroacetic acid.

5.5.2.4. Staining of Cellulose Acetate Strips

Celagram strips treated with trichloroacetic acid should be blotted lightly and immersed in stain for the detection of proteins.

(i) Naphthalene Black 12 B

Naphthalene black 12 B	0.2 % w/ v i.e. 200 mg
Acetic acid	10 % v/v.
Time	10 minutes
Destain	10 % w/v Aqueous acitic acid

(ii) Procion Blue H - 5 R

Procion Blue	0.2 % w/v i.e. 200 mg
Acetic acid	10 % v/v
Time	10 minutes
Destain	10 % w/v acetic acid

(iii) Azocarmine B

Azocarmine B	0.1 % w/v
Acetic acid	0.45 M containing
	0.45 Sodium acetate for 5 minutes
Destain	10 % w/v Acetic acid

(iv) Nigrosine

This is the most sensitive of all the protein stains and should not be used for zones containing more than 80 μg of protein. Stain is best carried out by immersing the strips overnight in a solution of

Nigrocine	0.001 % w/v
Acetic acid	2 % w/v Aqueus

After staining the strips are rinsed rapidly in tap water and air dried.

(v) Leuco Malachite Green (for haemoglobin)

Leuco malachite Green	0.1 5 w/v

Acetic acid	5 % v/v
Hydrogen peroxide	few drops
Destain	5 % Acetic acid then air dried

In some cases during the passage of current, electrolysis occurs at the electrodes resulting in pH changes. It can be minimized by isolating the electrode in a separate compartment from that of paper cellulose strip dips. These two compartments are connected by means of a paper wick, glass, fiber wick or gel bridge.

5.5.2.5. Factors Affecting the Separation

There are various factors which affect the movement of molecules and hence the separation become slow and resolution is low.

(i) Supporting Medium

The supporting medium such as (Paper, cellulose acetate strip, glass fiber, gels)are relatively inert hence they cause little effect to the material being separated. Paper is used for both high and low voltage and thin layer material for small amount of sample whereas gel is used for large molecule of the sample.

(ii) pH

At high pH value the migration of molecule will be faster because the ionization of the molecule depends upon pH and the molecule only migrates when it become ionized i.e. carries a charge.

(iii) Buffer

Buffer is a solution of weak acid and one of its salt, it resists change in H^+ and OH^- ion concentration and maintains constant pH. Each buffer has its own buffering capacity i.e. the rate of change of pH to the number of equivalents of acid or base added. It is helpful for maintaining pH and carrying currents. A wide variety of buffers are being used in electrophoresis. They should be inert in nature. Certain buffers such as borate can complex with a medium such as starch, thus influencing electrophoretic separation. Borate which which can complex with carbohydrate containing cis - hydroxy groups in general has been used to convert unchanged carbohydrates into complexes suitable for separation by electrophoresis.

The buffer should have good conductive properties and is usually used at a concentration of 0.05 - 0.10M i.e. buffer of high molarity results in sharper zone of separation than buffers of low molarity. Although the time of separation is longer in the former case, the conductivity of the buffer is determined by its ionic strength i.e.

$$\mu = {}^{1}/_{2}\,Mc^{2}$$

μ = ionic strength
M = molarity of ion
c = charge carried by ion

(vi). Voltage and heat effect : When the voltage (i.e. current) and heat of the apparatus is increased the rate of migration of charged particles will also be increased until equilibrium.

5.5.2.6. Advantages

- Time taken is less.
- Zones are sharper than normal.
- Several minor serum components which are not usually visible are detected by this technique.
- Due to small size of strip many samples can be applied simultaneously.

5.5.2.7. Electroendosmosis

Electrophoresis is frequently carried out on essentially inert media. But certain media used in electrophoresis themselves contain ionisable groups that are negatively charged in alkaline buffers e.g. Paper has a small but significant content of carboxyl groups. The negative charged ion moves towards anode but this is of course impossible since the media are stationary. To counter the force generated a movement of positively proptonated water molecules (H_3O^+) occur towards the cathode. This gives the effect of an osmotic movement of solvent towards the cathode, so that neutral molecule frequently appear to move towards cathode. This is why the electrically neutral γ globulin fraction of serum move towards the cathod during electrophoresis.

5.5.3. Gel Electrophoresis

Gel electrophoresis is a method that separates macromolecules either nucleic acids or proteins through a stationary (gel) material in an electric field on the basis of their size, electric charge and physical properties. The biological molecules such as amino acids, peptides, proteins, nucleotides and nucleic acids posses ionizable groups and therefore, they exist in the solution either in the form of cation(+) or anion (-) at suitable pH. These charged particles move towards cathode or anode depending upon their net charge. The positive charged particles move towards cathode while negatively charged particles move towards anode.

5.5.3.1. Principles of Gel Electrophoresis

- When ionized groups are placed in an electric field, they migrate towards either positive or negative pole according to their respective charges.
- Proteins and nucleic acids is electrophoresed within a matrix or Gel.
- The gel may be composed of agrose or polyacrylamide, which is used to perform a particular type of separation

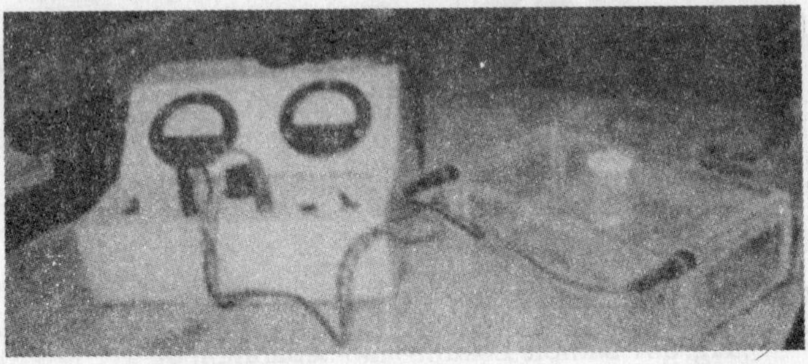

Fig. 5.6. Electrophoretic Apparatus

5.5.4 Agrose Gel Electrophoresis

Agrose gel electrophoresis is used for the separation of proteins such as enzymes, nucleic acids (DNA and RNA). Separation of molecule depends upon charge to mass ratio. Agrose is a linear natural polysaccharide derived from the agar of *Gelidium amansii* having a moleculer weight of 12,000 and made up of basic repeated unit agrobios that contains alternate units of galactose and 3,6 anhydrogalactose. It is generally used at concentration of 0.5 to 2 %. The gel is prepared by mixing agrose powder with buffer solution and melting it by heating until a clear solution is obtained. After cooling the solution to about 60 °C, it is poured on casting tray (plastic or glass) containing a sample comb and allowed to solidify at room temperature. The comb is removed after the gel solidifies. Now this gel plate is placed into electrophoretic chamber horizontally. The sample is mixed with loading buffer (Glycol) and then loaded in the sample well with the help of micropipette. When the current is applied the sample will migrate towards anode (as proteins are negatively charged particles). Bubbles on the electrode confirm the current supply. In case of DNA separation, ethidium bromide, the fluorescent

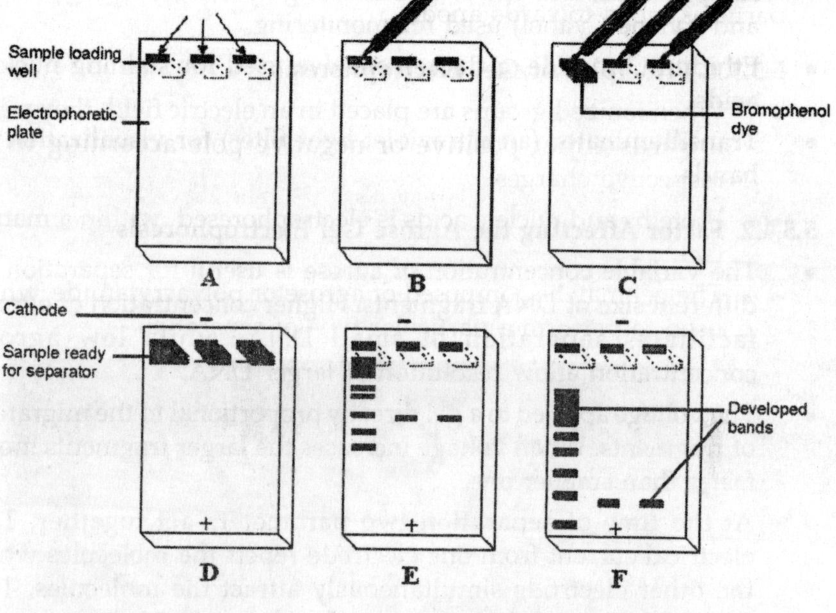

Fig. 5.7. Sample Loading and Separation through Agrose Gel Electrophoresis (A). Well formation in the gell; (B). Sample loading in the well; (C). Sample loading and Bromophenol dye mixing; (D) Plate ready for separation; E. Sample separated in bands; (F) Complete separation of sample into bands.

dye, helps in visualization of bands. If electrophoresis is carried overtime DNA or protein will diffuse within the gel. So observation or photography should be done shortly after completion of Electrophoresis.

5.5.4.1. Basic Requirement for Agrose Gel Electrophoresis

- An electrophoretic chamber and power supply.
- Gel casting trays, which are available in a variety of sizes and composed of UV – transparent plastic.
- Sample combs, around which molten agrose is poured to form sample wells in the gel, or wells may be prepared by removing gel with any sharp object.
- Electrophoresis buffer, usually Tris acetate- EDTA (TAE) or Tris borate is used.
- Loading buffer (glycol), which allow the sample to fall into the

sample wells, and one or two tracking dyes (Bromophenol Blue and Xylene Cyanol) used for monitoring.

- Ethidium bromide, a fluorescent dye used for staining nucleic acids.
- Transilluminator (an ultraviolet light filter) for visualization of bands.

5.5.4.2. Factor Affecting the Agrose Gel Electrophoresis

- The variable concentration of agrose is useful for separation of different size of DNA fragments. Higher concentration of agrose facilitates separation of small DNA, while low agrose concentration allow resolution of larger DNA.
- The voltage applied to a gel directly proportional to the migration of fragments. When voltage increases the larger fragments move faster than smaller one.
- At the time of separation two parameters act together. The electrical current from one electrode repels the molecules while the other electrode simultaneously attract the molecules. The frictional force of the gel material act as a "molecular sieve," and separating the molecules by size. Their rate of migration through the electric field depends on the strength of the field, shape and size of the molecules relative hydrophobicity of the samples, and on the ionic strength and temperature of the buffer in which molecules are moving.
- pH of the buffer changes with temperature variation.
- Ethidium bromide (a fluorescent dye) binding to DNA alters its mass and rigidity and therefore its mobility.

5.5.5 Polyacrylamide Gel Electrophoresis (PAGE)

The polyacrylamide gel electrophoresis (PAGE) technique was introduced by **Raymond and Weintraub (1959)**. PAGE is similar to agrose gel electrophoresis but their size of gel pores are very small providing slow down of the large proteins. Hence separation of molecules by charge to mass ratio is modified by sieving effect. Polyacrylamide is a cross linked polymer of acrylamide. The length of the polyacrylamide is decided by the concentration of acrylamide used (i.e. concentration between 3.5 and 20 %).The percentages of polyacrylamide may be 3 % to 30 % which is ideal range for gene sequencing, protein, polypeptide and enzyme analysis. Polyacrylamide gel casted in gradient provides continuous decrease in pore size from top to bottom of the gel, resulting in thin bands. In this the concentration of polyacrylamide gel is increased which decreases the size of pores in gel at the direction in which electrophoresis proceed. It separates the molecule on the basis of their size rather than charge. It can be used for the identification of native proteins of different sizes. When an electric field is applied to a pore gradient gel, the molecules begin moving at a speed determined by charge. But due to decreasing pore size the movement of larger molecules slow down and become immobilized where the pore size is very small. Therefore it leads to the formation of a molecule and also prevents from tailing edge, so that a narrow band is formed. On the other side the smaller molecules are weakly charged and move slowly. Therefore gradient gel provides a detailed genetic and molecular analysis of the material. It presents more resolution and sharper banding pattern than agrose gel electrophoresis. Care should be taken to prevent it from heating effect.

5.5.5.1. Procedure

For analyzing the mixture of proteins different samples are located in wells at the top of the polyacrylamide gel. When an electric current is applied, the protein moves into the gel. The gel minimizes convection currents caused by small temperature gradient, and it minimizes protein movement other than those induced by electric field. When migration of proteins are completed it can be visualized by treating with a stain like coomassie blue, which only binds to the protein but not to the gel itself. Each band on the gel plate represents a different protein or protein subunit. The smaller proteins are found near the bottom of the gel. Under electric field, these proteins move according to their molecular weight.

5.5.5.2. Separation of Haptoglobin by PAGE

Haptoglobin is an α_2 globulin that binds with free haemoglobin, when it is released into the serum by breaking of red blood cells. There are three main types of of haptoglobins known as Hp1 and Hp2 giving the homozygote Hp1-1 and Hp 2-2 and heterozygote 2-1.

Chemical requirements

HCl
Tris (Hydroxymethyl amino methane)
Acrylamide
Bis (N-N′ - methylene bis acrylamide)

Riboflavin
Ammonium per sulphate
TEMED
Sucrose
Glycerine

(i) Solution A

1N HCl	24 ml
Tris	18.3 gm
TEMED	0.12 ml
Distilled water	40 ml
pH	8.9

Cover it with 40 ml distilled water and finally make the volume 50 ml with distilled water.

(ii) Solution B

1N HCl	24 ml
Tris	2.99gm
TEMED	0.23 ml
Distiled water	40 ml
pH	6.7

Cover it up to 40 ml with distilled water and finally make the volume 50 ml with distilled water.

(iii) Solution C

Acrylamide	14 gm
Bis	0.36 gm

Cover it up to 50 ml with distilled water

(iv) Solution D

Acrylamide	5 gm
Bis	0.12 gm

Cover it with 50 ml distilled water

(v) Solution E

Sucrose	20 gm

Dissolve and cover it upto 50 ml with distilled water

(vi) Solution F

Riboflavin	4 mg in 100 ml water

(vii) Solution G

Ammonium per sulphate 140mg / 100ml water (freshly prepared)

1. Lower gel or Separating Gel

(i) Solution	**A**	**C**	**D/W**	**G**
	2ml	4ml	2ml	8ml

2. Upper gel (Stock gel)

(ii) Solution	**B**	**D**	**E**	**F**
	1ml	2ml	4ml	1ml

3. Sample buffer	**B**	**D/W**	**E**
	1ml	3ml	4ml

5.5.5.3. Method

Fill the tubes 2/3 with lower gel or separating gel, pour two drops of water from the sides of the tube so that separating gel will not be distributed (showing two different layers then polymerize 30-45 minutes). Afterwards fill the tubes with stock gel (leaving 1/2 cm for sample) again pour 2 drops of distilled water from the sides of the tube then polymerize for 30-45 minutes. Decant the distill water after polymerization in each tube. Now fix the tubes in the hole of disc of electrophoresis chamber. Now mix 1 drop serum + 2 drops sample buffers.

(i) Stock Tank Buffer

Tris	6.0 gm
Glycine	28.8 gm
Distill water	1 litre
pH	8.3

Working tank buffer 1:10 i.e. 1 ml tank buffer and 10 ml distilled water.

(i) Electrophoretic Run

Electrophoresis is carried out for 2 hours at a fixed voltage of 2 mA/ gel tube. A small amount of Bromophenol blue was added to one of the sample tubes as a marker dye to indicate the progress of separation.

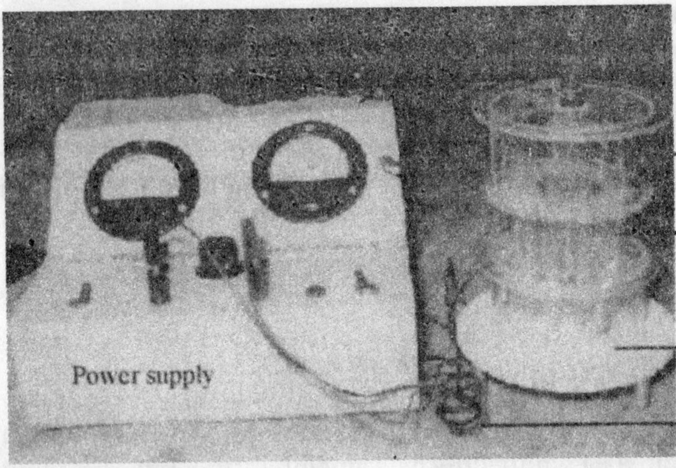

Fig. 5.8. Separation of Different Proteins by Electrophoresis

(ii) Staining of Gel

After electrophoresis the gel was removed from the tubes and directly expelled into test tube containing the benzidene solution. Then add 1-2 drops of H_2O_2 (30%), blue bands appear. Then transfer the gel into tubes containing distilled water.

Benzidine hydrochloride	1.5 gm
Acetic acid	13 ml
Distilled water	57 ml

or

Benzidine hydrochloride	1.0 gm
Acetic acid	2.5 ml
H_2O_2 (30%)	1 ml
Distilled water	500 ml

or

Dissolve 0.5 gm of amido black in 100 ml of 7 % acetic acid and stain it for 2-5 minute then destain with 7 % acetic acid.

5.6 Sodium Dodecyl Sulphate (SDS) Polyacrylamide Gel Electrophoresis (SDS-PAGE)

In 1967 **A. Shapiro, Edward Vinuela** and **Jacob Maizel** showed that the moleculer weight of most protein could be determined by measuring the mobility in polyacrylamide gel having the detergent Sodium Dodecyl sulphate (SDS).

This method was further improved by **Klaus Weber** and **Mary Osborn** and became a standard technique for the determination of molecular weight of single polypeptide chains. The sample to be analyzed is boiled with SDS and mercaptoethanol. The disulphide linkage of protein is reduced and broken by mercaptoethnol. The SDS binds with protein and denatures it. Now the protein acquires rod-shaped structure and an identical charge to mass ratio. This is because SDS molecule is bound to two amino acids of the residues. These SDS molecule develop the series of negative charges on denatured protein and prevent it from folding.

The high molecular weight protein separates from large pore size gel while the low molecular weight protein molecules separate from smallar pore size gel material. Sometimes an ionizable dye bromophenol is also added to the sample buffer for monitoring the separation. It changes its colour by changing pH. It indicates the electrophoresis front at the time of completion of separation.

5.6.1 Procedure

After pouring the gel into glass tray an additional layer of stacking gel is also poured to 1cm height on gel on which wells are formed for loading the sample. After loading the sample the current is passed through gel. The ionic species present in the sample and gel will move frequently at the same velocity and maintain the circuit. Movement

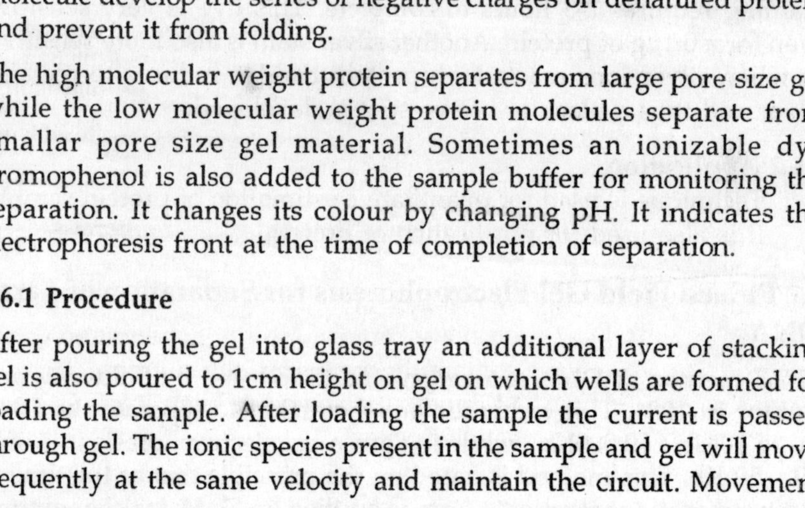

Fig. 5.9. (a) Denaturation of Protein (b) Loading of Sample

of glycinate ions in tank buffer is slower than SDS -protein complex while Cl^- ions in loading buffer move faster than SDS -protein complex. This results in the formation of Compact SDS - protein bands in-between Cl^- and glycinate ions. In an applied electric field SDS - protein complex move towards anode and proteins are separated according to their size and molecular weight.

When the separation is completed the slab is taken away from between the glass plates and stained by Coomassie Brilliant Blue R – 250 (CBB). Staining requires 2-3 hours to complete. This dye is very sensitive even for a 0.1µg of protein. Another silver stain is also more sensitive, as when silver ions reacts with protein band it reduces to metallic silver and thus a black or brown spot is developed.

5.6.2 Application

- Technique is used for quantitative estimation of protein sample.
- It is also used for purification of protein.

5.7 Pulsed Field Gel Electrophoresis for Separation of Large DNA

PFGE method of DNA separation was introduced by **Schwartz** and **Cantor in 1984**. This technique has the ability to separate the DNA up to 10Mb (10,000Kb), while in agrose gel electrophoresis it is only 30 - 50 Kb. This method is based on the principle that at the time of electrophoretic separation a force is applied on DNA for changing its direction from a single diffused band. So that separation will be achieved on a fine scale. Larger size DNA fragments are separated from smaller ones in the form of band. When the force is applied the smaller size DNA move quickly to change their direction with each reorientation angle to the electric field in relation to gel (reorientation angle may be 80ø, 90 ø or 120 ø).

5.8 Rotating Gel Electrophoresis

Rotating gel electrophoresis is the most commonly used recent techniques which provide various angle with homogenous electric field for the separation of larger DNA fragments (10,000Kb). In this method the electrodes are placed along opposite side of the buffer chamber having their fixed polarity. The gel is cast on a circular running plate instead of square plate and then placed in the buffer chamber. To overcome the problem of leakage the gel is coupled with magnetic drive beneath the buffer chamber. Migrating DNA can be forced into new direction by using the magnetic drive which simply rotates the gel into the new angle.

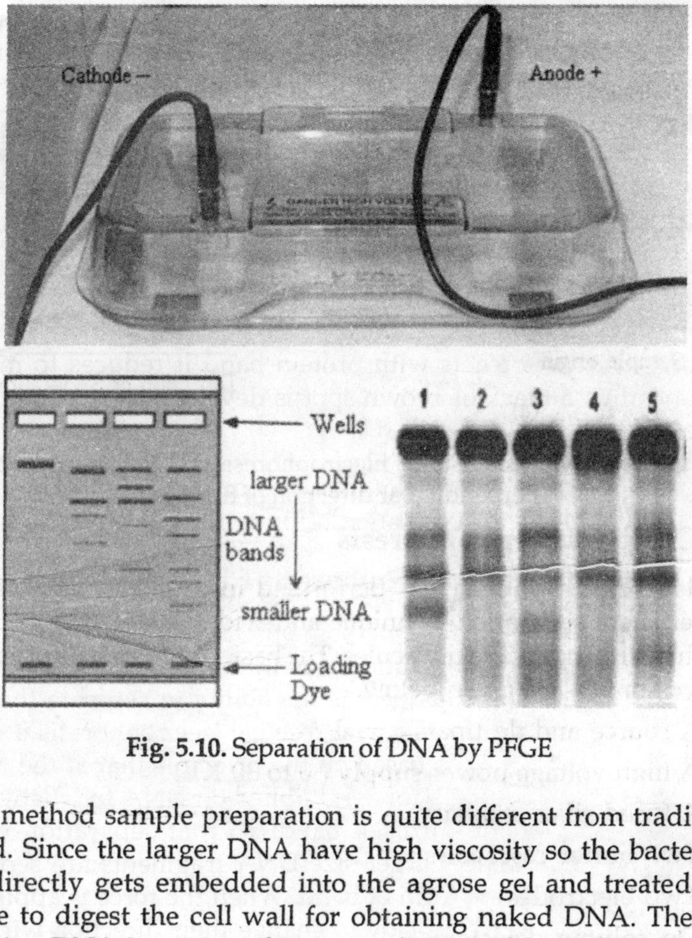

Fig. 5.10. Separation of DNA by PFGE

In this method sample preparation is quite different from traditional method. Since the larger DNA have high viscosity so the bacteria or yeast directly gets embedded into the agrose gel and treated with enzyme to digest the cell wall for obtaining naked DNA. Then the gel having DNA is cut into the required size and loaded into sample well to perform electrophoresis.

5.9 Two-dimensional Electrophoresis (Combined Electrophoresis)

Two-dimensional electrophoresis is the combination of two different separation techniques i.e. electrophoresis and chromatography which are involved in a single dimension. The sample is applied to a planer support (paper) and chromatography is performed in a particular dimension. Further electrophoresis is carried out in perpendicular direction. Normally chromatography is performed first than the electrophoresis. In this technique the same support is applied for both the separation (Fig. 5.11).

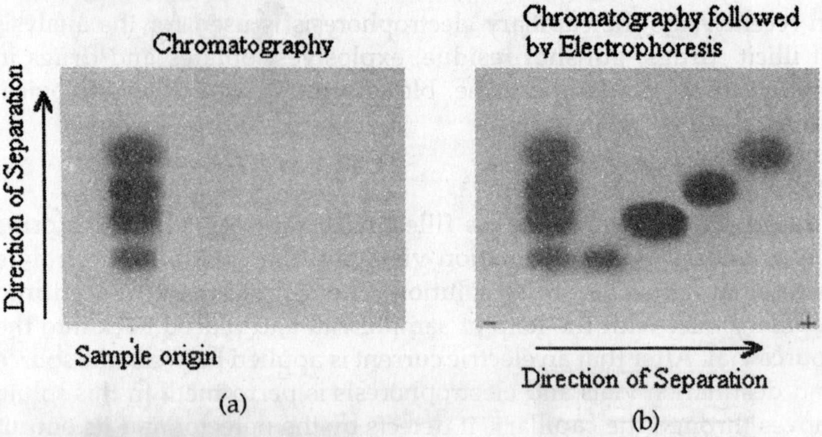

Fig. 5.11. Two Dimensional Electrophoresis (a) One direction (b) Perpendicular direction of first one

5.10 Capillary Electrophoresis

Capillary Electrophoresis is performed in capillary tube. It is the most efficient separation technique and widely used for the analysis of both micro and macro molecules. The basic requirements of capillary electrophoresis are given below:-

- A source and destination vial
- A high voltage power supply (0 to 30 KV)
- A fused silica capillary
- Two buffer reservoirs
- Two electrodes
- On-column detector
- Sample vial

For the capillary electrophoresis specific amount of sample is introduced by temporary replacment of one buffer reservoirs with a sample vial. The separation through Capillary electrophoresis provide high efficiency and sharp resolution. Electrophoresis can be conducted in free solution or in a solution containing non-conductive medium, such as gel. Usually the non-conductive medium is immersed in a conductive aqueous buffer solution, and an electric field is applied across the medium.

This medium may be paper, cellulose acetate membranes, agrose or polyacrylamide gels. As the process is done in capillary tube so it is referred to as capillary electrophoresis.

In recent years the capillary electrophoresis is used for the analysis of illicit drugs, gunshot residue, explosives, opiates and drugs in biological materials like urine, blood, viscera and other biological fluids.

5.10.1 Method

First of all the source vial is filled with sample, which performs electrophoresis and destination vials are filled with an electrolyte such as an aqueous buffer solution. The sample is introduced into capillary inlet with the help of sample vial and placed back into the source vial. After that an electric current is applied between the source and destination vials and electrophoresis is performed. In this solute moves through the capillary, it detects by the detector and its output is sent to an integrator or computer, this output is displayed in the form of electropherogram which is a plot of detector versus time (Fig. 5.12).

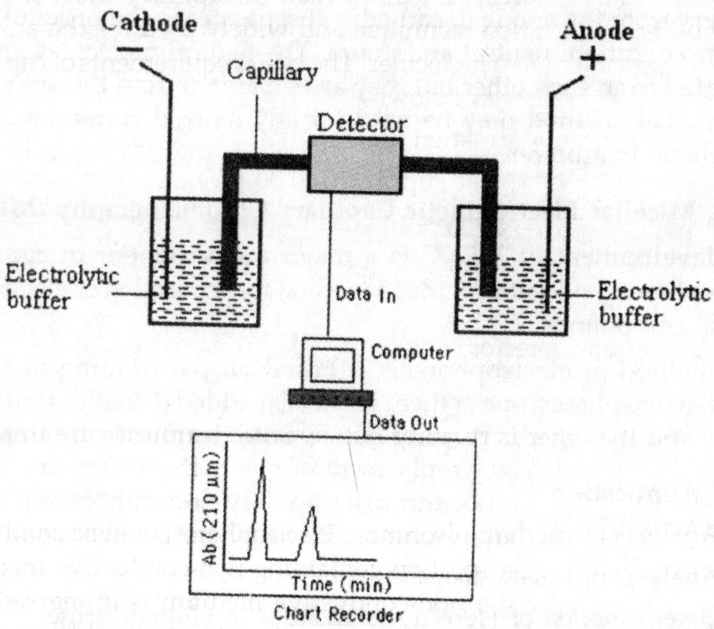

Fig. 5.12. Digramatic Representation of Capillary Electrophoresis

All these methods are the same as used in normal electrophoresis but the differences is that the process of electrophoretic separation is carried out in tiny capillaries generally made up of fused silica under high electric field.

5.10.2. Capillary Zone Electrophoresis

In this electrophoresis the separation occurs in a free solution so it is also known as free solution capillary electrophoresis (FSCE). This technique is used only for the separation of anion and cation, not the neutrals. For the separation, the capillary is filled with a buffer of constant composition and the source and destination vials are filled with the same buffer. Then the sample is injected into the capillary, which is filled with buffer.

Now the current is applied. Molecules of the solute migrate through the capillary and separated due to the differences in their rate of migration, which are dependent on their electrophoretic mobility. Electroosmotic flow facilitates the movement of solutes through the capillary from the anode to cathode. It separates in the order of their elution i.e. cation, neutral and anion. The neutral molecules are not separated from each other but they are separated from the anion and cations. The method may be used for any ionized compounds that are soluble in a buffer.

5.10.3. Micellar Electrokinetic Capillary Chromatography (MEKC)

The development of MEKC is a major advancement in capillary electrophoresis since it provides a method for separation of electrically neutral compounds.

This method of electrophoresis is based on partitioning of solute between two phases, one of them is Micellar added (Pseudo- stationary phase) and the other is running buffer. Both the phases are movable.

5.10.4 Application

- Analysis of methamphetamine by Capillary gel electrophoresis
- Analysis of opiate drugs in hair
- Determination of Heroin metabolities in Human urine
- Determination of LSD in blood
- Analysis of Forensic drugs like Caffeine, Morphine, Codeine, Cocaine, Diazepam and Narcotine etc.

5.11. Immunoelectrophoresis

Immunoelectrophoresis is also known as gamma globulin electrophoresis, immunoglobulin electrophoresis or agar gel electrophoresis. It is a method of determining the blood levels of three major immunoglobulins, IgM, IgG, IgA. Immunoelectrophoresis is an analytical technique with high resolving power as it combines separation of antigen by electrophoresis with immunodiffusion against an antiserum. Immunoelectrophoresis is used frequently to diagnose multiple myeloma, a disease affecting the bone marrow.

5.11.1 Principle

Immunoelectrophoresis combines two techniques to identify antigens in a sample i.e.

1. Electrophoresis
2. Immunodiffusion

Electrophoresis involves separation of protein in a sample (e.g. serum) according to their net charge. The sample is loaded on gel and this gel is connected with suitable electrolyte solution. Current is applied to the electrolyte solution. The positively charged antibodies migrate towards cathode (negative terminal) and negatively charged protein, such as albumin migrate towards anode (positive terminal). In Immunoelectrophoresis a gel is prepared in which wells and slots are cut alternately. The antigen mixture is placed in the wells. Then electrophoresis is performed. Later an antibody is added to the slots in the gel. Antigen and antibodies migrate towards one another and form precipitin arcs at the zone of optimal concentration.

To understand Immunoelectrophoresis well, it is essential to know the composition of blood and structure of antigen and antibodies.

5.11.2 Preparation of the Gel

For making 2 % Agrose gel 2 gm agrose and 100 ml Barbitone Acetate buffer is put in a conical flask and warmed in a bath for 35 - 50 minutes until it becomes completely transparent and bubble-free. The flask is taken out of the bath and cooled rapidly under running water (45°C-50°C). Now this solution is poured on a slide, already put on spirit labellar. After gelation the slides are kept in moist chamber at 40°C for 24 hrs to set.

5.11.3 Separation of Blood Proteins

It is highly complex mixture of cells, enzymes proteins and inorganic substances; it consists of 45 % RBC, WBC, platelets and 55 % plasma. Antigen are specific type of protein residing on the surface of RBC. It is these antigen that impart blood type characteristic to the red blood cells. More than 15 blood antigen have been identified but most important are A, B, AB, O, MN and Rh system.

As immunoelectrophoresis is also known as agar gel electrophoresis because agar is used to form slots. Agar is a polysaccharide derived by marine algae *Gelidium amansii* consisting of dextrose and Lavio units joined by 1 - 3 bands. They normally contains two distinct groups.

1. **Agrose** - It is practically neutral and used in electrophoresis. It decreases electroendosmosis and adsorption of sample.
2. **Agropectin** - It is negatively charged.

5.11.4 Buffers: for Immunoelectrophoresis

There are a series of buffers which vary in their ionic strength (μ) eg. separation of β globulin is improved at $\mu = 0.03$ while ionic strength $\mu = 0.05$ is best for protein.

1. Sodium Acetate, 0.1M, pH 4.0

Glacial Acetic acid	25.6 ml
Sodium Acetate	13.6 gm
Distilled water	1000 ml

2. Sodium Acetate - EDTA, 0.1M, pH 4.5

EDTA (disodium salt)	1.0 gm
Glacial Acetic Acid	125 ml
Distilled water	1000 ml

3. Sodium Phosphate Buffer 0.1M, pH 7.0

Disodium Hydrogen Phosphate anhydrous Sodium dihydrogen	36 - 92 gm
orthophosphate dehydrate	6.86 gm
Distilled water	1000 ml

4. Barbitone Acetate Buffer 0.1M, pH 8.6

Barbitone Sodium	10.0 gm
Sodium Acetate	6.5 gm

Hydrochloric Acid (0.1N)	64.4 ml
Distilled water	1000 ml

This is the most commonly used buffer system for the lipoprotein and serum protein separation.

5. Barbitone Calcium Lactate pH 8.6

Barbitone Sodium	12.8 gm
Barbitone	1.66 gm
Calcium Lactate	3.84 gm
Distilled water	1000 ml

Heating it to prepare the buffer.

6. Tris - EDTA Borate pH 9.0

Tris	60.5 gm
EDTA(Disodium salt)	6.0 gm
Boric Acid	4.6 gm
Distilled water	1000 ml

7. Glycine 0.1M pH 9.0

Glycine	3.0 gm
Sodium Hydroxide	0.82 gm
Sodium Chloride	4.68 gm
Distilled water	1000 ml

5.12. Isoelectro Focussing

Isoelectric focusing is one of the newest methods of separation based on the behaviour of molecules in an electric field. The first application of this principle was described by **Ikeda and Suzuki (1912)**. They separated glutamic acid from hydrolysates of plant proteins. After that **Williams and Waterman (1929)** clearly defined the principle of Isoelectro focussing.

The solution which contained both positively and negatively charged groups known as ampholytes (proteins are ampholytes). Ampholytes or Zwitterions have the property that their charge depends on pH i.e. they are positively charged at low pH (cathode) and negatively charged at high pH(anode). Each Ampholyte becomes uncharged at an existing pH. This is called the **isoelectric point**. At the isoelectric point, the ampholyte will not move in an electric field. If a proton solution is placed in a pH gradient, the molecule will move until they reach a point in the gradient at which they are uncharged, then will stop moving. When a mixture of different proteins are placed for the separation, then each type of molecule will come to rest at a point in the pH gradient, corresponding to its own Isoelectric point. This method of separating protein according to their isoelectric points in a pH gradient is called Isoelectric focusing. Thus the molecule having same isoelectric points are concentrated in a narrow band.

This technique is also known as Isoelectric fractionation, Isoelectric separation, Isoelectric condensation and Stationary electrolysis.

5.13 Isotachophoresis

The word Isotachophoresis is made of three words i.e. "Iso"- same- "tacho" - velocity and "phoresis" "to move". So it may be defined as the movement of sample molecules with the same velocity as electrolyte.

The special feature of this method is that there are two electrolytes - "leading" and "terminating". Leading electrolyte has high mobility ions whereas terminating electrolyte has low mobility ions and both are connected with anode and cathode respectivley.

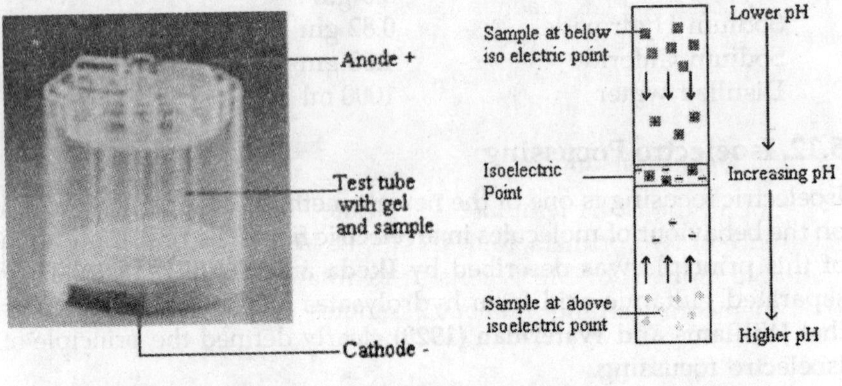

Fig. 5.13. Isoelectric Focusing Device and Separation through it

At the time of separation the negatively charged sample molecules move towards anode while positively charged molecules towards cathode. Thus the ions form a uniform layer within the ions form a uniform layer within the zone i.e. positively charged ions and at one end, negatively charged ions at another end and both charged ions in between them. In this method we find only sample molecules and counter ions at each zone (Fig. 5.13).

5.14 Polymerase Chain Reaction (PCR)

The technique of PCR was developed by **Kary Mullis** in 1985. It is an invitro method of nucleic acid (DNA and RNA) synthesis by which a small amount of DNA can be amplified into billions of copies. It includes two Oligonucleotide primer (amplifier) which flank the DNA molecule to amplified (not less than 20 base long), four deoxynucleoside Tri phosphate (dNTPs) [such as Thymidine Triphosphate (TTP), deoxycyctidine Triphosphate (dCTP), deoxyadenosine Triphosphate (dATP) and deoxyguanosine Triphosphate (dGTP)], DNA polymerase (Taq or Pfu Polymerase); these are heat stable enzymes obtained from different bacteria, another Pwo DNA polymerase also used having 'Proof Reading' activity. It removes and replaces incorrect nucleotides from a DNA strand during synthesis. All this process of PCR reaction takes place in **"Eppendorf tube"**. The following steps are involved for the synthesis of Nucleic acid (Fig. 5.14).

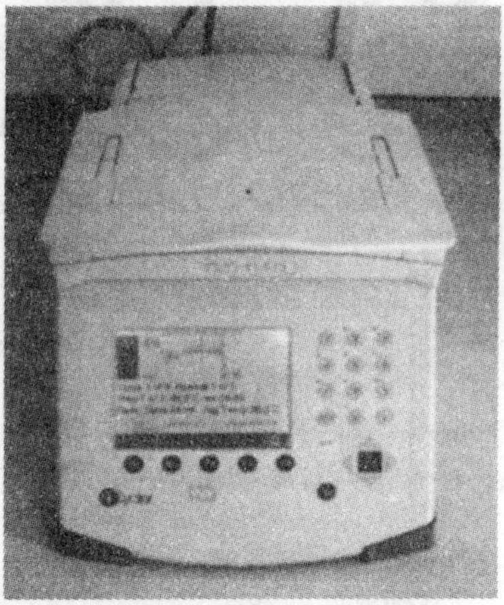

Fig. 5.14. PCR Appratus

5.14.1. Denaturation

First of all the DNA template is separated by heating at 94°C in the presence of two primers, four dNTPs, DNA Polymerase enzyme and suitable amount of Mg^{++} ions. It facilitates the separation of two complementary strand in about 2 minutes.

5.14.2. Annealing

Now the sample is cooled slowly to the temperature (45°C - 55°C) that allow to bind up primers with complementary strand of DNA. The enzyme DNA polymerase are required for this and the process will take about 1 minute.

5.14.3. Primer Extention

In this step the temperature is again increased to 72°C so that the DNA polymerase extend the primers creating a long complementary strand of DNA. This step will take about 1-3 minutes.

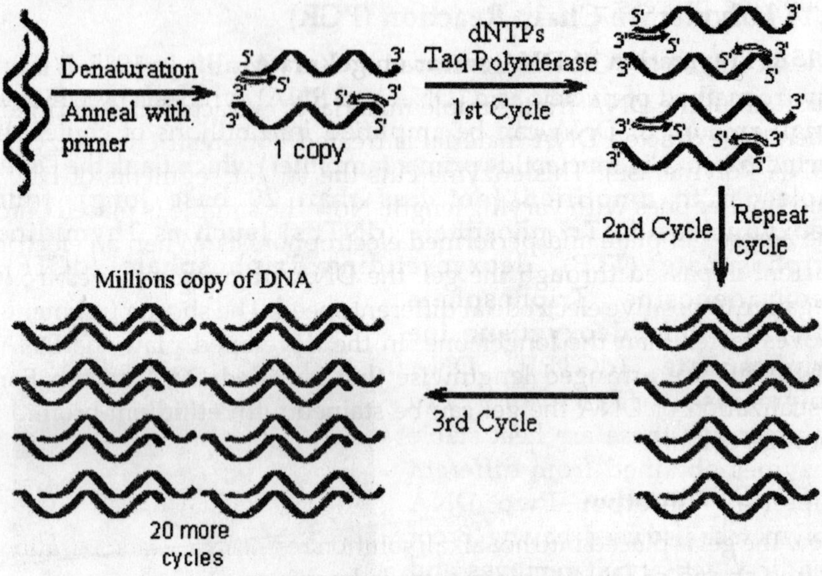

Fig. 5.15. Polymerase Chain Reaction

These steps can be repeated many times for obtaining a number of copies of DNA molecule (Fig. 5.15).

5.14.4. Application

- PCR can detect and identify bacteria and viruses that cause infections such as Tuberculosis, viral meningitis, viral Hepatitis, HIV etc.
- It is used to detect the presence or absence of a pathogen in a patient's blood or tissues.
- It is used in genetic testing for mutation and also in fossile preservation by preserving multiple copies of DNA.
- It is used to get information of evolutionary relation of an organism.
- It is helpful in Parental diagnosis i.e. in the detection of disease present in embryo.
- This technique is also used in genome mapping of different plants and animals.

5.15 Southern Blotting Technique

This technique was developed by **E.M. Southern (1975)** for detecting specific nucleotide sequences in DNA. This method includes the following process:-

5.15.1. Preparation of DNA smear on gel plate

First of all the DNA from sample material is extracted and purified. Then the extracted DNA material is treated with restriction enzyme (DNA Polymerase). This enzyme cuts the longer segments of DNA into smaller ones with varying length. Now the sample is placed onto the agrose gel plate and performed electrophoresis. When an electric current is passed through the gel, the DNA fragments moves from negative to positive electrode at different speed. The shorter fragments moves faster than the longer one. In the developed plate the DNA fragments are arranged lengthwise that is called DNA smear. For visualization of DNA the gel can be stained with ethidium bromide (orange colour).

5.15.2. Denaturation

Now the gel is placed into hot alkali solution resulting in the separation of two strand of DNA. This process is known as Denaturation.

5.15.3. Blotting

In this method the gel is placed on a filter paper. The upper surface of buffer is covered with nylon or nitrocellulose membrane. Filter paper draws buffer through the gel. The buffer carries DNA fragments upward and when it comes in contact with nitrocellulose membrane they get bound to it. Now the DNA smear is transfered on nylon membrane without disturbing its sequences. Then the membrane is washed and exposed to heat (about 80°C) or UV light for permanent fixing of DNA on to the membrane. The membrane is now a mirror image of the agrose gel (Fig. 5.16 & 5.17).

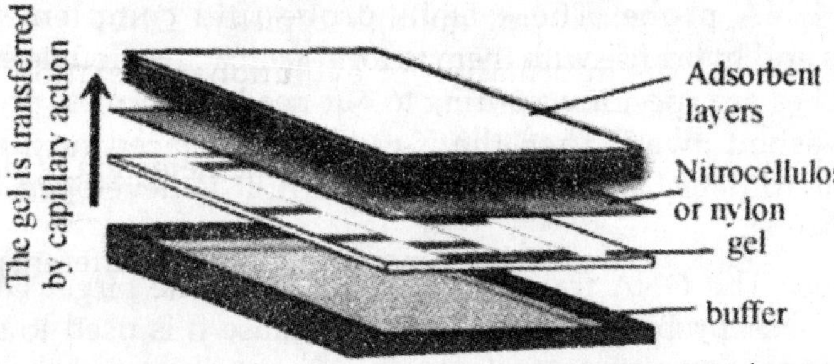

Fig. 5.16. Transfer of Blot on Nylon Membrane in the Presence of Suitable Buffer

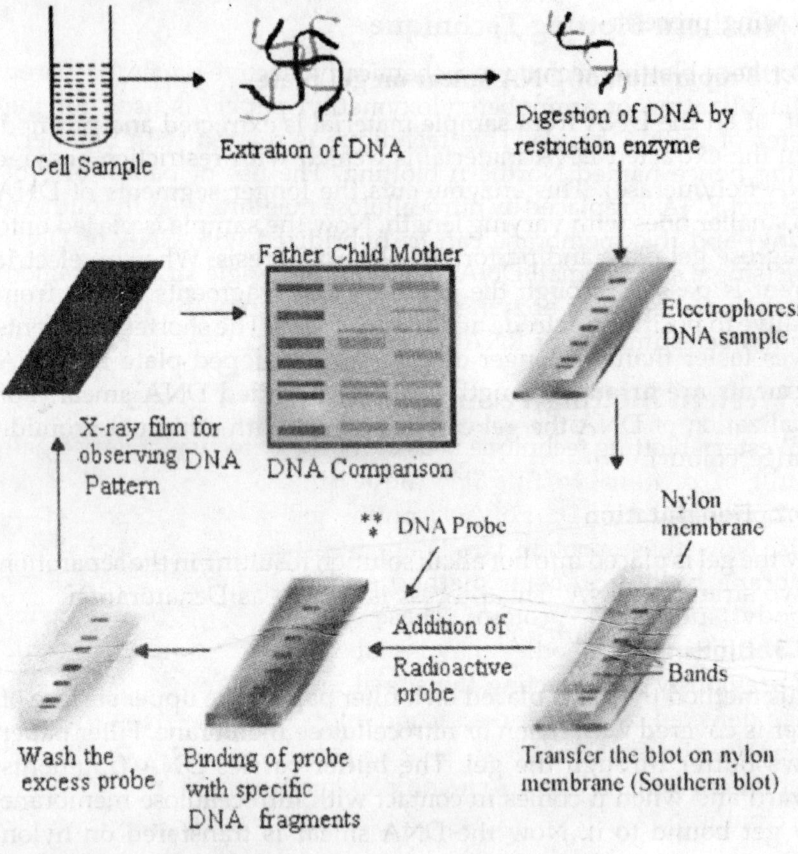

Fig. 5.17. Southern Blotting Method

5.15.4 Hybridisation of the DNA Probe with Target Sequence

The nylon membrane containing DNA smear incubated with radio labelled DNA probe. These DNA probe find complementary sequences and hybridise with them to form radioactive double strand. These probes are specific according to our need. The excess of probe can be washed away. Then the X-ray film is placed next to the membrane to detect the radioactive pattern. It is developed in the form of bands.

DNA Probe: The DNA fragment used to detect the target DNA is called as DNA probe. It is called probe because it is used to search out and detect complementary sequences amongst a number of non-complementary DNA sequences.

5.16 Northern Blotting Technique

In Northern blotting technique a chemically reactive paper (prepared by diazotization of aminobenzyloxymethyl paper) is used for the transfer of mRNA bands. This technique is related with Southern blotting hence named Northern blotting. The use of paper for blot transfer of RNA is replaced by nitrocellulose membrane (as in southern blotting) and this membrane can be hybridized with RNA or DNA probe (single strand small DNA) and then the single stranded region of probe washed with enzyme nuclease for removing it. Now the quantitative estimation of RNA can be done.

5.17 Western Blotting Technique

The Western blotting technique is used for the detection of very small amount of protein. In this technique first of all the protein is electrophoresed by SDS Polyacrylamide gel and obtained protein bands. Now these protein bands are transfered on Nitrocellulose membrane by blot transfer method and added specific labelled antibody (specific for protein). These antibody bind with protein, not hybridize it. Antibodies may be labelled with radioactive label (I^{125}) previously for detecting the signal in **Autoradiography.** It can also be detected by adding the second antibody with enzyme that is specific for the first antibody. This method is quite useful for the detection of proteins even from complex mixture. It is also used for gene cloning.

References

Anand, R., and Southern, E. M., (1990); Pulsed Field Gel Electrophoresis. In Gel Electrophoresis of Nucleic Acids: A Practical Approach. (D. Rickwood and B.D. Hames, eds.), pp. 101- 123. IRL Press at Oxford University Press, New York.

Birren, B., and Lai, E., (1993); Pulsed Field Electrophoresis: A Practical Guide. Academic Press, San Diego.

Birren, B., and Lai, E., eds. (1990); Methods: A Companion to Methods of Enzymology. Pulsed-Field Electrophoresis. Vol. 1, Number 2 Academic Press, San Diego.

Bisen, P.S., Mathur, S., (2004); Life Science in Tools & Techniques.

Cahill, Mathew, (1995); Handbook of Diagnostic Tests. Springhouse, PA, Springhouse Corporation.

Carle, G.F., Frank, M., and Olson, M.V., (1986); Electrophoretic separation of large DNA molecules by periodic inversion of the electric field. Science 232, pp. 65-68.

Clark, S.M., Lai, E., Birren, B.W., and Hood, L., (1988); A novel instrument for separating large DNA molecules with pulsed homogenous electric fields. Science 241, 1203-1205.

Dunn, M.J., (1993); Gel Electrophoresis : Protein Bios Scientific, Oxford.

Gemmill, R.M., (1991); Pulsed field gel electrophoresis. In Advances of Electrophoresis (A. Chrambach, M.J. Dunn, and B.J. Radola, eds.), Vol. 4, pp. 1-48. VCH, Weinheim, Germany.

Gray, P., (1964); Handbook of Basic Microtechniques, McGraw Hill Book Company, New York.

Hawcroft, D.M., (1996); Electrophoresis : The basics. IRL Press Oxford.

Jacobs, David S., et al.(1996); Laboratory Test Handbook. 4th ed. New York, Lexi-Comp Inc.

Mullis, K., Ferre, F. and Gibbs, R.A.(1994); The Polymerase Chain Reaction, Birkhauser, Boston.

O'Farell, (1975); Two-Dimensional Electrophoresis Technique. J. Bio. Chem.

Pagana, Kathleen Deska, (1998); Mosby's Manual of Diagnostic and Laboratory Tests. St. Louis: Mosby, Inc.

Robinson, J.W., (1976); Undergraduate Instrumental Analysis, Marcel Dekker, New York, U.S.A.

Schwartz, D.C., and Cantor, C.R., (1984); "Separation of yeast chromosome-sized DNAs by pulsed field gradient gel electrophoresis." Cell 37, pp. 67-75.

Southern, E.M., Anand, R., Brown, W.R.A., and Fletcher, D.S., (1987); A model for the separation of large DNA molecules by crossed field gel electrophoresis. Nucleic Acids Res. 15, 5925- 5943.

White, H.W., (1992); Rapid separation of DNA molecules by agrose gel electrophoresis: use of a new agrose matrix and a survey of running buffer effects. Biotechniques 12, pp. 574-579.

Wilson, K. and Walker, J., (2000); Practical Biochemistry : Principle & Techniques, Cambridge University Press.

CHAPTER 6

Basic Laboratory Instruments

6.1 Colorimetry

Colorimetry is the method which involves measurement of the intensity of a colour in a solution and relating it to the concentration of the biochemical compounds. Some materials are already coloured but colourless materials can be converted into coloured compound by adding some chemical reagents to them.

6.1.1 Principle

It is based on the principle of Lambert Beer's Law.

6.1.1.1 Lambert Law: When a ray of monochromatic light passes through an absorbing medium, its intensity decreases expotentially as the length of absorbing medium increases.

6.1.1.2. Beer's Law: When a ray of monochromatic light passes through an absorbing medium its intensity decreases expotentially as the concentration of the absorbing medium increases.

These two Law combined together are known as Lambert Beer's Law.

$$I \text{ absorbed} = I_0 - I_T$$

I Intensity of light

I_T Reduced intensity

I_0 Original Intensity

The measurement is based on the visual comparison of the intensity of colour to a set of colour standards which represents various concentrations of the biochemical compounds. A colorimetry may be used to get accurate and precise results.

6.1.2. Instrumentation and Methodology

It is a device consisting of the following equipments:-

6.1.2.1 A light Source: It is a tungesten bulb or filament which gives white light.

6.1.2.2 Device for Providing Beam of Light: It is a device which allows a narrow beam of light to pass.

6.1.2.3. Condenser: It is an optical lens which splits the white beam of light into parallel rays.

6.1.2.4 Sample Cell or Cuvette: This is a glass cell made of 1 cm^2 glass plate with their side focusing towards beam of light. It is filled with about 3 ml of sample solution.

6.1.2.5 Filter: It is made up of coloured glass placed after sample cell and allows maximum transmission of colour absorbed after selection by sample. The filter is of complementary colour depending on the nature and colour of sample solution. A yellow solution looks yellow because it absorbs blue light, so a blue filter should be used.

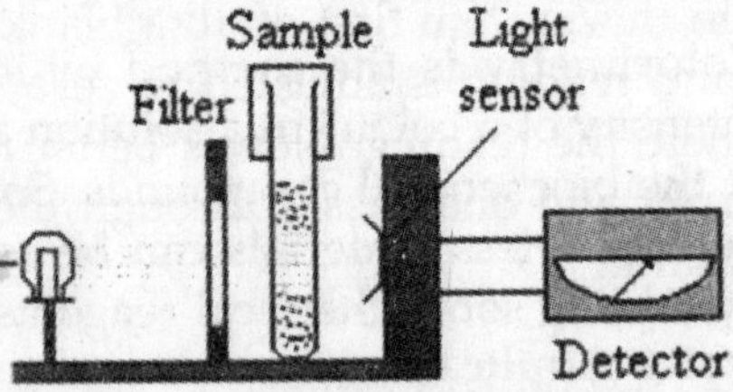

Fig. 6.1. Different Components of Colorimeter

In some instruments filter is placed before the absorption cell, and gives narrow transmission band. Therefore it is closely related to monochromatic light (Fig. 6.1).

Complementary filter and colour of the solution are given in following table :-

Table 6.1

S.No.	Colour of Filter	Colour of Solution
1.	Violet/Blue	Yellow
2.	Green	Purple
3.	Red	Green
4.	Red	Blue
5.	Green	Orange

6.1.2.6 Detector: Detector is in the form of photocell which converts light signals into electric signals and amplify it for detection. Electric current is directly proportional to the intensity of light falling on it.

6.1.2.7 Galvanometer: It is an electrical device with digital display which is calibrated with a logarthmic scale so as to indicate absorption readings of the sample.

6.1.3 Methodology:

The sample to be analyzed is filled in a sample cell. Beam of light is emitted from the tungesten bulb which passing through a slit and condenser lens, is split into parallel rays. Light falling on sample cell is absorbed according to its nature and colour. Later it is passed through a filter of complementary colour. Photocell detector converts the absorbed light into electric signals and amplifies it for detection by galvanometer

In this system first of all a blank solution is put into the colorimeter and reading is adjusted to zero then followed by test solution and note the reading. Now a better method is that the beam of light is split and one passes through the sample and the other through the blank.

6.1.4 Application

- It is used for the detection of Proteins lipids etc.
- It is used for the analysis of coloured organic substances.
- It is also used for the detection of biological fluids containing chromophores.

6.2 Balance

Balance is used for measuring accurate amount of chemical or biological materials. There are various types of balance according to the requirement and amount of material to be weighed, such as Single pan balance, Chemical or Analytical balance and Electrical balance. For the amount smaller than 1 gm, a digital electronic balance may be used but large amount (100g) should not be weighed in electronic balances.

6.2.1 Electrical Balance

For weighing any substance, two points are taken into consideration. First is the determination of weight of the desired chemical or materials and second one is keeping of materials. Therefore, the granular or paste like substances should not be directly placed on the weighing platform of the

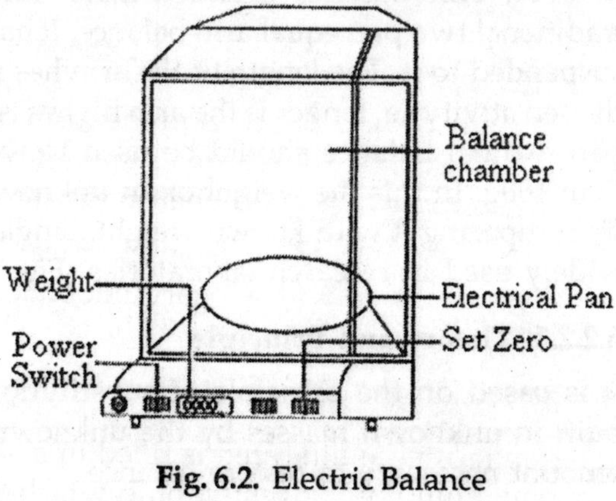

Fig. 6.2. Electric Balance

balance. It is necessary to use glazed paper for small amount (less than 15 gm) of material and a weigh pan or small glass vessel for weighing larger amount should be used. Glazed paper have light weight and it is subjected to negligible (Fig. 6.2).

The following steps are required for weighing:-

6.2.1.1 Initial step : Switch on of the device and set control to zero. If vessel or weighing pan is used set zero until it does. Then select the unit for which it is weighed (mg/ g).

6.2.1.2 Second step: Now place the chemical or biological material on to the pan with the help of glazed paper or vessel.

6.2.1.3 Final step: After placing the weight on to the pan a rapid change occurs on the digital display. It will stop at certain unit, then adjust the required weight and note the reading. Care should be taken that no fluctuations should occur in digital display at final stage. Now read the weight on digital display unit.

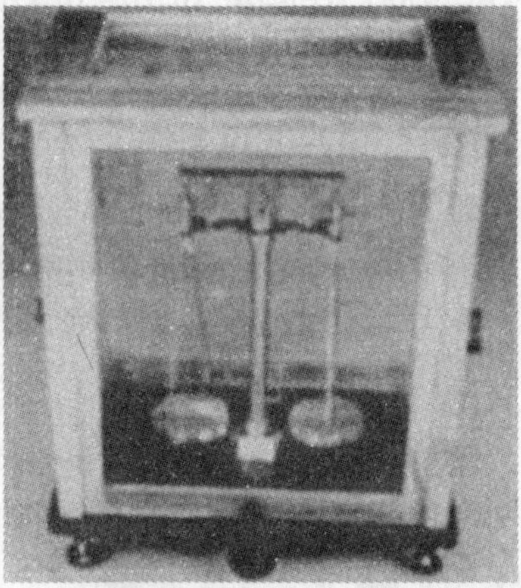

Fig. 6.3. Analytical Balance

6.2.2. Single Pan Balance

This type of balance was introduced commercially by **Erhard Mettler in 1946.** This balance is much faster and more convienient than traditional two pan equal arm balance. It has only one arm with a pan suspended to it. The length of the arm has a positive correlation with the sensitivity i.e. longer is the arm higher is the sensitivity. The Single pan manual balance should be used to weigh the amount of more than 100g. In this the weight of an unknown chemical is determined by comparing it with known weight. Single pan analytical balance is widely used in research laboratories (Fig. 6.4).

6.2.2.1. Theory and Principle

It is based on the principle of substitution weighing i.e. replacing built in unknown masses by the unknown object and removing an amount necessary to restore balance.

In this, the display system is operated mechanically by making a balance of shift of metallic weights already sets the balance. This balance can be used only with electric supply as light device display the weight on optical scale. The material to be weighed is placed on the pan and some removable known weight are lifted off the beam by internal lever so as to restore approximate balance. Any remaining imbalance tilts the beam slightly that is projected on the optical scale. The total weight of the unknown is equal to the weight removed plus the reading of the optical scale. A single pan balance can be used only with electric supply and it differs from double pan or equal arm balance in having a only one arm with a pan suspended to it.

6.2.2.3 Description

The balance case is made up of moulded plastic with an aluminium base plate. It measures 15.3″/4″ height, 8.1/ 4″ wide and 13.3/8″ deep. The balance has a capacity of 160g, a range of 1200 mg on the optical scale, an accuracy of ± 0.1mg.

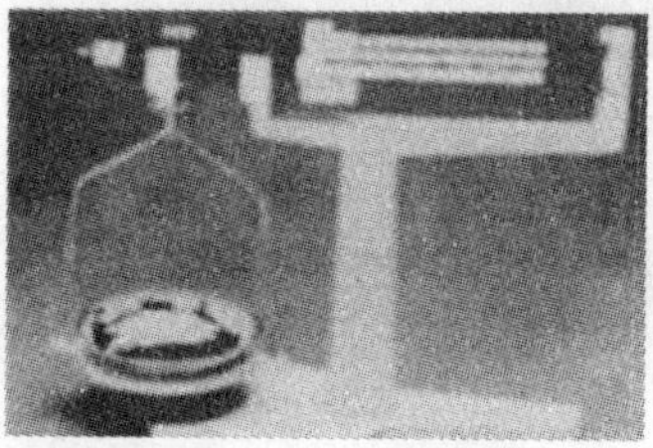

(a)

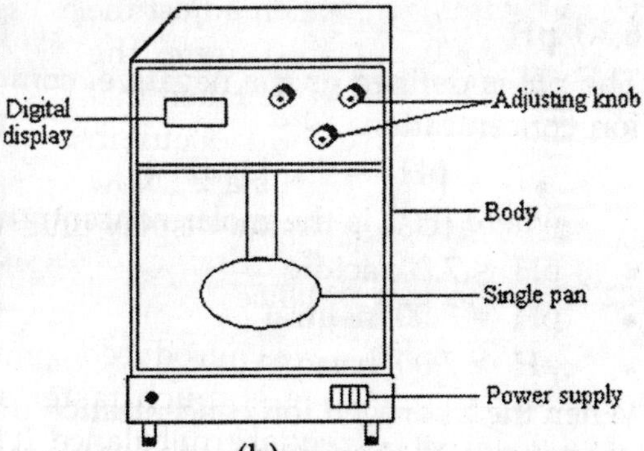

(b)

Fig. 6.4. (a) Single Pan Balance (b) Electronic Single Pan Balance

6.2.3 Triple Beam Balance

The Triple beam balance is the least sensitive balance commonly found in the chemical laboratory. It consists of a single pan on the left side of the beam. The right side of the beam is divided into three arms, each of which holds a rider. The two arms containing the larger riders are notched with the pan, the pointer should come to rest at the midway on the scale at the extreme right. The object to be weighed is placed on the pan. The heaviest rider (10 gm in this case) is moved to successive notches until the pointer drops to the bottom of the scale. The rider is then moved back one notch. The same procedure is then followed for the 1g rider. The 0.01 g rider is carefully moved along the arm until the pointer is midway on the scale. The weight of the object is then the total of the values on each of the arms.

6.2.4.1 Precautions

- There should be no vibration and disturbance on the bench at the time of weighing.
- Cleaniness is needed before and after use with the help of brush
- All parts must be arranged in a manner so that there is no friction or minimal friction would remain in the system.

6.3 pH Meter

The pH scale is a measure of acidity or the alkanity of a solution. If a solution having high concentration of hydrogen ion, it is acidic. In a neutral solution the concentration of hydrogen ion and hydroxyl ions are equal but in the alkaline solution the concentration of hydrogen ion is less than OH ion.

6.3.1 pH

The pH is defined as the negative common logarithm of hydrogen ion concentration.

$$pH = -\log [H^+]$$

where $[H^+]$ is the molar concentration of the hydrogen ion

- pH < 7.00, acidic
- pH = 7.00, neutral
- pH > 7.00, basic

When the hydrogen ion concentration decreases (eg: $[H^+]= 10^{-10}$) the pH value is 10 showing that the solution is alkaline. When it increases (eg: $[H^+]= 10^{-3}$), the pH value is 3 showing that the solution is acidic. According to Bronsted Lowary concept an acid is a donor of proton that is a hydrogen ion $[H^+]$, and a base is proton acceptor as OH^-. On the other hand the chemical that donate a hydroxyl ion $[OH^-]$ are said to be alkali, such as KOH, NaOH etc.

6.3.2 Measuring Method and Instrumentation

The measuring method for pH values includes using an indicator reagent, the metal electrode methods (Hydrogen electrode method, quinhydrone electrode method, and antimony electrode method), and the glass electrode method. The glass electrode method is considered to be the standard measuring method. In practice however, pH value are obtained from hydrogen ion activity (thermodynamic activity) rather than hydrogen ion concentration.

A pH meter consist of two electrode - the glass electrode sensitive to H^+ concentration and reference or calomel electrode. When two solution with different pH values exist inside and outside a glass membrane, electromotive force occur in electrode membrane in proportion to the difference between two pH values. This change is measured with a galvanometer calibrated for a pH scale. This whole unit is termed as pH meter (Fig. 6.5).

6.3.2.1 Glass Electrode

It is the most commonly used indicator electrode, consisting of an internal electrode of Silver - Silver chloride type in a reference solution of Hydrochloric acid (0.1M HCl) contained in a glass bulb which is made up of a thin glass membrane about 0.03 to 0.1mm thickness. It is usually made up of hydrated aluminosilicate containing sodium or calcium ions. When the electrode is placed in a solution, a potential is developed across the thin wall of the bulb relative to the hydrogen ion concentration present in the solution.

When the H^+ concentration changes in the external solution, it accompanies changes in the potential to the outside surface of the bulb is transmitted to the internal Ag/AgCl electrode. This electrode measures only H^+ activity not H^+ concentration (Glass electrode is sensitive to the hydrogen ion but the reference electrode is not). This potential difference can be measured against a reference electrode using a voltameter.

6.3.2.2 Reference / Calomel Electrode

It is commonly used as reference electrodes. It is usually a saturated calomel electrode which is filled with a standard solution of KCl in contact with a paste of mercurous chloride and mercury. The chlorine ions from KCl become saturated with mercury at the surface of the mercury. In such condition the electrode produces a constant reference potential to which the indicator electrode potential is compared. The calomel electrode is separated from the KCl salt bridge by a porous ceramic plug which reduces back diffusion and contamination. The most commonly used reference electrode is standard hydrogen electrode but due to inconvenience to use reference electrodes have substituted them. The two electrode namely the reference and indicator electrode are connected to a galvanometer calibrated for pH scale which measures the change in potential between them.

At present a combination of both the electrode i.e. glass electrode and reference electrode is available. The main purpose of the reference electrode is to complete the measuring circuit. It allows the pH value of the sample to be obtained by measuring the potential difference between the two electrodes with the potential difference meter. This measurement include two steps:-

- To standardize the instrument against a known standard buffer solution at the room temperature
- To measure the pH of the unknown solution

To calibrate the pH meter, a standard solution with a known pH value is used. As standard solution phthalic acid (pH 4.01), neutral phosphate (pH 6.86), and borate (pH 9.18) are mainly used.

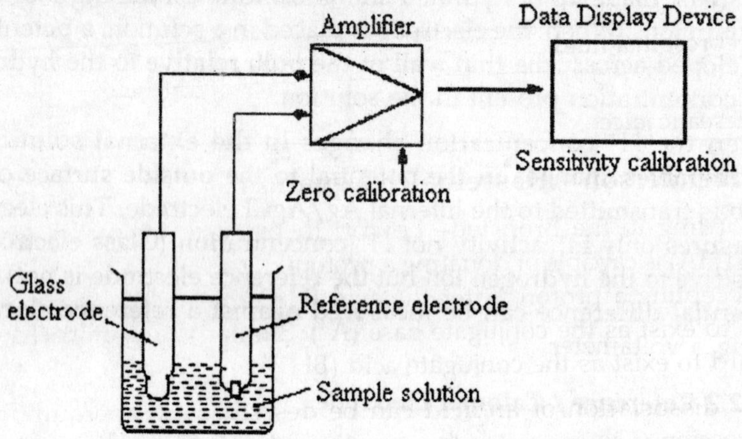

Fig. 6.5. Digramatic View of a pH Meter

6.3.3 Basic Procedure

It involves the following steps:-

- Switch on the Instrument.
- Set the temperature (according to room temperature or solution temperature).
- Clean the electrodes with distilled water and wipe with filter paper.

- Place both the electrodes in a standard known buffer solution
- Now set the meter reading to the standard pH by using standardization knob or adjusting button.
- After standardization, the instrument, the electrodes are put out and washed with distilled water and wiped with filter paper.
- Now place the electrode in the sample solution of unknown pH.
- Read the pH value on pH meter scale.

Table 6.2. pH Value of some of the Body Fluids and secretions

Body fluids/Secretions	pH
Gastric Juice	0.87
Urine	6.0
Milk	6.6 - 6.9
Saliva	7.2
Blood	7.4
Cerebrospinal fluid	7.4
Bile	7.8
Pancreatic juice	8.0

6.4 Henderson – Hasselbalch Equation

According to the Bronsted– Lowry theory of acids and bases, an acid (HA) is capable of donating a proton(H^+) and a base (B) is capable of accepting a proton. After the acid (HA) has lost its proton, it is said to exist as the conjugate base (A^-). Similarly, a protonated base is said to exist as the conjugate acid (BH^+)

The dissociation of an acid can be described by an equilibrium expression :-

$$HA \Leftrightarrow H^+ + A^-$$

Consider the case of acetic acid (CH3COOH) and acetate anion(CH_3COO^-)

$$\underset{\text{Acetic acid}}{CH_3COOH} \Leftrightarrow \underset{\text{Acetate}}{CH_3COO^-} + H^+$$

Acetate is the conjugate base of acetic acid. Acetic acid and acetate are a conjugate acid/base pair. We can describe this relationship with an equilibrium constant.

In this simulation, we will use KA for the acid dissociation constant. Taking the negative log of both sides of the equation gives

$$-\log K_A = -\log \frac{[H^+][A^-]}{[HA]}$$

This can be rearranged

$$-\log K = -\log[H^+] + \left(-\log \frac{[A^-]}{[HA]}\right)$$

By definition, pKA = - log KA and pH = - log [H⁺], So

$$pK = pH - \log \frac{[A^-]}{[HA]}$$

This equation can then be rearranged to give the Henderson - Hasselbalch equation:-

$$pH = pK + \log \frac{[A^-]}{[HA]} = pK + \log \frac{[\text{Conjugate base}]}{[\text{Conjugate acid}]}$$

The Henderson - Hasselbalch equation can be used to prepare buffer solutions and to estimate charges on ionizable species in solution, such as amino acid side chain in proteins. Caution must be exercised in using this equation because pH is sensitive to changes in temperature and salt concentration in the solution being prepared.

6.5 Autoclave

The word autoclave is said to be to sterilize and the dictionary meaning of autoclave is an apparatus which is used for sterilization by steam under pressure. The bacteria and other organism can be killed by using the heat action through gas or spirit flame or by hot air oven. But the spore of these organisms are resistant so that moist heat is used for sterilization in a closed system. This system is known as autoclave. It produces superheated steam under high pressure, and may generate temperature of above 100^{0}C. It is mainly used for decontamination and sterilization (Fig. 6.6).

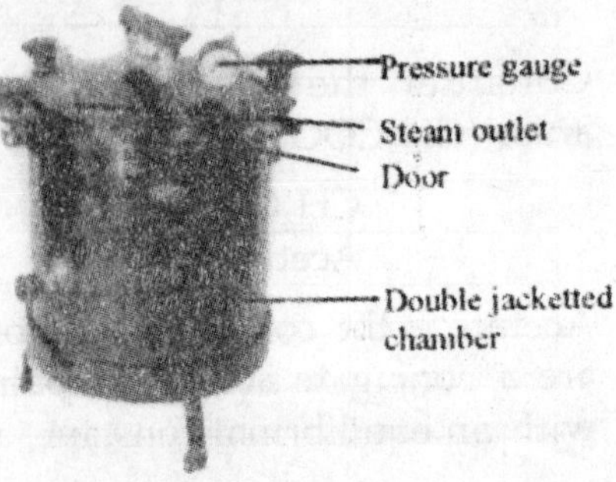

Fig. 6.6 An Autoclave

The effectiveness of sterilization depends upon the type of material to be used and the contact time. If the container is used it should have good permeability to steam.

There are various types of autoclave available in the market of different manufactures. These are designed according to the type of analysis or used.

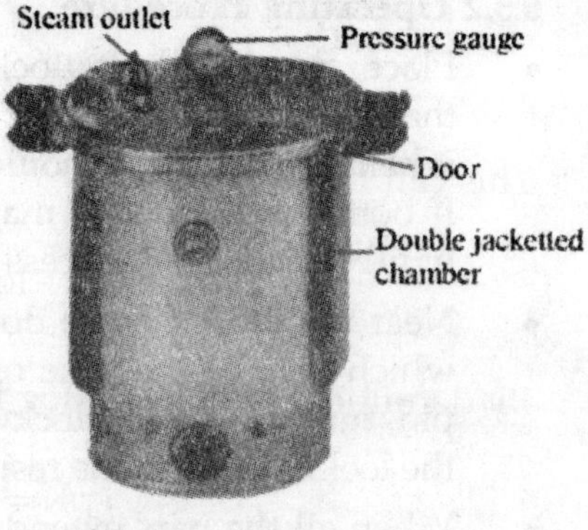

Fig. 6.7 Double-jacketed

6.5.1. Simple Autoclave

It is based on the principle of kitchen pressure cooker and made up of gun metal sheets which is supported in an iron case. The chamber of autoclave is partially filled with water and the material to be sterilized is placed in a tray inside the chamber. Then it is closed by swing door and tightened by radical bolts. When heat is generated water produces steam to a pressure higher than the atmospheric pressure and so the boiling temperature is also raised. The excess of steam passes out from the device through the valve after a certain pressure. The pressure inside the chamber is recorded by the pressure gauge on the device and can be regulated by the pressure meter. It consists of safety valve that guards against the accident. The relationship between temperature and pressure is shown in the following table:

Table 6.3. Relation between temperature and pressure

S.N.	Steam Pressure (psi)	Temperature°C
1.	0	100.0
2.	3	105.3
3.	5	108.4
4.	7	111.3
5.	10	115.2
6.	12	117.6
7.	15	121.0
8.	17	123.0
9.	20	126.0
10.	22	127.8
11.	25	130.4
12.	27	132.1
13.	30	134.5

6.5.2 Operating Procedure

- Place items to be autoclaved inside the chamber, make sure that there is no plastic or melting material. If the liquid material is being sterilized, it should be placed in a stainless steel container. If bottles are capped, make sure that the caps are screwed on lightly so that any excess pressure can escape.
- Near the center of the door, there is a locking wheel and a pin which help at the time of locking the door. After engaging the pin, turn the wheel clockwise by about 1/8 of a turn to insert all the locking bars in the respective slots on the rim of the autoclave.
- When all the bars extend securely through the slots release the pin so that the door locking wheel is now free to spin. Rotate the wheel clockwise until it is hand tight, then apply pressure to the door to seal it air tight so that steam pressure can be built up inside the chamber. Engage the pin to lock the wheel.
- Turn selection valve on top of the autoclave to the sterilized position (STER) so that steam enters into the chamber from the jacket.
- Now wait for chamber pressure for 5 minutes. This marks the starts of the autoclave and the temperature can be read with the help of the gauge (Fig. 6.8).

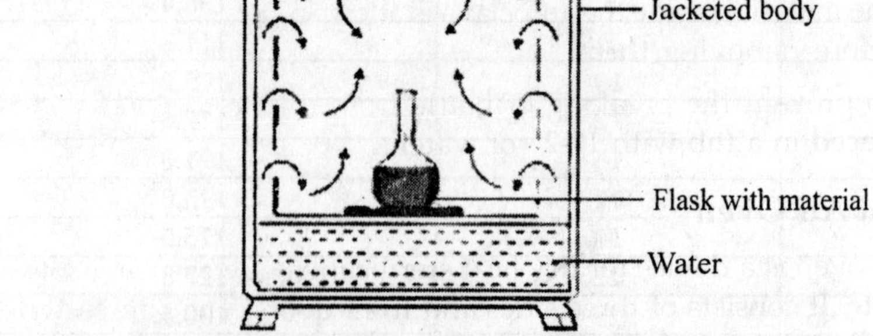

Fig. 6.8. Digramatic View of an Autoclave

- After autoclaving for 20 – 30 minutes, terminate the autoclaving cycle by shutting off steam to the chamber and venting it slowly to the ambient pressure. It takes about 3 – 5 minutes to vent the excess steam. It is safe to open the door when pressure is marked around zero psi.
- Open the door on the autoclave slowly and cautiously. Take out all the items from the autoclaving runs.

Table 6.4. Average liquid sterilization time

Liquid	Time
500 ml	30 minutes
500-1litre	40 minutes
2 litre - 4 litre	55 minutes
4 litre -	1 hour

6.5.3 Precautions

The following precautions are to be taken:-

- The air should be completely evacuated from the autoclave and the steam must have access to the material to be sterilized.
- Sealed container should never be placed in the autoclave.
- The volatile or corrosive chemicals such as phenol, trichloroacetic acid, chloroform etc. and radioactive materials should not be autoclaved.
- After starting autoclave, its processing time should be noted when it reaches normal operating conditions (i.e. 121°C and 15 psi pressure).
- Before opening the door make sure that pressure in the autoclave chamber is near zero.
- The material inside the autoclave is allowed to cool for 10 minutes before removing them.
- To prevent the breaking of bottle from the bottom, it must be placed in a tub with 1″-2″ of water.

6.6 Hot Air Oven

Hot air oven is a device for dry heat sterilization of glasswares, metal items etc. It consists of three sides and front doors. The gap between two walls is insulated. There is a heating device on the bottom or in between the side walls of the oven. A convection current travels a

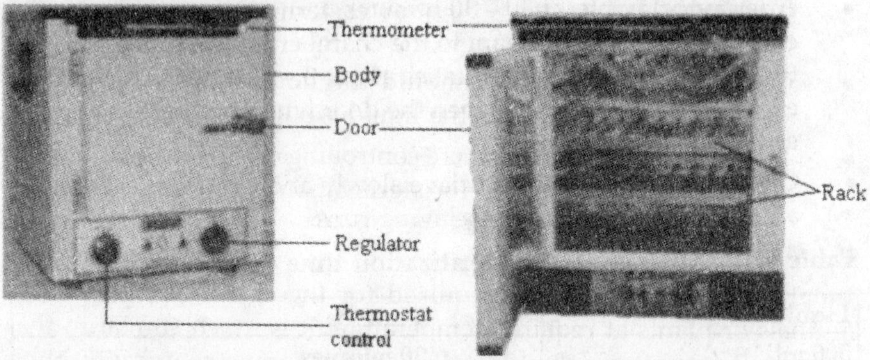

Fig. 6.9. (a) Hot Air Laboratory Oven (b) Open view

complete circuit through the wall space and interior of the oven. The temperature inside the oven is controlled by thermostat (Fig. 6.9).

6.6.1. Basic Principle

In hot air oven the sterilization is accomplished by dry heat or hot air. It is operated at a temperature of 160ºC to 180ºC for a period of one and a half hour (at 180ºC the period should be 30 min). The hot air sterilizer is used for sterilizing all kinds of laboratory glassware, such as test tubes, petri dishes, pipettes, flasks, bottles etc. The material which will not be burnt at high temperature may be sterilized by this. The glass material should be wiped and dried before keeping inside the chamber in the oven, otherwise it may break. The air within the oven, should be circulated by a fan to keep the hot air circulation at a constant temperature and a thermometer is fitted for recording the temperature of the oven.

6.6.2 Application

- It is mainly used for sterilizing laboratory glassware such as test tubes, petri dishes, pipettes, flasks, bottles, and other material which will not be burned at higher temperature.
- It is also useful for the activation of TLC plates and for drying the plant material to make it powder form for X-ray diffraction analysis.

6.6.3 Precautions

- After the holding time is over, the glassware should not be taken out immediately.

- It is important to check the proper temperature at which the materials are sterilized.
- Under no circumstances should the hot air oven be used to sterilize culture media, as the liquid would boil to dryness.
- There should be a temperature controlling device for maintaining the temperature required for sterilization.

6.7 Incubator

Incubator is an equipment required for the culture or growth of animals or plants at required temperature. It is much similar to that of oven. It consists of a double walled steel or copper chamber through which hot air is circulated by an electric device. Its temperature is controlled by a themostat. It may be set at required temperature and cuts off the supply if temperature exceeds the set temperature or maintaned if temperature is below the required temperature. It has perforated shelves so that uniform temperature may be mentioned inside the chamber. Latest models of incubators are equipped with controlled humidity and oxygen supply (Fig. 6.10).

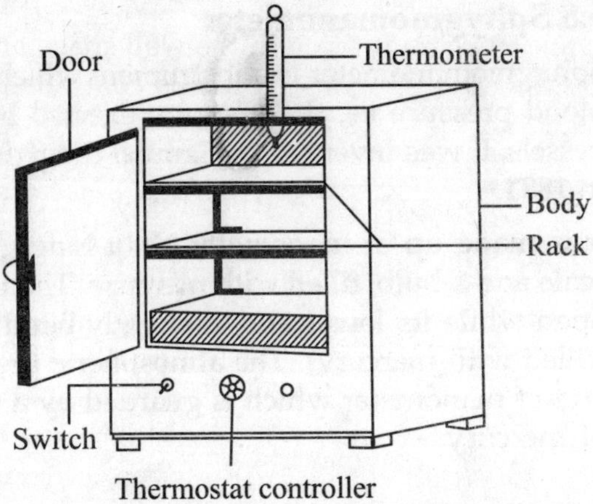

Fig. 6.10. An Incubator

6.7.1 Principle

An incubator functions on the basis of temp regulating device. It may control the temperature variation of about ± 2°C. If temperature increases more than required it maintains by circulating water around through an ice chest.

6.7.2 Precautions

- Beakers or petridishes should be kept covered with lid and test tubes should be tightened with cotton plugs to avoid dehydration.

- If incubation time is long i.e. 2-4 hours or more, vessels should be closed otherwise it will dry the culture media.
- Excessive dryness may be avoided by keeping moist cotton or water filed beaker into incubator.
- To mentain the required temperature inside the incubator, its door should be opened only when necessary.

6.7.3 Uses

An Incubator is used for the culturing of micro-organisms at a constant temperature favourable to the growth and development of various micro-organisms.

6.8 Sphygmomanometer

Sphygmomanometer is a instrument which is used for measuring the blood pressure i.e. the pressure exerted by blood against the blood vessels. It was invented by **Samuel Siegfried Kari Ritter Von Bascsh in 1881.**

It is made up of manometer i.e. a long glass capillary tube with a scale and a bulb, filled with mercury. The upper end of manometer is open while its lower end is slightly bend and connected with bulb (filled with mercury). The atmospheric pressure is exposed to upper end of manometer which is guarded by a valve to check the spilling of mercury.

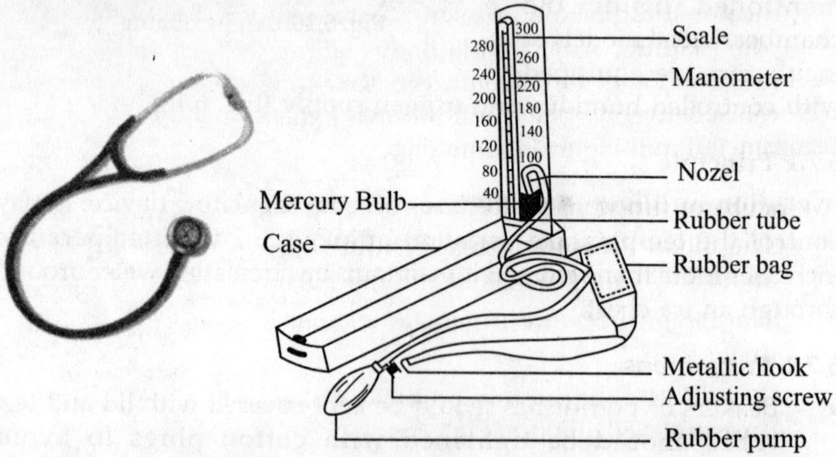

Fig. 6.11. Different Parts of a Sphygmomanometer and Stethoscope

The upper end of bulb joined with nozzle which is further connected with a rubber tube of narrow lumen that connected with a rubber bag enclosed in cuff. The fabric cuff is better than that of leather one. This fabric cuff is used for wrapping around the arm. It is joined with a pumping bulb (made up of rubber) with the help of rubber tube. The pumping bulb is equipped with a screw when screw has tightened the air flows into the fabric cuff known as inflation whereas the untightened screw facilitates flow of air outside the cuff, known as deflation (Fig. 6.11).

6.8.1 Method

First of all untighten the screw for removing the air from cuff and rubber tubes. The armlet (cuff) is wrapped around upper arm above the bend of elbow and the sphygmomanometer is placed about the level of heart. The care should be taken that the rubber tubes attached with cuff is facing towards the lower end.

Now tighten the screw of pumping bulb and pump the air by pumping it rapidly. It will raise the Hg, up to 110-120 mm Hg that is seen on monometer scale. At this time stethoscope is used to observe the arterial blood, it is short and sharp sound, associated with first heart sound and indicates systolic pressure. After that this sharp sound disappear and note the reading (after closing the screw). Then again pump the air slowly and observe the sound. That is accompanied by a loud clear sound which becomes distant and disappears after some time.

It indicates the diastolc pressure. Now close the screw and again note the reading. After taking both readings untighten the screw, remove all air, open the cuff and keep it at a suitable place. The pressure difference between systole and diastole indicates pulse pressure that is about 110 mm Hg to 140 mm Hg.

Variation in Blood Pressure

- The Blood Pressure increase with the age. At advance age it is about 80-90 mm Hg distolic and 130-150 mm Hg systolic pressure.
- The blood pressure in female is about 5-10 mm Hg less than male.
- In childhood the diastolic pressure is 60 mm Hg while the systolic pressure is 80-100 mm Hg.
- After exercise, food and in emotional state the blood pressure should rise.

6.9 Khymograph

Kymograph is an instrument used to record the temporal variations in heart beat and muscular twitch (Physiological process). It mainly consists of a revolving drum (made up of brass) and a record sheet (that is usually a smoked paper) on which a stylus or penpoint travels to and fro at right angles to the motion of the cylinder. The drum is rotated and the information registered on the paper sheet. In some cases the record sheet surrounds the drum, which rotates spirally and allows a continuous record at different levels of the sheet (Fig. 6.12).

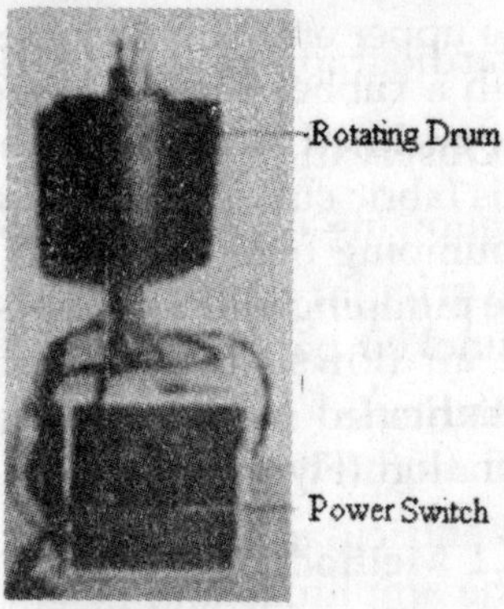

Fig: 6.12. Khymograph

6.9.1 Preparation of Smoked Paper

It consists of placing a blank sheet of paper over a petroleum lantern fumes. Then the smoked paper is wrapped around the drum that is ready for the touch of the inscriber. As the drum rotates the signal marker contacts the drum leaving a line record.

6.9.2 Method

For recording the heart beat of frog first of all destroy its nervous system (by pithing its brain) then expose the heart carefully in situ condition. Then by adding 0.65% Sodium Chloride solution, a hook (small pin) is passed through the apex without injuring the vertical cavity. The heart is gently lifted by a thread attached to the hook. The free end of the thread is tied to the heart lever by a screw. Then the pointer of the lever is adjusted just to touch the smooth surface of the drum containing smoked paper.

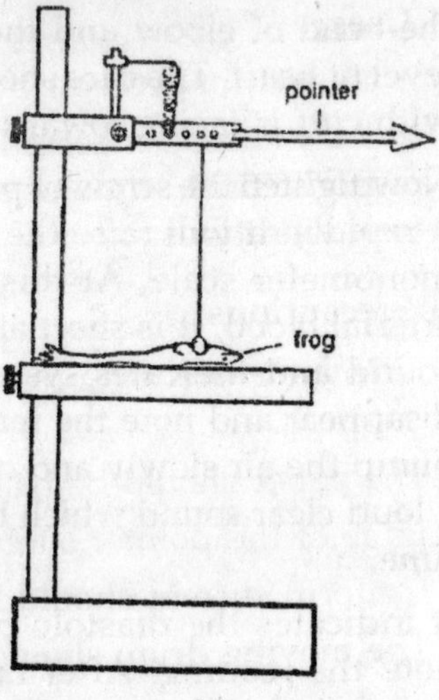

(a)

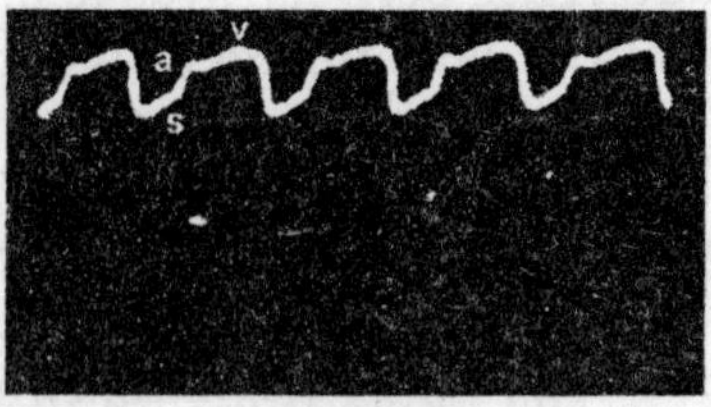

(b)

Fig: 6.13. (a) Recording of Heart Beat of Frog (b) Khymograph. Contraction of Auricle (a); Contraction of Sinus (s); Contraction of Ventricle (v)

The cardiograph records on the surface of the paper (Fig. 6.13).

6.9.3 Observation

The following observations are obtained by the Cardiograph.

1. **Auricular Contraction:** It shows downward facing on the smoked paper.
2. **Auriculo - Ventricular pause:** It is in the form of a small straight or slightely inclined line.
3. **Ventricular Contraction:** It is same as auricular contraction but the amplitude and height of contraction of downward record is much longer than auricular contraction.

6.9.4 Uses

- It is used for recording blood pressure.
- It is also used for recording various time-related events such as response time, stimulus presentation, muscle exertion and tuning fork vibrations.

6.9.5 Precautions

The following precautions should be taken at the time of using Khymograph.

- The paper should be blackened well.
- Edge of the pointer should be accurate.
- Uniform current should flow from the electric device.
- The moving drum should not be fast.

6.10 Camera Lucida

Camera Lucida is an optical instrument invented by **William Hyde Wollaston (1807).** It is used to sketch the accurate diagram or sketch of an object.

6.10.1 Structure and Principle

It consists of a prism with one reflective surface mounted on a stand above the sheet of paper. It works on a simple principle of light refraction. On observing into the prism from right angle, it will produce two images. One of the objects to be sketched, the other of the pencil and paper with which we can draw the diagram. As a result an eye percieves the object as if it is actually on the paper. Thus we can trace the object on paper.

6.10.2 Mechanism

Light rays passing through the prism are reflected at an angle of 90°. These rays are further passed in the same line of sight as the paper and pencil. Our eye allows the image of the object to enter the upper part and image of the paper and pencil to the lower part. Both of them are perceived simultaneously in the same plane.

6.10.3 Sketching through Camera Lucida

The instrument should be attached to the edge of the table, we are working on. The bar of the prism holder should be horizontal and the main telescoping rod should be fixed in a convenient position with the lever at the base.

The prism holder should be opposite of both the centre of the object and paper on which drawing is to be made. This may be adjusted by changing the inclination of rod or lowering the prism holder (Fig. 6.14).

6.10.4 Viewing in Camera Lucida

It takes some time to adjust our eyes in Camera Lucida. If eyes are too far from the prism, only the subject is visible. If our eyes are not over the prism, only paper and pencil will be seen. So our eyes must

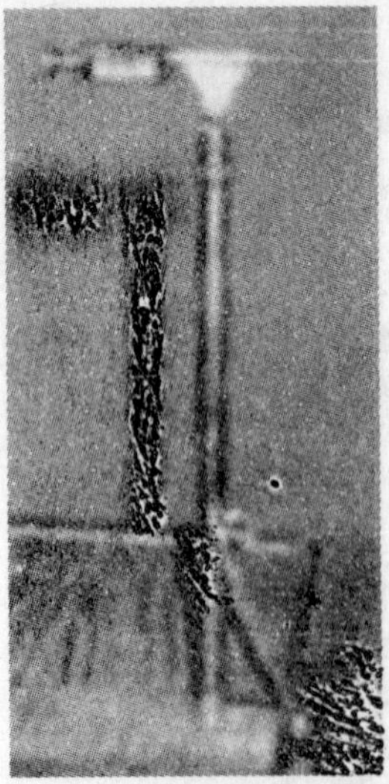

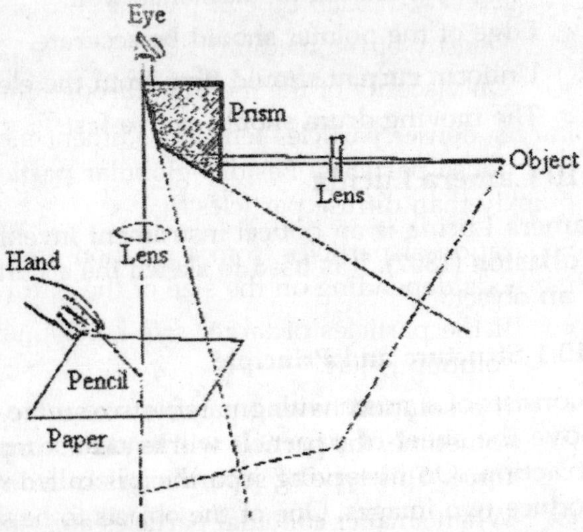

Fig. 6.14. (a) Camera Lucida (b) Diagramatic Respresentation of Working of Camera Lucida

be just at the edge of the prism only then can we see both images. It requires uniform lighting on the object and paper for maximum sharpness. Size of the image on the paper may be reduced or enlarged by changing the distance between prism, paper and pencil.

6.11 Centrifugation

Centrifugation is a technique that separates a heterogeneous mixture into liquid and solid phase on the basis of particle size and density difference between them. It is a technique for separation of crystalloid as well as colloidal solution. In biochemical, cytological, cytochemical, molecular and biotechnological studies, we need to separate certain components.

Centrifugation technique is based on the behaviour of solute particles. It basically increases the rate of sedimentation of the solid phase by spinning a solid liquid mixture at high speed creates a centrifugal force that acts on the particles and accelerates the settling of particles. The solid precipitate settles to the bottom of the test tube, called pellets while upper solution is called centrifugate, which lies as supernatant liquid. The rate of sedimentation depends on the following factors:-

- Shape of the particles
- Size of the particles
- Density of each type of particle
- Density of the medium
- On viscosity of the medium through the particles are spin

Larger denser particles tend to sediment more quickly than smaller less dense particles. Besides globular particles will sediment more quickly than diffuse particles.

Separation of particles from a solution may occur through different methods depending on the size of the particles.

- If the particles of larger size i.e. 200 μm are in a solution and solution is left.
- If a solution having particle size more than 200 μm is left for sometime, the particle will tend to sediment under gravitational force. This type of separation is called sedimentation.
- When smaller colloidal particles are separated from crystalloids by selective diffusion through a semi permeable membrane, the process is called dialysis. While spinning, the particles are

subjected to a centrifugal force created by the spinner rotor. The magnitude of the force is dependent upon the speed of the spin and radius of the rotation (i.e. the distance between sample container and center of the rotor). This force can be expressed as :

- The relative gravitational force
- Revolutions per minute (rpm)

6.11.1 Principle of Centrifugation

It is based on the following principle

$$G = V_2r$$

V = angular velocity in radius per second

r = radius of rotations in centimeters

Speed of the centrifuge may be observed as revolutions per minute.

$$\text{Relative Centrifugal Force (RCF)} = G = \frac{2\pi\ (\text{rpm})2r \times g^{-1}}{60}$$

2p = one revolution of the rotor

g = radius per second

The particle will sediment only if their mass is greater than the solvent displaced.

$$\text{Net Force} = (mp - ms)\ V_2\ r - fv$$

mp = mass of particle

ms = mass of equal volume of solvent

fv = frictional force

Particles may be arranged according to their rate of sedimentation per unit centrifugal field, which is also known as sedimentation coefficient (s). A svedberg unit(s) is defined as sedimentation coefficient of 1x 10^{-13} second.

6.11.2 The Instrument

Basically a centrifuge consists of a rotor designed to hold the tubes of the material to be separated. The rotor is filled on top of the device shaft that is in turn attached to a motor when the centrifuge is turned on. The device shaft rotates and the containers spin very fast exerting a force which cause the sample particles to sediments.

6.11.3 Types of Centrifuge

There are different types of centrifuges designed for different purposes. Generally 4 types of centrifuges are required in most of the laboratories.

6.11.3.1 Clinical Centrifuges

They are also known as Table top or Bench centrifuges. They are inexpensive and can run at a speed of up to 3000 – 7000 rpm. They can pellet (sediment) cells but not organelles or biomolecules. They are good for sedimentation of erythrocytes, yeast cells and other coarse precipitates.

Some smaller model called Microfuges which may rotate at 8000 – 13,000 rpm and generate a centrifugal field of about 10,000 g. They are very useful for the sedimentation of small quantities 0.25ml to 1.5ml of sample. Microfuges can pellet nucleic acid and denatured proteins.

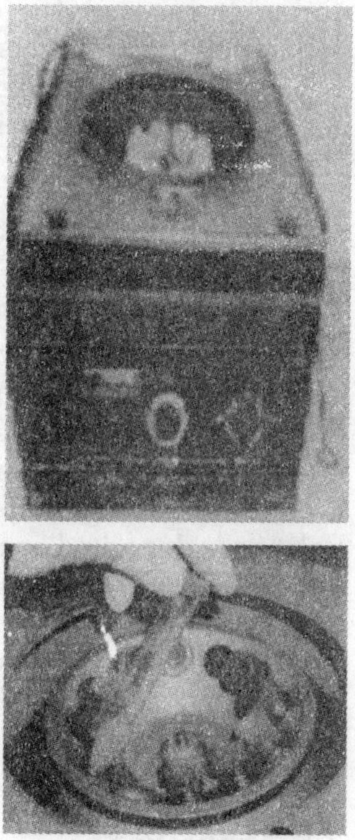

Fig. 6.15. A Centrifuge Commonly used in Laboratory

6.11.3.2 High Speed Refrigerated Centrifuges

They are high speed centrifuges and rotate up to 25,000 rpm. Centrifugal field of 6000 g. They have interchangeable swinging bucket with fixed angle rotors. It is used to separate microorganism, cell organelles and protein precipitates. They cannot separate nucleic acids.

6.11.3.3 Large Capacity Refrigerated Centrifuges

They rotate at 6000 rpm and 6500 g and are used to separate out protein molecules. In these type of centrifuge, the rotor chamber is refrigerated so that proteins are saved from being denatured due to its high speed. Rotor angles are fixed with interchangeable swinging buckets. Sample tubes of 10, 50, 100 ml capacity may be used. This type of centrifuge is used to separate nuclei, chloroplast, yeast, RBCs etc.

6.11.3.4 Super Centrifuge

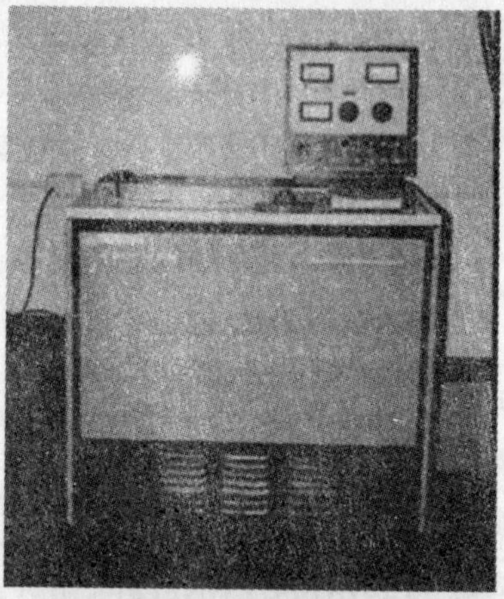

Fig. 6.16. Super Centrifuge

Super centrifuge is very high speed tabular bowl centrifuges, which generates 13000 times more centrifugal force than gravitational force. It is used for continuous separation of two immiscible liquids having different specific gravities. It is also used for clarification of liquids.

(i) Functioning of Super centrifuge

Two immiscible liquids are separated by this centrifuge. The mixture continuously enters through an inlet at the base of the machine into hollow cylindrical rotor. The speed of rotor is 15,000 rpm and generates a centrifugal force of 13,000 times the force of gravity. This force separates the two liquids according to their specific gravities into concentric cylindrical layers and the solids are deposited against the rotor wall. The separated liquids are displaced by the incoming mixture and discharged through their outlets at the top of the rotor. The deposited solid on the wall of the rotor is cleaned out when the centrifuge is shut down. In this type of centrifuge the rotor is designed to separate two liquids so it is also known as a "Separator". If it is designed to remove only suspended solids from a single liquid it is called "Clarifier".

(ii) Application

The open type of Super centrifuge is used in

- Grinder and Fruit juices
- Dehydration of animal fats
- Water gas Tar
- Ball pen ink
- Preparation of blood plasma
- Preparation of sugar syrups

It can be supplied with special covers for dealing with viscous liquids such as –

- Gum Arabic

- Gum thicker
- Chewing Gum
- Wool grease etc.

In factories Super centrifuge is used with little modification for treatment of various industrial oils, such as

- Hydraulic oil
- Cutting oils
- Engine test bed oil
- Rolling mill lubricants
- Wire drawing lubricants

6.12 Haemocytometer

Haemocytometer is an instrument used for counting RBCs, WBCs and bacterial cells etc in a unit volume of blood or fluid.

6.12.1 Instrument

The instrument includes two pipettes, one bearing red bead used for RBCs count and the other with white bead, used for WBCs count and a specific slide. The slide has certain grooves and gratieuls. Pipettes

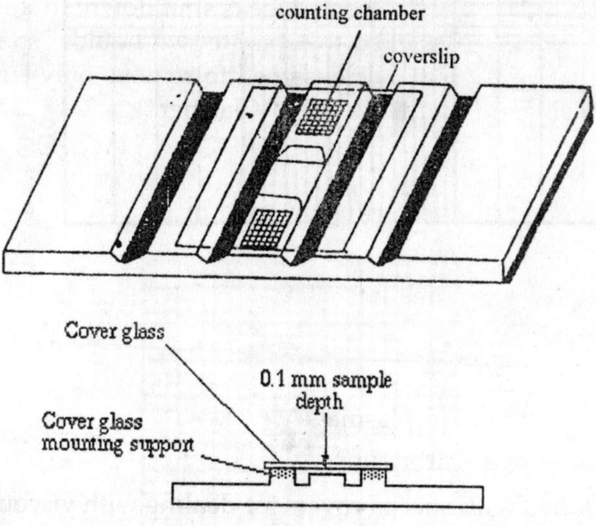

Fig. 6.17 Haemocytometer Counting Grid

are graduated at three points. RBC pipette is marked 0.5, 1 and 101 while WBC pipette has 0.5, 1 and 11. Glass slide is very thick measuring 7.5 cm long by 3.75 cm wide (Fig. 6.17).

Slide

- 7.5 cm x 3.75 cm
- There are two counting chamber with a coveslip
- The chamber has a grid etched onto it, which can be seen under the microscope.

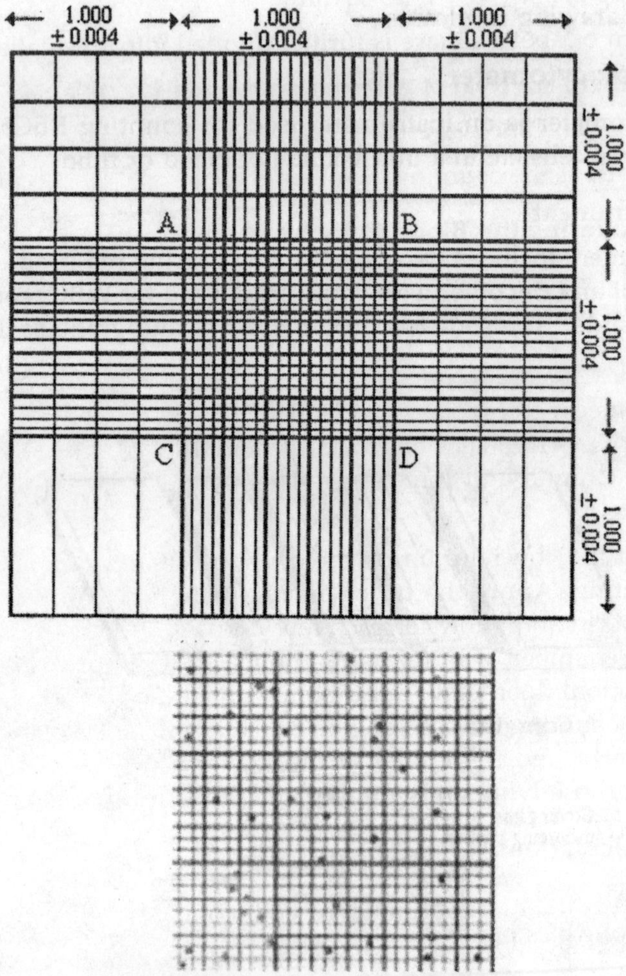

Fig. 6.18. Haemocytometer Counting Chamber

- The grid is made of squares rather like graph papers.
- On both sides of the central platform, are lateral platforms, demarcated by lateral grooves.
- Each counting chamber is formed by several straight perpendicular and horizontal lines forming squares of various measurements as follows :-

(i) The biggest square is 3 x 3 mm = 9 sq mm.

(ii) Each is divided into 9 squares of 1 x 1 mm

(iii) The central square is again divided into 25 smaller squares. Each measuring 1/5 x 1/5 = 1/25 sq. mm

(iv) Each of above square is further divided into 16 smaller squares.

(v) So there are total of 400 squares to each 1 sq.mm.

(vi) Thus each one has an area of 1/400 sq.mm.

(vii) Depth of the counting chamber is 0.1 mm.

6.12.2 Counting the Blood Cells by Haemocytometer

For preparing blood suspension of human prick the finger tip with the sterilized (with spirit) needle. Now take the micropipette washed with alcohol and dried. Suck the blood up to 0.5 mark avoiding the air bubbles. Excess blood sticking to outside should be cleaned. Now transfer the micropipelte to container of Hayem's solution and suck up to 101 mark. Shake or rotate the micropipelte well, keepin g between thumb and fore finger. This makes the dilution of blood 200 times.

Put the coverslip up on the counting chamber, before starting the counting. Apply the tip of micropipette between the coverslip and platform and allow to reach few drops of cell suspension to the counting chamber, wait for a few minute so that RBCs setlled down on the bottom floor. Now put the slide under the microscope carefull and start counting the cells only in 5 smaller squares. The RBCs lying on the lower and right sides of the square are to be added in the total, but those lying on the upper and left sides should be rejected.

6.12.3 Calculations

$$\text{Number of RBCs per} = \frac{\text{Number of cells counted X dilution x 4000}}{\text{No. of small squares counted}}$$

Suppose total number of RBCs for 5 smaller squares are equal to

A+B+C+D+E

$$\therefore \text{RBCs in the smallest square} = \frac{A+B+C+D+E}{80}$$

∴ RBCs in 400 smallest square = 5 (A+B+C+D+E)

But the height of blood film = 0.1 mm and dilution of blood is 200 times . So the number of RBCs in 1 cubic mm of blood will be

200 x 10 x 5 (A+B+C+D+E) RBCs

= 10,000 (A+B+C+D+E) RBCs

6.12.4 Application

It is used to measure the density of cells in liquid (means the number of cells per unit volume of liquid) eg. RBC in blood, density of bacteria in Milk, population of Paremecium or other Protozoans in water.

6.12.5 Precautions

Cells will invariably be found on the lines dividing the cells. In order to make our result standardized, we should include any cells found on the left and top lines, and ignore any cells found on the right and bottom lines of each other.

References

Atlas, R.M., (1995); Microbiology. William C. Brown, UK.

Bowen, T. J., (1970); An Introduction to Ultracentrifugation. Wiley Interscience, New York.

Bradshaw, L.J., (1992); Laboratory Microbiology. Harcourt Brace, San Diego, California

Clydesdale, F.M., (1976); Instrumental Techniques for colour Measurement of Foods @ Food technology : 52

Cowdry, E.W., (1952); Laboratory Techniques in Biology and Medicine 3rd ed. Baltimore, Williams and Wilkins.

Ford, T.C. and Gragam, J.M., (1991); An Introduction to Centrifugation, Bios Scientific, Oxford.

Francis, F.J. and Clydesdale, F.M. (1975); Food Colorimetery : Theory & Application (Westport, Connecticut : the AVI Publishing Company, Inc.),v - vii

Handbook of Phycological method ; pg. 203

Kupper, Walter E. "Balance" in Mc Graw Hill Encyclopedia of Science and Technology 8th ed. V2 McGraw Hill, New York pg.486.

Robyt, J.F. and White, B.J., (1987); Biochemical Techniques. Brooks/Coles.

Thomas, B., Greenslade, Jr. (1989) "Nineteenth Century Textbook Illustrations XLV III: The g 45 Camera Lucida", *Phys.Teach.*, 27, 48-49.

Titchener, E.B., (1918); Experimental Psycology, a Mannual of Laboratory Practice : Volume I, Quantitative Experiments, Part II, Instructor's Mannual. New York ; Macmillan. pp. 172 - 176.

CHAPTER 7
Immunological Techniques

Immunology is the branch of science which deals with immunity and immune system of our body. The word immunity has been derived from a Latin word "Immunis" meaning 'to safe' or 'free from' (i.e. freedom). Actually our body has a self-defence system which is able to protect us from microorganisms i.e. viruses, bacteria and fungi etc. Immune system also protects our body from any type of foreign toxins. Such a capacity of the body is called "Immunity"

7.1 Immune System

Immunity forms the defence system of the body against any pathogenic activity. Such a protective system is called immune system.

7.2 Immunology

The study of immune system and its related aspects are called immunology. There are three pathways of defence which prevent the disturbance of immune system.

Ist pathway of defence: It is actually innate immunity which is perceieved from parents. Any foreign particle, which tries to enter the host body, is checked by this pathway. Skin, Lysozyme in Saliva, HCl and digestive enzymes in stomach etc. forms the first pathway of defence.

2nd pathway of defence: It is formed by circulating WBCs and macrophages.

3rd pathway of defence: It consist of antibodies, produced by B lymphocytes cells and activated T lymphocyte cells.

7.3 Types of Immunity

In broad terms immunity has two types of origin.

7.3.1. Innate or Inborn Immunity

It is parental immunity and includes the following forms:-

(a) Skin and mucous membrane act as barrier. They entrap the foreign particles and prevent their entry into the body.

(b) If the pathogen enters the body the physiology of the body prevents the growth of the foreign pathogen. It includes, temperature, pH, and enzymatic secretion in the body. It also produces interferon that is responsible for killing the viruses.

(c) The body contains specialised phagocytic cells in the blood known as WBC or leucocytes. These cells selectively entrap the pathogen and phagocytise them.

(d) The damaged mast cell secretes histamine and antibacterial fluid which helps to kill the pathogens.

(e) There are a group of more than 30 amino acids which forms a complement system and help in immunity.

7.3.2. Acquired Immunity

This immunity is acquired by the organisms after their birth. It forms antibodies and lymphocytes to destroy the pathogens. The actively acquired immunity is generated in responce to an antigen, which may be natural or artificial (by vaccination) whereas in passively acquired immunity the already made antibodies are injected into the body to produce immune responce.

On the basis of type of cells and physiological responce acquired immunity may be divided into two classes:-

7.3.2.1. Cell Mediated Immunity

This type of immunity is produced by T lymphocyte cells that is generated in response to antigen. It is also called cellular immunity because it occurs inside the cell or nearby the cell. These T cells are of various types known as effector T cells (Cytotoxic T lymphocyte and Delayed type Hypersensitivity Lymphocyte), Helper T cells, Supresser T cells (T8 cells), Killer T cells and Memory T cells. When an antigen enters the body, it is swallowed by a macrophage (a monocyte cell) and alters the activation of T cells into a blast cell and also produce several daughter cells known as regulatory and effector cell.

7.3.2.2. Humoral Immunity

This type of immunity is developed by B cells. B cells can bind with antigen only in the presence of helper T cells. B cells after binding with antigen, produce B memory cells and plasma cells. These plasma cells further produce antibodies. Antibody binds the antigen and neutrilizes it. This antigen antibody complex is phagocitized by macrophages.

7.4 Antigen

Any foreign substance capable of inducing immune responce in the host cell is known as antigen or immunogen. The high molecular weight (more than 10,000) macromolecule such as carbohydrate, protein, lipids and nucleic acid can act as antigen. It may also be dust, smelled material, pollen grains and medicines. Antigen must posses two properties due to binding of it with two components such as lymphocytes and antibodies.

(i) Immunogenicity: It is the ability to induce a humoral and cell mediated immune responce (i.e. formation of antibodies in the host cell).

(ii). Antiginicity or Specificity: It is the ability to combine specifically with final products of the immune responce (i.e.with antibody or cell surface receptors).

7.4.1 Properties of Antigen

There are various properties of antigen. Some common ones are given below:-

- It possesses immunogenic property
- It has high molecular weight not less than 1000 Dalton e.g: Penicillin, Progestron, Dinitrophenol etc.
- Substances must be over 10,000 dl in molecular weight are considered to be good antigen, whereas substance like insulin and histone with approximately 6,000 dl molecular weight are poor antigen.

7.4.2 Molecular Complexity

Proteins are polypeptide chain which is made up by 20 different amino acids. These amino acids change their sequence and are responsible for producing different types and forms of proteins such as primary secondary and tertiary, hence different types of antigen are formed, and show molecular complexity.

7.4.3 Major Classes of Antigen

1. Carbohydrates
2. Lipids
3. Protein-more the degree of complexity more will be the immunogenic property.
4. Nucleic acid

7.4.4 Haptane

Haptanes are small organic molecules that are antigenic but not immunogenic. It cannot cause production of immune lymphocyte or antibodies but can react with preformed antibodies. If they are coupled with a large carrier molecule, they give the property of immunogenicity, carrier molecule may be globulin or synthetic polypeptide. It may be simple or complex.

7.4.5 Epitope

Epitopes, are also called antigenic determinant group. Epitopes are sites either on or within the antigen with which antibody react. They consist of six amino acids or carbohydrate residue. So it may be said that haptanes are artificially added to molecule, while epitopes are the integral part of molecule.

7.4.6 Complement

These are proteins which are present at the time of Antigen-Antibody reaction without which reaction does not occur.

7.4.7 Adjuvant

These are substance, which induce its immune responce, when mixed with Antigen.

7.4.8 Antigen Antibody Reaction

Antigen and antibodies interact by spatial complementary actions. Antibody recognizes antigen through its complementary shape. The combination of Ag-Ab to form an AgAb complex is termed as **primary reaction.**

7.4.8.1 Affinity

The strength of attraction between Ag and Ab is known as affinity (i.e. to bind up). It is affected by dilution. High affinity antibodies closely fit to antegenic determinant and are not easily dissociated.

$$Ag + Ab \rightarrow AgAb \text{ (complex)}$$

7.4.8.2 Avidity

Strength of AgAb bond after formation of complex AgAb termed as avidity.

$$Ag + Ab \rightarrow AgAb \text{ (complex)}$$

It can be measured by degree of dissociation of AgAb complex to free Ag and Ab.

7.4.8.3 Secondary Reaction

1. It includes preparation of AgAb complex.
2. Aggulination of Ag containing particles by Ab.
3. Lysis of Ag containing cells or organisms.
4. Complement fixation.

The antigen - antibody reaction may be of the following types:-

(i) Precipitation

It involves the reaction between soluble antigens with antibodies to form precipitation (precipitin). The antigen - antibody reaction may be performed in any semi solid medium i.e. agrose gel. The reaction depends on buffer electrolytes, pH of medium, temperature and relative concentration of antigen and antibody. When antigens and antibodies are in optimal ratio, a precipitin ring or band is formed which is known as zone of equivalence (Fig. 7.1).

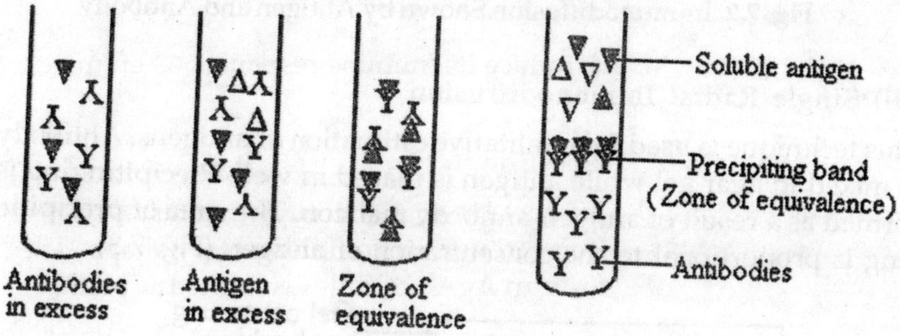

Fig. 7.1. Precipitin Reaction

(ii) Immunodiffusion or Agar Gel Diffusion

Agar gel diffusion is the most common test performed in laboratory to show antigen - antibody reaction. "Ouchterlony's test" is the diffusion in agar coated slides in which both antigen and antibodies are free to move towards each other and precipitate. Pour 2 % Agar gel on glass slides and allow them to cool and harden. Now punch the wells in gel, a few millimeter apart, fill the wells with antigen and antibody samples in opposite direction. Antigen and antibodies will diffuse radially in a moist compartment and a precipitin band develops within 12-18 hours. Precipitin band is stained with comassie brilliant blue and preserved.

This method may be used to recognize more than one antigens at a time. The precipitin band formation may be achieved within 45 minutes to 1 hour by applying electric current in buffer of appropriate pH. This method is used to detect antigen in the clinical materials (Fig. 7.2).

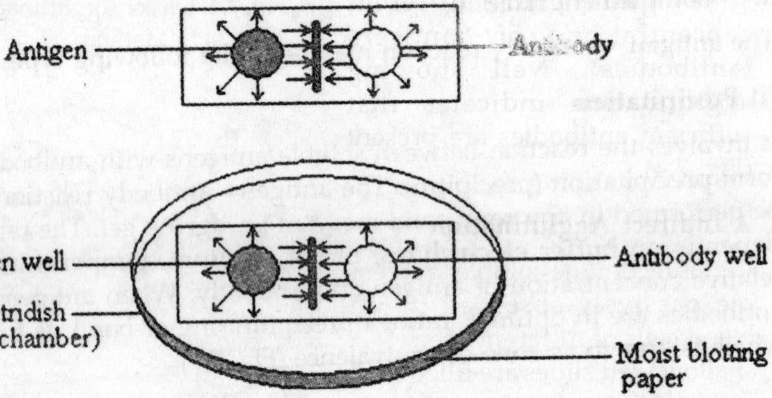

Fig. 7.2. Immunodiffusion Shown by Antigen and Antibody

(iii) Single Radial Immunodiffusion

This technique is used for qualitative estimation of antigens. Antibody is mixed in agar gel while antigen is placed in well. Precipitin ring is formed as a result of antigen-antibody reaction. The area of precipitin ring is proportional to the concentration of antigen (Fig. 7.3).

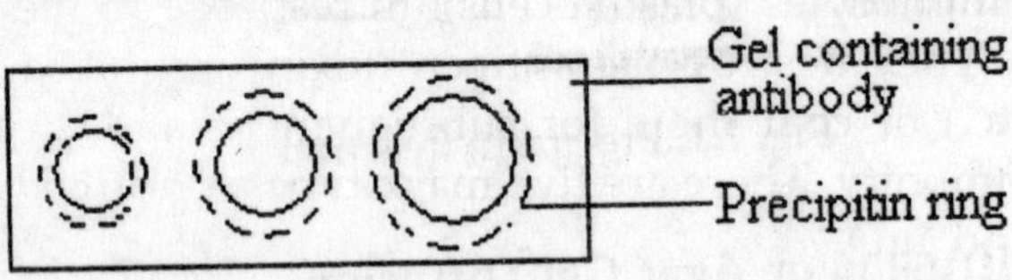

Fig. 7.3. Single Radial Immunodiffusion

(vi) Agglutination

Agglutination is the process of cross-linking of soluble antigens by antibodies resulting in the formation of visible lump or aggregates. Agglutination reactions are visible and highly sensitive. Technique is useful for detection of a variety of substances. Agglutination reactions are of two types.

1. Direct Agglutination

In this technique any cell or antigen may be agglutinated, directly by antibody. Bacterial agglutination with specific antibody may help in their diagnosis. Concentration of serum antibody may also be measured. Put equal amount of antigen in the shallow well of slide and pour different concentration of antisera (antibodies), well showing agglutination indicates that sufficient antibodies are present (Fig. 7.4).

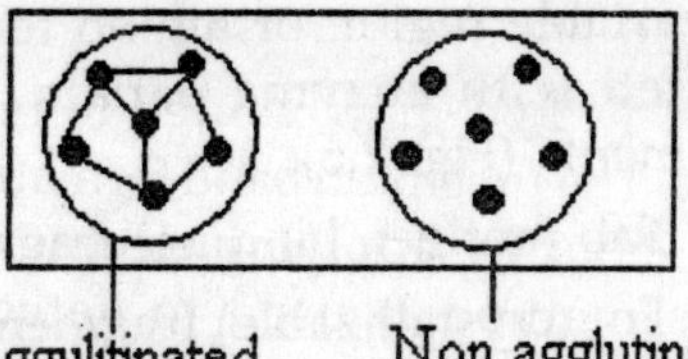

Fig. 7.4. Direct Agglutination Method

2. Indirect Agglutination

In this technique soluble antigens are passively absorbed to red blood cells of different species. A shallow well slides are filled with different concentration of serum. Fixed amount of absorbed antigen is added to each well. After few hours positive agglutination occurs which indicates antigen-antibody reaction (Fig. 7.5).

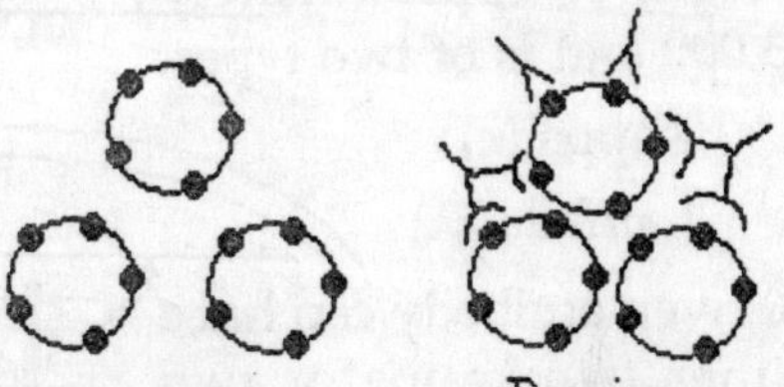

Fig. 7.5 Indirect Agglutination Method

7.5 Antibodies (Immunoglobulins)

These are certain specific glycoprotein molecules, which are produced by the B lymphocytes (plasma cells), in response to the infection by an antigen. They destroy the antigen (toxin) produced by invaders (bacteria etc.) or coat them for subsequent phagocytosis. It forms humoral immunity. There are five major types of antibodies IgG, IgM, IgA, IgE, and IgD.

7.5.1 Structure

The basic unit of antibody is a four-chain monomer. These four polypeptide chains consist of two identical heavy chains and two identical light chains. These chains are held together as a tetramer by disulphide bonds forming Y-shaped structure. Each polypeptide chain contains an amino terminal (variable region) and carboxy terminal (constant region) hence light chains have variable VL and constant CL region and heavy chain have variable VH and constant CH region.The portion of the antibody that binds the antigen is known as variable region or amino termines. If an antibody molecule is treated with enzyme papain, the Ab is cleaved into 2 types of fragments (Fig. 7.6).

1. Fab (antigen binding) fragments
2. Fc (crystallizable) fragments

The light chain of antibody consist of about 200 amino acids with molecular weight of approximately 23,000 and is of two types.

1. Kappa (κ)
2. Lambda (λ)

A given antibody can have either two kappa or two lambda chain, but never a mixture of both. The heavy chain of antibody consist of 400 amino acids with a molecular weight of about 50,000. It is of five types, known as α, β, μ, δ and ε.

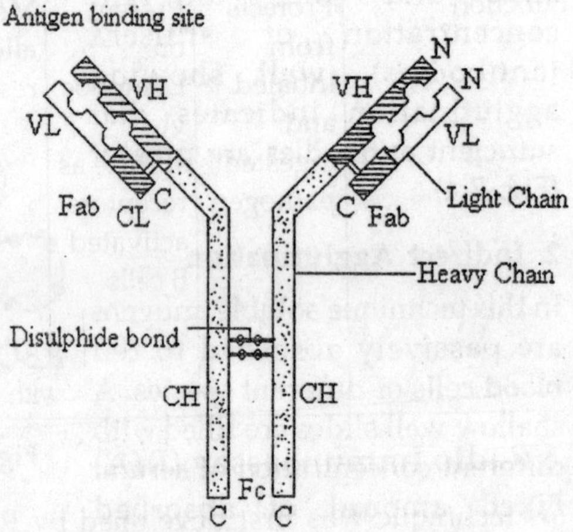

Fig. 7.6. Structure of an Antibody

These are responsible for five classes of Immunoglobulin i.e. IgA, IgB, IgM, IgD and IgE.

Table.7.1 Different types Antibodies and their properties

Characterstic Feature	IgG	IgM	IgA	IgE	IgD
Heavy chain	γ	μ	α	ε	δ
Light chain	k or γ	k or γ	k or γ	k or γ	k or γ
Presence in Milk	–	–	–	–	–
Cross through Placenta	+	–	–	–	–
Binding to Phagocyte	+	–	–	–	–
Present on B Lymphocyte cell	–	+	–	–	+

Characterstic Feature	IgG	IgM	IgA	IgE	IgD
Half life	23	5	6	2.5	3
Molecular Weight (dalton)	150,000	900,000	150,000-600,000	190,000	150,000
Function	Protects from inhaled and ingested pathogen	Present on Lymphocyte surface as receptors, activated B cells	Mediator in allergic responces	Stimulation of Phagocytes and complement system, provides passive immunity to the foetus	Activates B cells

7.6 Radio Immunoassay (RIA)

This technique was first developed by **Rosalyn Yalow** and **Samual Berson**. RIA was first carried out for quantification of Insulin in diabetic patient. It is quite useful for quantitative measurement of drugs, steroids and harmones. It is more sensitive and specific than chemical method for the analysis of clinical and biochemical fluids.

7.6.1. Basic Principle

It is based on the principle of interaction of unlabelled antigen (i.e. test sample) with a fixed amount of corresponding labelled antigen. It is used for a fixed amount of antiserum with limited number of antibody binding sites. At the time of reaction when it reaches to an equilibrium, the bound and free forms of the labelled antigen are separated from each other. As the concentration of unlabelled antigen in the sample increases the amount of labelled antigen bound to antibody will decrease.

$$12Ag + 4Ag^* + 4Ab \rightarrow Ag^*Ab + 3AgAb + 3Ag^* + 9Ag$$

12Ag: unlabelled Antigen — Variable amount

4Ag*: labelled Antigen — Fixed amount

Ag = unlabeled Antigen

We can determine the amount of antigen in the sample simply by using the amount of unlabelled antigen and fixed amount of antibody and labelled antigen. It can be done by plotting a calibration curve between unlabelled antigen added and bound labelled antigen.

7.6.2. Labelling of Antigen and Technique of Assay

The basic requirements of RIA are pure antigen (for standard sample) labelled antigen and specific antisera. The antigen for this purpose is obtained by extraction from tissue and purified. This purified antigen is labelled with suitable isotope. Most commonly used isotopes are carbon 14, tritium and iodine isotopes 125 and 131. The labelled antigen is immediately separated from unreacted iodine and any denatured protein is removed by gel filteration. Care must be taken to ensure the specificity and avidity of the antiserum produced. Thus from the amount of labelled antigen measured out at different antibody concentration, a curve is constructed. A linear curve obtained over a relatively limited range. Hence antibody sample is diluted.

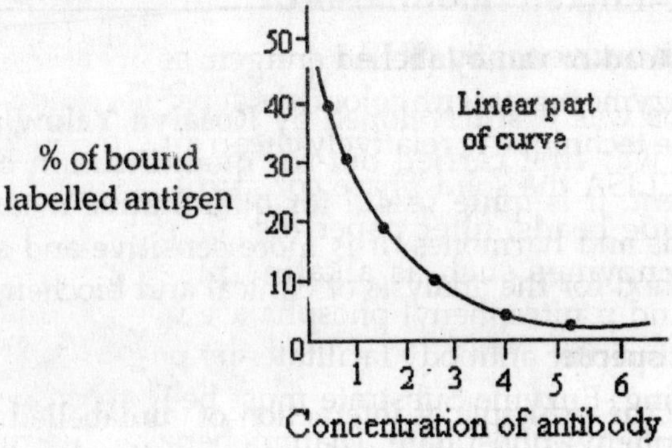

Fig. 7.7. Calibration Curve between Unlabeled Antigen added and Bound Labelled Antigen

Whenever RIA is being carried out it is essential that a number of standards should be assayed under identical standards and sample should be in duplicate. The technique is carried out at room temperature and incubated time exceed 6 hour. The temperature 4°C is used to prevent proteolysis and microbial growth. In solid phase RIA antigen or antibody is incorporated in single phase matrix.

Table7.2. Commonly used Isotopes in RIA and their Emission

S.N.	Isotope	Half life	Emission
1.	Carbon - 14	560 a	β
2.	Hydrogen-3	12.26 a	β
3.	Iodine - 125	60 d	β & γ
4.	Iodine - 131	8.04d	β & γ

7.6.3 Application

- It can detect any compound which is available in pure form, radiolabelled and immunogenic.
- It provides high specificity and sensitivity.
- The technique may be used to detect even a small amount of antigen from unknown source.

7.7 Enzyme-Linked Immunosorbent Assay (ELISA)

In ELISA instead of radio labelled antigen, easily assayed enzyme is used. This enzyme reacts with colourless substrate producing coloured products. The technique is relatively cheap and free from radiological hazards. In ELISA the solid phase consist of cross linked dextron or polyacrylamide beads, filter paper disc or polypropylene tubes. A number of enzymes such as alkaline phosphatase, horseredish peroxidase and p nitrophenyl phosphatase may be used. Binding of antigen with specific antibody facilitates by passive adsorption or co-valent coupling. Enzyme Substrate must be inexpensive, stable and safe. P-nitrophenyl phosphate, Diaminobenzene 5 amino salicylate and O-Phenylediamine are common colourless substrate. They are converted into coloured products by the reaction with enzyme. For the assay of specific antibody indirect method is applied. Calibration curve should be prepared.

7.7.1 Competitive Method

In this method the mixture of unknown amount of enzyme labelled antigen and mixture of known amount of unlabelled antigen (sample) react with specific antibody attached to a solid phase and make a complex. This complex washed with buffer (triton X-100) followed by adding enzyme substrate and measure the enzyme activity. It is proportional to the labelled antigen in the mixture of antigen i.e. sample (Fig. 7.8).

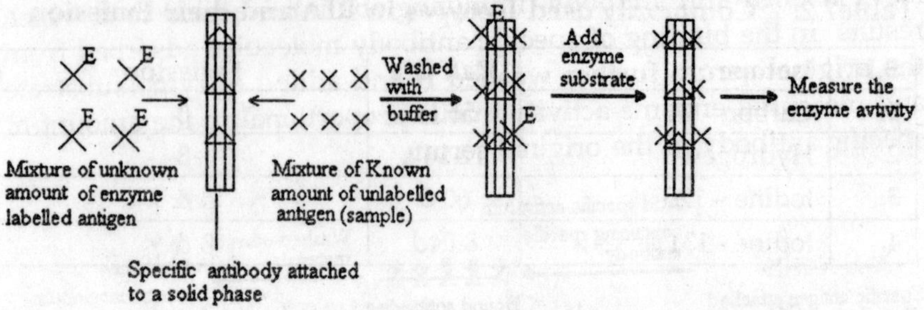

Fig. 7.8. Competitive Method of ELISA

7.7.2 Sandwich or Double Antibody Method

In sandwich method the antigen become sandwiched between specific antibody and antibody enzyme conjugate. The set of unknown antigen react with specific antibody attached to solid phase. Washed and treated with enzyme labelled antibody then further wash and added enzyme substrate. Now the enzyme activity is measured directly. It is proportional to the amount of antigen present in original solution. (Fig. 7.9)

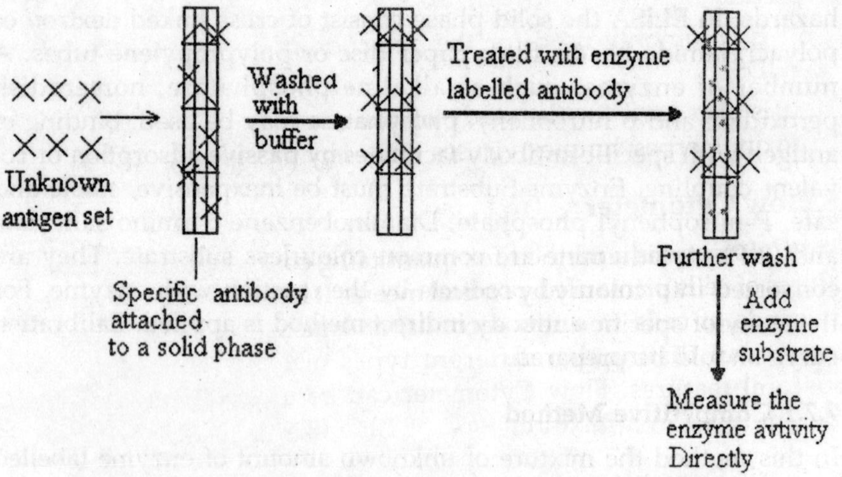

Fig. 7.9 Sandwich or Double Antibody Method of ELISA

7.7.3 Indirect Method

This method is used for assaying specific antibody and to measure level of antibody. The specific antiserum containing specific antibody is added into specific antigen attached to a solid surface then the antigen and antibody bind up and other materials are washed out.

Now labelled anti antibody (immunoglobulin) is added to it which results in the binding of specific antibody molecules adsorbed from the original serum further washed it and added enzyme substrate and measured enzyme activity that is proportional to the amount of specific antibody in the original serum.

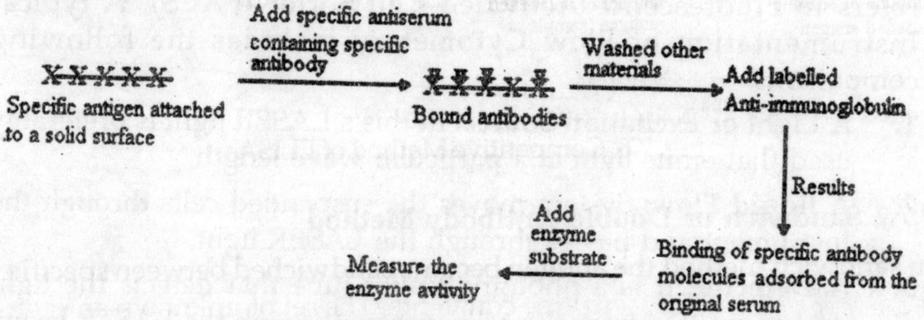

Fig. 7.10 Indirect method of ELISA

7.7.4 Application

1. The ELISA technique is mainly used for the assaying of antibodies in infectious disease having antiviral antibodies such as *Candida species.*
2. It is commonly used for the detection of HIV + ve or -ve for AIDS.
3. It is also used for the study of various infections like bacterial toxin, Herpes simplex viruses and Hepatitis B etc.

7.8 Flow Cytometer

Flow Cytometer is a method for quantitaing component or structural features of cells primarily by optical means. It has a capacity to process thousands of cells in a few seconds, and measure on one cell at a time. It can distinguish different types of cells by quantitating structural features. Flow Cytometer can be used to count cells of different types in a mixture.

7.8.1 Basic Principle

Flow Cytometer is based on the principle of light scattering, excitation and emission of flurochrome molecule to generate specific multiparameter data from particles and cells in the size range of 0.5 µm and 40 µm diameter. Cells are hydrodynamically focused in a sheath of PBS before intercepting an optimum focused light source. Laser light source is frequently used in flow cytometery.

When cells which is to be analyzed is passed through the light source they scatter light and flurochrome are excited to a higher energy state. This energy is released as a photon of light with specific spectral lines unique to every flurochrome.

Flow Cytometer is a technology to count and sort cells and sometimes refers to Fluorescence Activated Cell Sorter (FACS). A typical Instrumentation of Flow Cytometery includes the following components:-

1. **A Light or Excitation Source:** In this a LASER light is preferably used that emits light at a particular wave length.
2. **A liquid Flow:** System moves the suspended cells through the Instrument and passes through the LASER light.
3. **A Detector:** It is a photomultiplier tube that detects the light flashes emitted from the cells, passes through the LASER beam.

In a Flow Cytometer, single cell move past the excitation source and the light hitting the cell is either scattered or absorbed and then re-emitted (fluorescence). This scattered or re-emitted light is collected by the detector (Fig. 7.11).

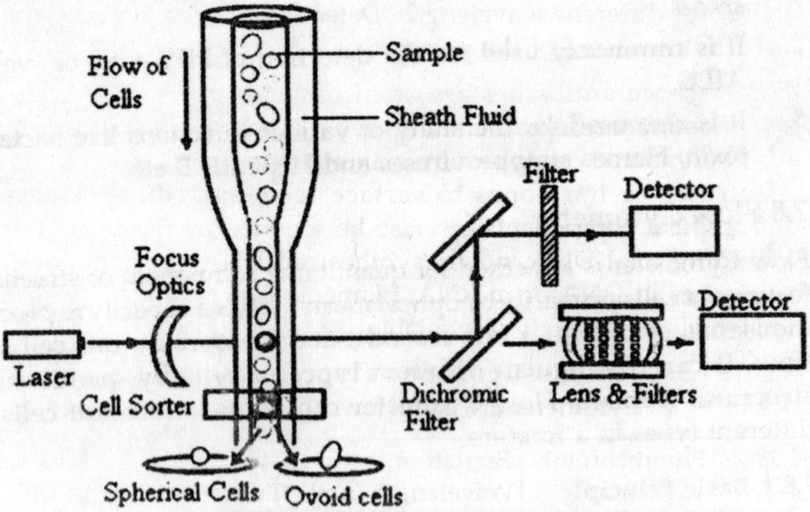

Fig. 7.11. Diagramatic Representation of Flow Cytometer

7.8.2 Light Scattering

When light beam come in contact with cell it is scattered. Which results in either reflected or refracted light reaching the detector. The pattern of light scattering is dependent on cell size and shape. It is commonly used to exclude dead cells, cell aggregates and cell debris from the fluorescence data. It is sufficient to distinguish lymphocytes from monocytes and granulocytes in blood samples.

The process of light scattering is quite useful, in this cell can be sorted on the basis of size or shape into different collection tubes by using a technique known as electrostatic deflection, which employs charged plate to change the path of the cell.

7.8.3 Fluorescence

Fluorescence based detection depends on the absorption of light by the cell and the subsequent re-emission of this light at a different frequency. Flow cytometers make use of this technology by employing filters to block the original light source from reaching the detector, while the fluorescence emission is allowed through it for detection.

It allows only a very low background of stray light to reach the detector. Fluorescence probes (dye) are used to report the quantities of specific components of the cells. These fluorescent probes are usually a type of dye, which fluoresce only when light of the appropriate wavelength hits them, causing the emission of secondary light of a different wavelength. Detection of second wavelength is used as a measure of the presence of dye on the cell.

Fluorescence antibodies are often used to report the densities of specific surface receptors and thus helpful to distinguish subpopulation of differentiated cell types. By making them fluorescent, the binding of viruses or harmones to surface receptors can be measured. Intracellular components can also be reported by fluorescent probes including total DNA, newly synthesized DNA, specific nucleotide sequences in DNA or m RNA, filamentous actin and any structure for which an antibody is available

Table 7.3. The most common fluorescent dyes used in Flow Cytometer are as follows :-

S.N.	Fluorochrome	Excitation Wavelength (nm)	Wavelength Emission	Emitted colour
1.	Texas Red	488 nm	615 nm	Red
2.	Phycoerythrin	488 nm	575 nm	Green
3.	Fluorescein Isothiocynate	488 nm	525 nm	Green

At the time of measurement the material is passed through a laser beam by continuous flow of a fine stream of the suspension. Each cell scatters some of the laser light, and also emits fluorescent light excited by laser. The cytometer typically measures several parameters simultaneously for each other.

- Low angle forward scatter intensity, approximately proportional to cell diameter.
- Orthogonal (90°) scatter intensity, approximately proportional to the quantity of granular structure within the cell.
- Fluorescence intensities of several wavelength.

7.8.4 Detector and Data output device

Flow Cytometers involves sophisticated fluidics, laser optics, electronic detector, analog to digital converter and computer. The amount of a cell scatter or fluoresces light is measured by the detector and subsequently needs to be displayed for interpretation. These profiles of cells are normally displayed as dot plots or histograms. In dot plot displays the X and Y axis measure the different emission, displaying a dot for each of the cells that show that particular emission.

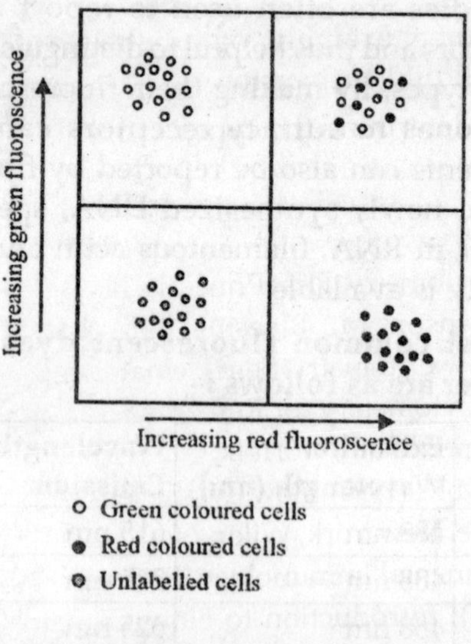

Fig. 7.12. A Dot Plot Representation Showing Different Colour of Fluoroscence at 'X' and'Y' Axis.

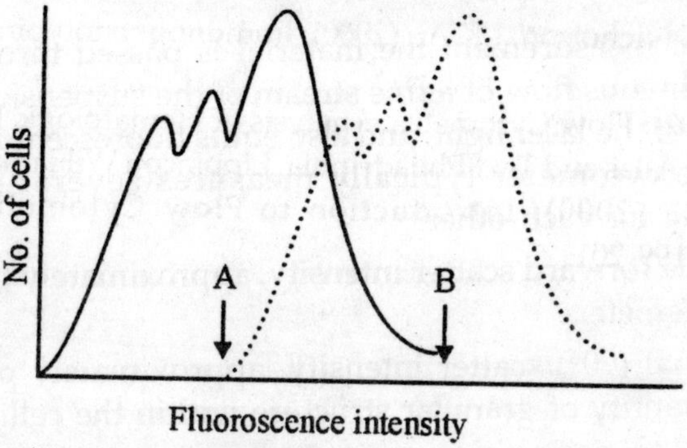

Fig. 7.13. Histogram showing Fluroscence Intensity at 'X' Axis and Number of Cells at 'Y' Axis. Histogram shows the Shift in the Fluroscence Intensity of the Sample Cells.

7.8.5 Application

- Flow cytometer mainly used for the diagnosis of diseases and research.
- It is used in various field i.e. immunology, pathology, plant breeding and medicinal.
- D.N.A contents in cell easily determined by flow cytometer.
- It can be used to select and purify a specific group of cells within a population.
- It provides the measurement of biochemical properties of individual cell in liquid suspension.
- It is also used to determine the types of markers and receptors on cells surface.

References

Givan, A., (2001); Flow Cytometry, First Principle. New York, Wiley-Liss.

Marti, G.E., Steler-Stevenson, M., Bleesing, J.J., Fleisher, T.A., (2001); Introduction to Flow Cytometry. Sem Hematology 38 (2): 93-9.

Nunez, R., (2001); Flow Cytometery for Research Scientist : Principles and Applications. Wymondham, Norfolk, UK . Horizon Press. pg 110.

Owens, M.A. and Loken, M.R., (1995), Flow Cytometery: Principles for Clinical Laboratory Practice. New York, Wiley-Liss.

Paul, W.E., (1984); Fundamental Immunology, Raven Press, U.S.A.

Recktenwald, D.J., (1993); Introduction to Flow Cytometery: Principles, Fluorochromes, Instrument Setup, Calibration. J Hematotherapy 2 (3) : 387-94.

Stewart, C.C., Nicholson, J.K.A., (2000); Immunophenotyping. New York: Wiley-Liss.

Tsien, S., (2002); Flow Cytometric Analysis of Hematologic Neoplasm: A Colour Atlas and Text Philadelphia, Lippincott Williama and Wilkins.

Weaver, J.L., (2000); Introduction to Flow Cytometry. Methods 21 (3): 199-201.

CHAPTER 8

Radioisotope Technique

Radioactivity may be defined as spontaneous emission of suitable particles and electromagnetic radiation by unstable nuclei. The process of natural radioactivity was discovered by a French Scientist, Prof. Atoine Henri Becaquerel (1896) in uranium mineral. He found that uranium salts emit some invisible radiations. These radiations were originally called Becquerel rays. The substances which posses this type of property are known as radioactive and the rays emitted by them are called radioactive rays. Radioactivity does not depend on any external factor like temperature, light, electricity, magnetism and chemical substances. The element having atomic number greater than 83 are radioactive.

8.1 Units of Radioactivity

There are several units of Radioactivity.

8.1.1. Curie (ci): It is defined as the amount of any radioactive substance which produces 3.7×10^{10} disintegration per sec. (dps) i.e.

1 ci = 3.7×10^{10} (dps)

8.2.2. Rutherford: It is defined as the amount of radioactive substance which produces 10^6 dps.

i.e. 1 rd = 10^6 dps

1 ci = 10^4 rd

8.2 Radioisotopes

The isotopes of an element have the same number of proton but different number of neutrons due to difference in mass. (i.e. same atomic number but different atomic mass). Radioisotopes are artificially produced unstable atom of an element. These can be manufactured by neutron activation in a nuclear reactor. The nuclei of Radioisotope usually become stable by emission alfa (α) and beta (β) particles. This process is known as Radioactive decay.

Many Radioisotopes used in medicine are known as Radiopharmaceuticals.

Table 8.1. Some common Radioisotopes used in medicine

Radioisotope	Half life	Uses
Chromium 51	28 days	To label R.B.C. and quantify gastrointestinal protein loss
Cobalt 60	10.5 month	For external beam Radiotherapy
Copper 64	13 hours	To study genetic disease
Iodine 125	60 days	To evaluate the filteration rate of kidney and in cancer brachytherapy
Iodine 131	8 days	In treating Thyroid cancer and treating abnormal liver function
Iron 59	46 days	To study the Iron metabolism in urine
Rhenium 186	3.8 days	Used for pain relief in bone cancer
Sodium 24	15 hours	To study the electrolyte within the body
Thallium 201	73 hours	Used for the diagnosis of coronory disease

8.3 Radio-Tracer Technique

In Radio-tracer technique the metabolites or substance which is to be studied is labelled with the help of Radioisotopes and then study the path of that metabolites into the organism (either plant or animal) or any process. The commonly used Radoisotopes are C^{14}, P^{32}, S^{35}, H^3 etc.

8.3.1 Principle

The Radioisotope material in sufficient physical or chemical form is injected into the examining material. Thus a portion of the material becomes labelled and follows the behaviour of that material. Its movement can be monitored by using radiation detector (Fig. 8.1).

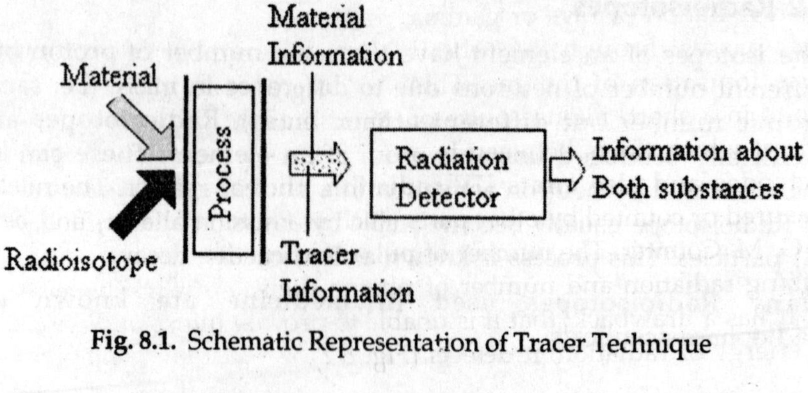

Fig. 8.1. Schematic Representation of Tracer Technique

8.3.2 Uses

1. This technique is used to determine the permeability of cells and cell organells.
2. It is used to know the metabolic pathway of different compounds such as glucose containing C^{14} Radioisotope.
3. The rate of growth, decaying and their proper order can be determined by studying the amount of Radioactivity in different parts.
4. N^{15} Tracer technique is used to determine the root production and mortality in plants.

For measuring the radioactivity of the substance two type of apparatus are used as follows :-

8.4 Gieger-Muller Counter (G. M.Counter)

G. M. Counter was invented by **Johannes Wilhelm Hans Gieger** and **Walther Muller in 1925**. This apparatus consist of a glass tube filled with gas (Neon or Argon) at low pressure and two electrodes. Cathode is in the form of hollow metal cylinder while anode (a wire) placed along the central axis of the cathode. These two electrodes are joined with the adjustable high voltage source called the G. M. amplifier.

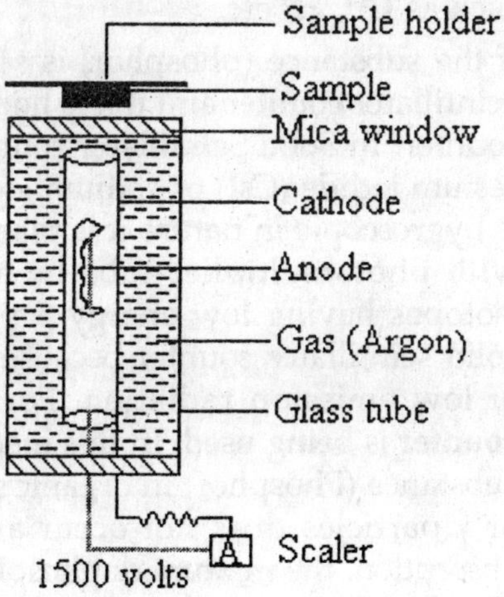

Fig. 8.2 Diagramatic Representation of G.M. Counter

When radiation (X-rays or gamma rays) passes through the tube it cause ionisation of the gas. This results in a short, intense pulse of current which flows between two electrodes and also emits UV radiation, this pulse of current is measured or counted by other parts (such as Photomultiplier tube) of the G. M. Counter. The number of pulse/sec indicate the intensity of ionizing radiation and number of photon (light) crossing the tube/sec. It has a drawback that it is unable to provide information about the energy of radiation, it detects (Fig. 8.2).

8.5 Scintillator Counter

The G. M. technique is rapidly replaced by an alternate method known as Scintillation counting. In this method the energy of radiation is used for producing pulses of light which can be measured or counted. Scintillator counter usually consist of

1. Scintillator material (crystal)
2. Photomultiplier tube
3. Analog to Digital converter (Scaler)

When the radiation of alfa (α), Beta (β), Gamma (γ) rays falls on a substance (Scintillators) it produce light by the use of phosphor (an aromatic compound which produce light by absorbing radiation from radioactive compounds). These Scintillation (flash of light) are converted into electric pulses by photomultiplier tube (see in UV visible Spectrophotometery) and measured by scaler. This technique is quite useful for the detection of isotopes which emits low energy β particles such as C^{14}, H^{3} etc.

If the substance (phosphor) is solid the technique refers to as Solid Scintillator counter and if it is liquid, it is known as Liquid Scintillator counter. In Solid Scintillator counter method a single large crystal of cesium iodide (CsI) or sodium iodide (NaI) is used. Since NaI crystal is hygroscopic in nature it is placed in an aluminium box and joined with photomultiplier tube by a transparent slit or window. The isotopes having low energy β particles cannot be detected by this solid scintillator counter because aluminium box inhibit the passing of low emission radiation. For this purpose **Liquid Scintillator counter** is being used. In this method the isotopes are dissolved with substance (Phosphor) in organic solvent (toluene). So absorption of β or γ particles does not occur and emission will transfer without absorption. the mixture of phosphor and organic solvent is known as "**Cocktail**".

8.5.1 Method: The radiation from the sample interact with their surrounding material and cause excitation of the sample molecule. When this excitation energy falls on phosphor it emits photon of light by the process of emission. A photomultiplier tube converts this photon of light into electric signal that can be counted by scaler. It suffers a major drawback of quenching of light flashes due to the presence of various chemical compounds in biological sample (Fig. 8.3).

We can use the Scintillator counter to measure the energy of any particle even in the similar energy range.

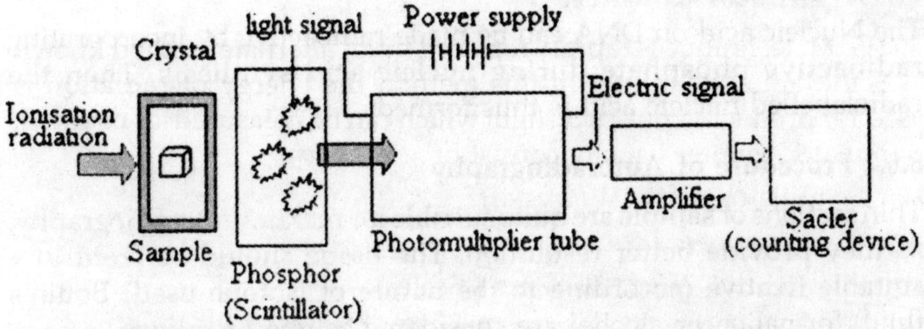

Fig. 8.3. Diagramatic Representation of Scintillator Counter

Table 8.2 Some Common Radioisotopes and their properties

Compound	Isotope	Half life	Type of Radiation	Energy of Radiation
Hydrogen	H^3	12.5 years	β radiation	0.018
Carbon	C^{14}	5760years	β radiation	0.155
Sulphur	S^{35}	87.1 days	β radiation	0.167
Potassium	K^{42}	12.5 hours	β radiation	3.550
Calcium	Ca^{45}	152 days	β radiation	0.255
Phosphorus	P^{32}	14.3 days	β radiation	0.171
Iodine	I^{131}	8.1 days	γ radiation	0.280

8.6 Autoradiography

Autoradiography is a technique by which we detect the radioactivity of a test material with the help of photographic emulsion and radioactive tracer. A photographic film of the test material is obtained and this film is known as autoradiograph. After development the irradiated areas appear on the film as dark areas corresponding to the distribution of the tracer.

8.6.1 Principle

It is based on the principle that if a photographic emulsion is brought into contact with radioactive material the ionic radiations will convert the emulsion as dark spots of silver at certain points. Radioactive substances are introduced to test material in two forms:-

1. Direct in chemical form

2. Tagged with metabolic precursors

The Nucleic acid on DNA can be made radioactive by incorporating radioactive phosphate during nucleic acid synthesis. Then the radiolabelled nucleic acid is thus formed.

8.6.2 Procedure of Autoradiography

Thin sections of sample are quite suitable for making autoradiography, as they provide better resolution. The tissue should be fixed in a suitable fixative (according to the nature of isotope used) Bouin's fluid, formalion or alcohol are considered as good fixatives.

After fixation, the tissue should be dehydrated and processed for histological preparation. Thin section of the tissue should be transfered on glass slide and subjected to photographic emulsion.

Follwing steps are performed for making a good autoradiograph.

- Remove the wax of paraffin section by placing it in petroleum.
- Cut the photographic emulsion film with the help of razor or scissor in size of 1" x 1".
- Take one piece of above film and float it on distilled water ($23^o \pm 2$) in a container. Care should be taken that emulsion side should face downwords.
- Now place the slides, mounted with deparaffinized sections, in distilled water, section should be facing upwords.
- Lift the slide upwords and bring it near the film so that it covers the specimen.
- Dry the slide with hot air blower or in fan.
- Keep this slide in dark at low temperature (4°-6^oC) for exposure.
- Proceed for photographic processing and wash with distilled water.

A photographic emulsion consists of crystal of Silver bromide and small quantities of Silver sulfide and colloidal silver mounted with gelatin in a glass or flexible support. When photographic is emulsion is imposed with radioactive emission then this emission cause ionisation and sets electron free in the ionic Silver bromide lattice. These electrons migrate over short distance to the sensitivity speck's area which are probably composed of Silver sulfide and these in turn become negatively charged. This charge attracts interstitial silver ions and upon reaching the speck they are neutralized to silver and forming latent image. Thus the growth of metallic silver occurs and its amount is being dependent upon the amount of radiation received.

At the time of development of the film the developers supplies electrons and causes the reduction of silver ions to metallic silver atoms and these are responsible for visible image. Then the fixer solution is applied in which thiosulphide removes unexpected Silver bromide and hence stabilizes the image.

References

Boyd, G.A., (1955); Autoradiography in Biology and Medicine., New York, Acad. Press.

Boyd, G.A., (1955); Autoradiography in Biology and Medicine., New York, Acad. Press.

Chapman, J. M. and Avery, G., (1981); The use of Radioisotopes in the Life Sciences. George Unwin, London.

Francis, G.E., Mulligan, W., Wormall, A., (1954); Isotopic Tracer. The Athlone Press, London.

Plummer, D.T., (1987); An Introduction to Practical Biochemistry, 3rd ed., McGraw-Hill, London

Slater, R.J., (2000); Radioisotopes in Biology. A Practical Approach 2nd ed.

Wang, C.H., Wills, D.L., (1965); Radiotracer Methodology in Biological Science. Prentice Hall, New Jersey.

CHAPTER 9

Histological Technique

Generally in the laboratory study of plant or animal material, microscopical preparation are required. Stepwise procedure for such microscopic study is known as histological microtechnique. Students of life science such as microbiology, biotechnology and embryology are expected to know these techniques. A number of steps are involved for detailed histological studies.

9.1 Fixation

Animal or plant material in living condition may be studied but their detailed cellular structure can be studied only by fixing them. The first steps in histological preparation for microscopic studies is fixation which has the following purposes:-

- Fixation checks postmortem decay.
- It provides a harder consistency to many tissues.
- It preserves the cellular structure by interrupting cell activities.
- Fixation precipitates the cell proteins thus structural details are fixed and preserved.
- Fixation favours least alternation in structure and chemical composition of the living tissue.
- Fixation and hardening of the tissue depends upon the proper ratio of fixing and hardening agents.

A good fixative should have the following qualities:-

1. It should stop postmortem changes
2. It should have good penetrating properties.
3. It should precipitate the cell protein in such a way that tissue acquires a hard texture for good sectioning.
4. It should preserve the shape and size of the tissue or cell as such.
5. Fixatives should fix the cell components in such a way that they are not disturbed by further processing
6. Fixative should be removed easily and not interfere in further staining.

The main substance which is required to be fixed are lipoprotein, Cytoskeletal fibrous protein, fiberous glycoprotein, globular protein and nucleic acids etc. A good fixative should also preserve the histochemical properties.

There are many methods of fixation:-

9.1.1. Physical Method of Fixation

9.1.1.1. Heat

Heat application helps to coagulate the proteins and melt lipids. Large specimens are exposed to boiling saline containing formaline. Recently microwave is used at controlled temperature for fixation.

9.1.1.2. Freezing

The technique is generally known as freeze drying. But specimen should be frozen in such a way that minimum ice crystals are formed. Cryoprotective agents such as Dimethylsulphoxide (DMSO), Glycerol propylene glycol and 10 -20 % sucrose may be used to reduce ice formation. In freeze drying, frozen material is transferred to a chamber at 40ºC, after removal of water vapour the material should be infiltered with paraffin wax and sectioned in a usual way.

9.1.2. Chemical Method of Fixation

Generally liquid chemical fixatives are used which penetrate the tissue according to their nature. Rapid penetrating agents require less time for fixation than slow penetrating agent.

9.1.2.1. Individual Fixative Agents

(i) Mercuric Chloride

Mercuric chloride is a very good fixative for fixation of smear of micro-organism. Solution contains $HgCl_2$ molecules which insolubilize proteins. It penetrates the tissue quickly and staining results are bright. It has one drawback, that a brown precipitate is deposited in the tissue which may be removed by treating it with a solution of Iodine followed by sodium thiosulphate.

(ii) Acetic Acid

Acetic acid is a suitable fixative to preserve chromosomes and chromatin materials of nuclei. It inhibits the shrinking action of ethanol and picric acid. It is a powerful penetrative and coagulates nucleic acids but does not fix the protein of cytoplasm. It is used with other fixatives.

(iii) Ethyl Alcohol (C_2H_5OH)

Ethyl alcohol is used directly as fixatives it shrinks and hardens the tissue. It precipitates the cytoplasmic proteins but does not fix chromatin. Its mixture with acetic acid gives good penetration.

(iv) Chromic Acid (CrO_3)

Chromic trioxide (strong oxidising agent) dissolved in water form deep Red-orange chromic acid in ionized form ($HCrO_4^-$, $Cr_2O_7^{2-}$)

$$CrO_3 + H_2O \rightarrow H^+ + HCrO_4^-$$
$$2HCrO_4^- \leftrightarrow n\ Cr_2O_7^{2-} + H_2O$$

It is a good fixative for chromosomal studies, but its penetrating power is slow and hardens slowly. Nuclei are stained brightly. It should not be mixed with reducing agents such as formalin until immediately before use. Tissue fixed in fixative containing chromic acid must be washed for 12 - 24 hours in running tap water before dehydration to remove insoluble precipitate.

(v) Osmium Tetraoxide (OsO_4)

It is a non ionic, solid volatile at room temperature. Its penetrating power is slow. It is used for preservation of fine structures in electron microscopy and is effective for small specimen. Tissue should be washed thoroughly after fixation, as it reduces to form precipitate during dehydration

(vi) Simple Organic Coagulants

This group include acetone, ethyl alcohol and methyl alcohol that are able to replace water from proteinaceous materials by breaking hydrogen bonds causing denaturation. Methanol, Ethanol and Acetone are used alone for fixing films, cell smear and cryostat section.

(vii) Formaldehyde (HCHO)

37 - 40 % w/v in water is formaline. It is good fixative for plant and animal specimens.

$$\underset{\text{formaldehyde}}{HCHO} + H_2O \rightarrow \underset{\text{Methylene hydrate}}{HOCH_2OH}$$

For 4 % Formaldehyde

100 ml of 40% formaldehyde

900 ml Distilled water

4 gm Sodium phosphate (monobasic)

6.5 gm Sodium phosphate (dibasic anhydrous)

It is most commonly used routine fixative for paraffin embedded section. Penetration is moderate. It is also used in histochemistry. It preserves most lipids but does not react significantly with carbohydrates.

(viii) Formol Acetic Alcohol (F.A.A)

Formaline (40%)	5 ml
Glacial acetic acid	2.5 ml
Ethyl alcohol	42.5 ml

It is used for the fixation of Nematodes and some plant materials. It is also good fixative for polysaccharides and nucleoproteins.

(ix) Mayer's Albumin

White of egg	20 gm
Glycerin	50 ml
Sodium salicylate	1 gm

Mix all the material gently, stir and filter. This fixative is used to stick the ribbons of microtomy, contain thin section. It is also used to stick small micro-organism such as protozoans on the slide.

(x) Picric Acid

It is a trinitrophenol which is very strong acid in aqueous solution. In dry condition it is explosive so it should be stored in water. A saturated solution of picric acid forms picrate salt with basic group of proteins. To remove these picrate salts, wash the tissue in 70 % alcohol containing a pinch of ammonium acetate. Its penetrating power is slow but does not harden the tissue. Picric acid together with acetic acid serves as good fixative and predisposes the tissue to bright staining with acid dyes.

(xi) Potassium Dichromate ($K_2Cr_2O_7$)

It is a good fixative for lipids but does not precipitate proteins. It penetrates well but tissue is not hardened due to which section cutting becomes difficult. It is a good fixative for mitochondria. After fixation, tissue should be washed well to remove the precipitate of Cr_2O_3.

(xii) Altmann Fixative

Potassium dichromate	5 %	20 ml
Osmic acid	2 %	20 ml
Fixation time		12 - 20 hours

After fixation material should be washed in running tap water for 12 hours.

9.1.2.2. Non-aqueous Fixatives

Some fixatives are used in mixtures for general histology, preservation of nucleic acid and carbohydrates.

(i) Clark's Fluid: It is very good for microanatomical fixation.

Absolute alcohol	75 ml
Glacial acetic acid	25 ml

Both the ingredients must be mixed just before use.

(ii) Cornoy's Fluid: It is good fixative for cytological materials.

Absolute alcohol	60 ml
Chloroform	30 ml
Glacial acetic acid	10 ml

Ingredients should be mixed just before use. It is rapidly penetrating, coagulating protein and nucleic acid. Tissue of moderate size (2 - 5 mm thick) may be fixed for 4-8 hours and then transferred to 95 % alcohol.

(iii) Alcohol - Formaline - Acetic Acid Mixture

Ethyl alcohol	95 %	85 ml
Formaline	30-40 %	10 ml
Glacial Acetic acid		5 ml

All the chemicals are mixed before use.

It is a good fixative for general morphological studies, nucleic acid and carbohydrates. Penetration is rapid. Smears for the whole mount require 15 - 35 minutes. After fixation, specimen are transferred to 95 % alcohol.

9.1.2.3 Aqueous Aldehyde Fixatives

(i) Formal Saline

Formaline	30-40 %	100ml
Sodium Chloride		9 gm
Water		To make 1000 ml

The solution should be made a day before using, may be kept for several months.

Fixation time 24 hours to 70 hours.

(ii) Neutral Buffered Formaline (R.D. Lillie)

Phosphate buffer neutralize the acidity of formaline thus pH of solution becomes stable for many months.

Sodium Phosphate Monobasic ($NaH_2PO_4H_2O$)		4.0 gm
Sodium Phosphate Dibasic (Na_2HPO_4)		6.5 gm
Formaline	30 - 40 %	750 ml
Water	Make up to 1000ml	

(iii) Formal Calcium

Formaline	30-40 %	100 ml
Calcium acetate $(CH_3COO)_2Ca.H_2O$		20 gm
Water	Make it to	1000 ml

In this fixative, acetate ion neutralize acidity of formaline, Calcium ion insolubilize phospholipid prior to cutting frozen section. Fixation time 1-3 days

9.1.2.4 Other Aqueous Fixatives for general Histology

Table 9.1

Fixatives	Requirement	Amount	Uses
1. Bouin's Fluid	Saturated aqueous Picric acid Formaline Glacial acetic acid	90 ml 30 ml 6 ml	It is most commonly used for general histological work in the laboratory. It preserves nuclei and connective tissue, show rapid penetration, little shrinkage. Paraffin sections are easily cut, multiple staining results bright and differentiated colours.
2. Alcoholic Bouin (Gendre's Fluid)	Saturated alcoholic Picric acid Formaline 40 % Glacial acetic acid	400 ml 75 ml 25 ml	It may be kept for a long time. Penetration is better. Fixation time is 4 hours and then tissue should be washed in 70 % alcohol.
3. Rossman's Fluid	100 % ethanol saturated with picric acid Neutralize commercial formaline	45 ml 5.0 ml	Tissue should be fixed for 12 - 24 hours and then wash several times in 95 % alcohol.

Fixatives	Requirement	Amount	Uses
4. Heidenhain's (SUSA)	Mercuric Chloride ($HgCl_2$) Sodium Chloride (NaCl) Trichloroacetic acid Glacial acetic acid Formaline 40 % Distilled water (To make 100 ml)	9.0 gm 1.0 gm 0.4 gm 0.8 ml 40 ml 160 ml	It is a good fixative for histology of tissue. Fixation time is 24 hours then tissue should be transferred to 95 % alcohol.
5. Zenker's Fluid	Mercuric Chloride Potassium dichromate Glacial acetic acid Distilled water	25 gm 12.5 gm 25 gm 475 ml	This fixative is excellent for analytical work. After fixation material should be washed 12-24 hours in running water for removal of Mercury. Acetic acid in this fixative should be mixed immediately before use which improves its solubility due to low pH.
6. Helly's Fluid	**Solution A** Distilled water Potassium Dichromate Sodium Sulphate Mercuric Chloride **Solution B** Formaldehyde 40 %	 1000 ml 25 gm 10 gm 50 gm 50 ml	In this fixative formaline is added immediately before use. It is mainly used for fixation of mitocondria, bone marrow, spleen, lymph etc. Fixation time is 12-24 hours. Material should be washed overnight in running water to remove mercury deposits.
7. Elfman's Fluid	Mercuric Chloride Potassium Dichromate Water	5 gm 2.5 gm 100 ml	It is used for the fixation of frozen section containing lipids, Proteins, amino acids
8. Flemming's Fluid	2 % Osmium tetraoxide 5 % Chromium trioxide Glacial acetic acid Water to make	4.0 ml 3.0 ml 1.0 ml 20 ml	Solutions mix before using. It is a good stain for fixing the material to study meiotic and mitotic cell division.

9.1.3 Processing of hard Tissue

9.1.3.1 Decalcification

Hard tissue such as bone or teeth can be softened after fixation by removing its hardening substance. The material to be decalcified is kept in the decalcifying fluid i.e. Hydrochloric, nitric and formic acid. Calcium from the tissue is removed as calcium ions. Decalcifying fluid is changed frequently. Completion of decalcification is recognized, if calcium ion are not detected in chemical test.

9.1.3.2 Decalcification by Chelating Agents

A chelating agent is an organic compound which can combine with a metal ion to form metal chelate. Ethylene Diamine Tetraacetic Acid (EDTA) is commonly used as chelating agent. Its ion combine with calcium ion to form stable, soluble chelates. But decalcification process is very slow.

9.1.3.3 Decalcification by Acid

Formic acid (pH 1.5 - 3.5) is most commonly used for decalcification. Acetic acid and citric acids are also used as acid reagents cause protein hydrolysis and tissue swelling, addition of chloral hydrate and alcohol. Check the swelling of tissue (by increasing osmotic pressure of the fluid)

(i) Formiç acid

Formic acid	5.0 - 25.0 ml
Formalin	5.0 ml
Distilled water	100.0 ml

(ii) Nitric acid

Formalin	10.0 ml
Nitric acid 68- 70 %	5.0 ml
Distilled water	85.0 ml

(iii) Kristensen fluid

8 N Formic acid	50.0 ml
1 N Sodium formate	50.0 ml

Material should be exposed to the reagent for at least 24 hours, then it should be washed in running water and then transferred to 70 % alcohol.

9.1.4 Bleaching of Tissue

Sometimes certain tissues like skin or chitinous exoskeleton of insects or the animals are darkly coloured and create problem in staining. So they have to be bleached before dehydration.

9.1.4.1 Chlorine Bleach (for skin and pigmented tissues)

Potassium Chlorate	0.2 mg.
Concentrated HCl	Few drops
70% Alcohol	20 ml - 40 ml

Immerse the material in this mixture for 24 hours till it is destained.

9.1.4.2 Bleaching of Chitinous material

Immerse the tissue in 1 % aqueous solution of potassium permagnet then transfer it to 5 % aqueous solution of oxalic acid till it is bleached completely. Lastly wash it thoroughly and proceed for dehydration.

9.2 Dyes and Stains

Dye is a coloured compound that binds with a substrate. In histological preparation of tissue and specimen dyes are used to stain the tissue and differentiate their different components. Any dyes has two parts. Chromogen is its coloured part and auxochrome attaches to the substrate. Colour of the dye is due to some unsaturated group such as carboxyl, azo, nitroso, nitro, quinoid, and ethylene etc. Azodyes are the largest group of dyes (-N = N-). They may contain mono, di, tri or tetra azo groups. There is a long list of different groups of dyes: Few commonly used dyes are given below.

9.2.1 Commonly used Dyes and Stains

Table 9.2

Name of the Dye	Nature	Composition	Use
1. Orange G (Anionic azodye)	Cytoplasmic stain, very soluble in water	80 % anhydrous dye in 95 % alcohol	Used in counterstain
2. Bismark brown (cationic azo dye)	Soluble in water and alcohol but insoluble in acetone	45 % anhydrous dye in 95 % alcohol	Used in counterstain
3. Acid fuchsin (anionic azo dye)	This is sodium, calcium or ammonium salt of trisulphonic acid, derivative of basic fuchsin, very soluble in water	Acid fuchsin 0.5 gm Distilled water 100 ml	Used to stain chitinous tissue

Name of the Dye	Nature	Composition	Use
4. Basic fuchsin (cationic azo dye)	It is a mixture of triphenyl methane dye	Basic fuchsin 2.0 gm Distilled water 200 ml boil, add 30 % aqueous ferric chloride 25 ml, boil for 5 minutes dry and dilute with 200 ml of 95 % alcohol and add 4 ml of concentrated HCl	Used to stain elastin, cartilage etc.
5. Light Green	---	Light green 0.5 gm 95 % alcohol 100 ml	Used to stain cellulose wall, chromatin, lignified walls etc.
6. Fast green	This is bluish green anionic triphenylmethylene dye	Fast green 1 gm 90 % alcohol 100 ml	It is commonly used as counter stain, cellulosic cell wall, cytoplasm and connective tissue staining
7. Methyl blue or aniline blue (anionic dye)	It is very soluble in water but insoluble in alcohol	Methyl blue 1 gm 1 % aqueous in 95% alcohol	Good stain for connective tissue
8. Eosine (alcoholic)	It is soluble in alcohol but least soluble in cold water. It binds with cationic group of protein molecules	Eosine yellow 1.0 gm 90% ethyl alcohol 100 ml Glacial acetic acid 5.0 ml Dilute with equal amount of 90 % alcohol	Cytoplasmic stain. Used as counter stain in double staining
9. Eosine (aqueous)	Soluble in water	Eosine 1.0 gm Distilled water 100 ml	Used for staining animal tissue
10. Methylene blue	It is freely soluble in alcohol but less soluble in water	Methylene blue 78 % by weight	Used in bacteriology and hematology
11. Safranine	It is soluble in water and alcohol	Safranine 1.0 gm Distilled water 100 ml	Commonly used for the plant tissues chromosomes and proteins

Name of the Dye	Nature	Composition	Use
12. Crystal violet	These are violet cationic dyes, soluble in water and alcohol	Crystal violet dye 14.0 gm 95% ethanol 100 ml	Used to stain bacteria and protozoans
13. Indigocarmine	It is blue anionic dye soluble in water but insoluble in alcohol	80 % dye by weight is used in aqueous solution	Used for staining connective tissue
14. Picro-Indigocar-mine	Soluble in alcohol	Alcoholic picric 10.0 ml acid solution (in 90% alcohol) Indigocarmine 20.0 ml saturated solution in 70% alcohol	It is good stain for hard and chitinous structure
15. Cango red	It is more soluble in water than alcohol	Cango red 0.5 gm distilled water 100 ml	Used for staining cellulose wall of Plant cell
16. Borax carmine	Soluble in water and alcohol both	Borax 2.0 gm Carmine 1.5 gm 70% alcohol 50 ml Distilled water 50 ml mix all the ingredients and boil for 30 minutes then allow to stand for 2-3 days and then add equal volume of 70% alcohol, filter and store	Commonly used for cytoplasmic stain
17. Acetocarmine	---	Glacial acetic acid 45 ml carmine powder 1.0 gm Distilled water 55 ml, mix glacial acetic acid and water, heat it to boil, then add Carmine powder shake well and filter	Used for chromosomal staining

9.2.1.1 Haematoxylin

This dye is obtained from a tree *Haematoxylon campechianum,* log wood tree fauna in south and Central America. It is equally soluble in water and alcohol, **"Haematein"** is the active ingredient of the dye. Stain may be prepared by oxidising (ripening) it slowly in the air but its rapid oxidation may be achieved by adding an oxidizing agent such as sodium iodate or ferric ions (ferric salt). So there is no need of ripening if it is iron haematoxylin mixture. There are different mixtures of haematoxylin used for different purposes as follows:

(i) Delafied Haematoxylin

Haematoxylin	4.0 gm
Absolute alcohol	25 .0 ml
Ammonium alum (saturated aqueous)	400.0 ml
Glycerine	100 ml
Absolute methyl alcohol	100 ml

Dissolve Haematoxylin in ethyl alcohol and mix it gradually into ammonia alum solution. Keep the mixture in the light for 7 days. After filtering the mixture, add glycerine and methyl alcohol. Now keep this solution for ripening for one and a half month.

(ii) Ehrlich Haematoxylin

Haematoxylin	2.0 gm
100% Alcohol	100 ml
Glycerol	100 ml
Glacial acetic acid	10 ml

Aluminium potassium sulphate in excess

It is mainly used for the staining of nuclear materials.

(iii) Heidenhain's Iron Haematoxylin

It consist of solution A and B where A is mordant solution.

Solution A

Ferric alum	44.0 gm
Distilled water	100.0 ml

Dissolve by shaking

Solution B

Haematoxylin	10.0 gm
95 % ethyl alcohol	100.0 ml

Mix both ingredients and leave to ripen for 3 - 5 months. Add 100 ml distilled water to this stock solution before use.

A is mordant and should be added before use.

(iv) Mayer's Haematoxylin

Haematoxylin	1.0 gm
Sodium iodate	0.1 gm
Potassium alum	50.0 gm
Citric acid	1.0 gm
Chloral hydrate	50 gm
Distilled water	1000.0 ml

Dissolve haematoxylin in 1000 ml of water with gentle heating and add sodium iodate and potassium alum then add citric acid and chloral hydrate. Allow to ripen 6 - 8 weeks.

9.2.2 Double Staining

It involves staining of nucleus by one stain (aqueous haematoxylin) and staining of cytological organelles by another stain (alcoholic eosine). The process involves the following steps:-

- Place the slide in xylene filled vessel for dewaxing (In case of paraffin sections.)
- Proceed through descending series of alcohol for hydration as follows:

Xylene
(2-3 minutes)
↓
Absolute alcohol + Xylene
(1:1, 2-3 minutes)
↓
Absolute alcohol (2-3 minutes)
↓
Absolute alcohol (1-2 minutes)
↓
90 % alcohol (2-4 minutes)
↓
70 % alcohol (2-4 minutes)
↓
50 % alcohol (2-4 minutes)
↓
30 % alcohol (2-4 minutes)
↓
Running water (5 minutes)
↓
Stain in Haematoxylin 2 minutes

- Proceed the slide in counterstain (eosine - if aqueous)
- Proceed the slide to ascending series of alcohol for dehydration as follows:

30 % alcohol (3-5 minutes)
↓
50 % alcohol (3-5 minutes)
↓
70 % alcohol (3-5 minutes)
↓
90 % alcohol (3-5 minutes)
↓
Counter stain (if it is alcoholic eosine)
↓
Absolute alcohol (2-3 minutes)
↓
Absolute alcohol + Xylene
(1:1, 2-3 minutes)
↓
Xylene (2 - 5 minutes)

- Mount the slide in DPX mount

Under microscope nuclei show blue stain and cytoplasmic structures show pink colour.

9.2.3 Triple Staining:

Triple staining is an exclusive method for microtomy slide. It provides better differentiation for different cell organelles. It is used for connective tissue, bone marrow, muscle, nuclei, chitin, bone matrix, collagen etc.

9.2.3.1 Mallory's Triple Stain

Solution A

Acid fuchsin (1 % aqueous)	10 gm
Distilled water	100 ml

Solution B

Orange G	2.0 gm
Phosphomolybdic acid (1 % aqueous)	2.0 gm
Aniline blue WS	2.0 gm

Distilled water	100 ml

Solution C

Phosphomolybdic acid	2.0 gm
Distilled water	100 ml

Sample is stained in solution A, B and C followed by rinsing in distilled water after each stain. Then dehydrate and mount the slide. Hyaline substance shows blue colour. Yolk, myelin and R.B.C. shows yellow to orange whereas nervous tissue, muscles and other cytoplasmic structures shows red to orange colour.

9.3 Specific Staining Method

9.3.1 Gram Stain

This is a common stain used for bacterial staining. The technique involves trapping of an insoluble derivatives of a dye. Steps are as follows:-

1. Stain the slide with crystal violet.
2. Treat the slide with an aqueous solution of iodine and potassium iodide. Tri iodide solution (I_3) present in the reagent, forms a water insoluble complex with the dye.
3. Now slide should be treated with an organic solvent such as ethanol, acetone or aniline to extract the dye iodine complex.

The solvent extracts the dye from gram negative bacteria but leaves gram positive bacteria as such (stained). A second dye of different colour (red cationic dye) is applied to stain the gram negative bacteria. Some bacteria have very thick outer membrane and could not be stained with crystal violet so they are gram negative.

(i) Hucker's Crystal Violet

Crystal violet	2.0 gm
95 % ethanol	20 ml
Ammonium oxalate $(NH_4)_2 C_2O_4H_2O$	0.8 gm
Water	80 ml

First dissolve the dye in ethanol and ammonium oxalate in water then mix both the solutions.

(ii) Gram's Iodine

Potassium Iodide	2.0 gm
Iodine	1.0 gm

Water	100 ml

(iii) Extracting Solvent

95 % ethanol	95 ml
Water	5 ml

(iv) Counter Stain

Safranine	0.25 %
Ethanol	9.5 %
Water	9 volume

9.3.1.1 Procedure

- Stain the slide with crystal violet
- Rinse with water 2 - 3 times
- Put the slide in Gram's Iodine
- Wash with water
- Pour the extracting solvent slowly on slide (30 second)
- Wash quickly with water to stop destaining
- Now pour the counterstain on the slide
- Rinse with tap water, blot with blotting paper.
- Smear slides should be observed under oil immersion microscope.
- Section should be cleaned in xylene and then mount in DPX

9.3.2 Endocrine Gland Staining

9.3.2.1 Aldehyde fuchsine - Haematoxylin - Light Green - Orange G for Pituitary Gland

(i) Solution A

Aldehyde Fuchsin	HCl	1 ml
	Para-aldehyde	1 ml
	0.5 % basic fuchsin (in 70 % alcohol)	100 ml

Keep at room temperature until solution turns deep violet from reddish colour (24 hours)

(ii) Solution B

Phosphotungstic acid	0.5 gm
Acetic acid	1 ml
Orange G 2 %(aqueous)	50 ml

Light Green SF 1 %	20 ml
Distilled water	30 ml

First of all stain the section in 3 - 10 days old solution A for 2-10 minutes then proceed for in 2 changes of 95 % alcohol for 5-10 minutes after that rinse in 70 % alcohol and in distilled water. Now stained the section stained in Ehrlich haematoxylin stain for 3-4 minutes, rinse with distilled water and differentiate in 0.5 % acid alcohol. Now counter stain in solution B, rinse quickly in 0.2 % acetic acid in 70 % alcohol, dehydrate and mount.

9.3.3 Polytene Chromosomes Staining in Chironomous Larva

(i) Acetocarmine (stock solution)	Carmine	0.5 gm
	.Acetic acid	45 ml
	Distilled water	55 ml

Boil it for 2-5 minutes. After cooling at room temperature filter it.

(ii) Aceto-orcein solution	Orcein	1-3 gm
	Hot Acetic acid	45 ml
	Distilled water	55 ml

Method

- Take the Chironomous larva and put it on a clean slide with a few drops of cold blood saline.
- Now with the help of forceps hold the posterior end of the larva and pull away the mouth parts by dissecting needle.
- The salivary glands will now be clearly visible as two translucent bodies on each side of the oesophagus.
- Remove the mouth parts and fix the glands in aceto alcohol for 2-3 minutes. Hydrolyse in 1N HCl at 57° for 1-2 minutes.
- Then transfer the glands on to the slide having drop of stain for 5 minutes.
- Place a coverslip on the gland and press it firmly with the help of blotting paper and repeat this process with another blotting paper.
- For making permanent slide it must be coated with albumin before squashing.

Acetocarmine stain shows red colour while aceto-orecin shows dark purple colour.

9.3.4 Staining of Nerve Fibres with Methylene blue

It is a cationic dye (pH 5.0 - 7.0) and stains living or freshly removed nervous tissue. It takes about 30 minutes to stain fresh tissue. Generally the stain is used during dissection of nervous system of insects or vertebrates.

9.3.5 Preparation of Blood Smears

Blood films of fresh blood of human may be prepared directly but if blood has to be kept for sometime, anticoagulant must be used.

Anticoagulant

Sodium citrate	25 mg
or	
EDTA	0.5 mg

Should be added for 1 ml of blood.

9.3.5.1 Procedure

- Take a clean glass slide, (degreased in alcohol) and put a drop of blood on it.
- Put another glass slide on the blood at 45° angle and spread it as shown in fig. The film is allowed to dry (Fig. 9.1).

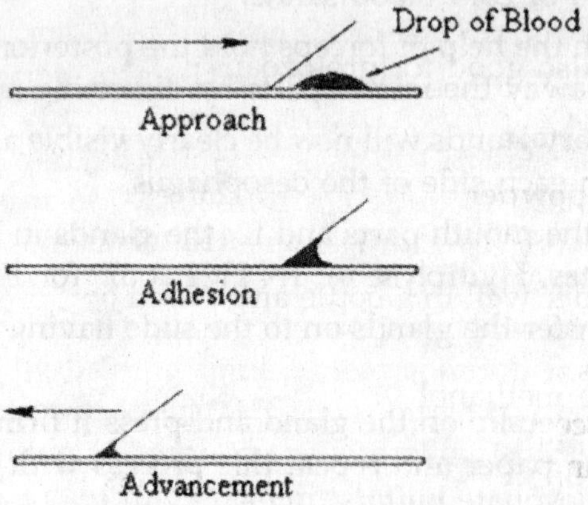

Fig. 9.1. Technique for Preparation of Blood film

If the slide is not stained within few hour, it should be fixed with 95 % alcohol for 5 minutes, rinsed in water, air dried and then stored.

(i) **Leishman Stain**

Leishman stain	0.15 gm

Absolute alcohol	100 ml

Shake well and leave for two days

A. Procedure

1. Place the slide on a horizontal staining rack over sink.
2. Put sufficient amount of **Leishman's stain or Wright's stain** (1 min).
3. Add buffer solution (pH 5.5) in sufficient quantity (3 minutes)
4. Wash the slide with water till violet colour is drained.
5. Drain the water and dry the slide.
6. Mount it and observe under microscope.

B. Observation

Erythrocytes	Pink colour
Nuclei of Leucocyte	Deep purple
Cytoplasm of agranular Leucocyte	Pale blue
Basophils	Blue
Neutrophils	Purple
Eosinophils	Red
Platelets	Blue

The stain is also good for protozoans

(ii) Giemsa's stain

Giemsa powder	2.0 g
Glycerol	132 ml

Mix the powder well in a bottle and put in oven at 60°C for 2 hours. Then add

Absolute methanol (mix gently)	132ml

Acetate or phosphate buffers (pH 4.0 - 7.0) are required.

Composition of buffer, as follows:-

Stock Solution

Solution A - 0.1 M

Sodium Dihydrogen Phosphate	12.0 gm

Water	1000ml
Solution B	
Disodium hydrogen	
Phosphate	14.20 gms
Water	1000 ml
Take solution A	188 ml

Solution B - 120 ml

A. Procedure

1. Hydrate the paraffin section
2. Put the slide in buffer (pH 4.0)
3. Transfer the slide in diluted Giemsa stain (stain 1 vol. : buffer 50 vol.) 40 minutes.
4. Rinse the slide with buffered wash
5. Dehydrate the slide in absolute alcohol (3 times)
6. Clean in xylene and mount.

B. Observation

Nuclei	Blue
Erythrocyte	Pink
Basophils	Deep purple

9.4 Physiological Solutions

Physiological solutions are actually balanced salt solutions. They keep the tissue unchanged for several hours after removal from the body. They have similar osmotic pressure and ionic concentration

9.4.1 Normal Saline

Sodium Chloride	8.5 gm
Water	to make 1000 ml

It is a good isotonic solution for mammalian and avian cells but for cold blooded animals, the concentration of NaCl should be 0.65 %

9.4.2 Ringer's Solution

Sodium chloride	9.0 gm
Potassium chloride	0.25 gm

Calcium chloride	0.30 gm
Sodium bicarbonate	0.5 gm
Glucose	10 gm
Water	to make 1000 ml

9.4.3 Acid Alcohol

70 % alcohol	100 ml
Concentrated Hydrochloric acid	1 drop

9.4.4 Acid Water

Concentrated Hydrochloric acid	1 drop
Distilled water	100 ml

9.5 Microtomy

Microtomy is the process of studying histological, histopathological and histochemical details of the tissues. The process involves thin section cutting of the organ or tissue for its detailed study. Thin histological section helps in diagnosis of disease and identification of peculiar cell types. Technique for histological preparation involves the following steps:-

1. Fixation of Tissue
2. Washing
3. Dehydration
4. Cleaning
5. Infiltration or impregnation
6. Embedding
7. Block preparation
8. Trimming of blocks
9. Section cutting
10. Stretching of Ribbon
11. Slide preparation

9.5.1 Fixation

Fixation is the first step in any histological preparation which has greatest effect on final result.

So the following factors should be considered.

- Type of the tissue to be fixed

- Density of the tissue
- Size of the tissue (smaller tissue need slow penetrating fixative while larger tissue require fast penetrating fixative).
- Penetrating power of the tissue

Aqueous fixation fix lipids while alcoholic fixatives dissolves them.

Volume of the fixative should be 30 to 40 times more than that of tissue volume. Fixation time depends on the kind of fixatives, penetrating power and size of the tissue. Excess time of tissue in the fixative causes its hardening and distortion.

9.5.1.1 Method of Fixation

Slide bearing film or smears should be immersed in buffered formaldehyde or absolute ethanol or methanol.

Tissue should be fixed as follows:

- Sacrifice the animal (Vertebrate or invertebrate in normal saline or aqueous bouin's fixative)
- Remove the tissue separately and wash in physiological saline
- Transfer it quickly in appropriate fixative
- Small and soft animal should be fixed as such but larger tissues should be cut into 2-4 mm thick pieces.
- Tissue should be cut with sharp blade

9.5.2 Washing of the tissue

After fixation (24 hours), tissue should be washed under running water for several hours. Tie the mouth of the bottle or vessel with a clean muslin cloth and put it under tap (running water). Continue washing till yellow colour of the fixative (picric acid) is removed completely. When tissue is cleaned completely it should be proceeded for dehydration (Fig. 9.2).

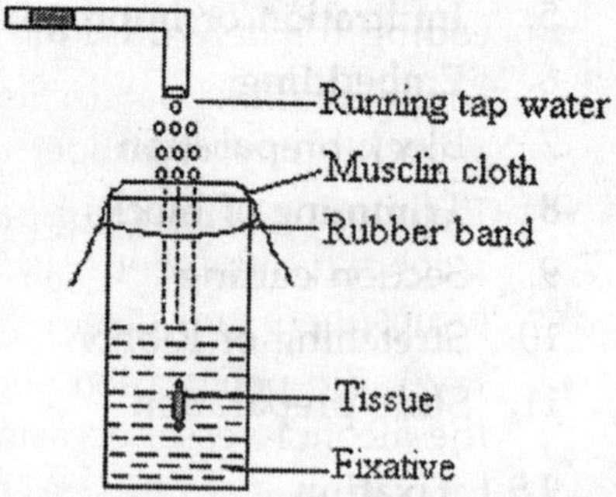

Fig. 9.2. Washing of Tissue under Tap Running Water

Note: Tissue fixed in alcoholic Bouin's fixative should be washed only with 70 % ethyl alcohol for 4 - 8 hours or till the supernatant is clear. Picric acid retained in tissue interfere during infiltration and creates problem in section cutting.

9.5.3 Dehydration

Dehydration is an important step in histological techniques which means "removal of water" from the tissue. Actually tissues fixed in aqueous fixatives retain water within them which is not miscible with cleaning agent so it is important to remove water before proceeding for clearing.

Dehydration is a successive process because gradual replacement of water with dehydrating agent, saves the tissue from shrinking and deforming. Then successful removal of water involves stepwise treatment (gradual) of tissue with dehydrating agent. Series of alcohol (30 %, 50 %, 70 %, 90 %, absolute alcohol) serve the purpose well. Later dehydrating agents should be substituted by clearing agent to make the tissue transparent. Xylene, chloroform and paraffin are used for cleaning and embedding the tissue.

9.5.3.1 Dehydrating agents

(i) Ethyl alcohol

This is the most commonly used reagent which removes the water gradually from the tissue. The tissue is passed from different grades i.e. 30 %, 50 %, 70 %, 90 % and absolute alcohol. The tissue should be immersed twice in absolute alcohol for complete removal of water. Time required in different grades of alcohol depends on the nature and size of the tissue. It may vary from 10 minutes to 1 hour for 2mm to 6mm thick tissue.

The following points should be taken into consideration before proceeding for dehydration:-

- There should be sufficient alcohol in the vessel (10 - 30 times more) to ensure proper dehydration.
- Dehydration should be proceeded in closed jars or tubes, because alcohol has the tendency to absorb humidity and water from the atmosphere and it may also get evaporated in open tubes.
- For rapid penetration and homogenous grade, keep on shaking the alcohol vessel occasionally.
- The tissue should not be left in alcohol beyond the required time because it will macerate or harden and will create difficulty in section cutting.
- Precaution should be taken in proceeding the tissue from lower to higher grade of alcohol.

Use blotting paper for checking the contamination of water.

(ii) Preparation of Alcohol Series

Grade of Alcohol	Volume of absolute alcohol	Volume of distilled water
30 %	31.5 ml	68.5 ml
50 %	52.6 ml	47.4 ml
70 %	73.6 ml	26.4 ml
90 %	94.7 ml	5.3 ml

(iii) Ethylene Glycol Monoethyl Ether

It may be used in place of alcohol because it is less hygroscopic than ethyl alcohol. It is also less volatile and does not evaporate rapidly. Dehydration may proceed in open vessel but one drawback makes its utility limited i.e. in bulk it may cause distortion of protoplasmic cells due to its rapid penetration activity. Thus it is good for paraffin embedding.

(iv) Isopropyl Alcohol

It is a better dehydrating agent, as it takes less time than ethyl alcohol. But it has certain disadvantages i.e. it is insoluble in nitrocellulose so may not be used in tissues that have to be embedded in nitrocellulose.

(v) Dioxane

It has similar dehydrating properties as ethyl alcohol. It takes less time for dehydration and never makes the tissue brittle or hard but it is not used very commonly because stain and dyes are less soluble in it.

9.5.4 Cleaning of Tissue

After dehydration, the tissue has to be made translucent and its alcohal (any dehydrating agent) should be replaced by a solvent which is immiscible with alcohol as well as wax. A good clearing agent substitutes dehydrating agent, cleanses and prepares the tissue for infiltration. There are a number of cleaning agents used for wax microtomy.

9.5.4.1 Xylene, Benzene and Toluene

These three hydrocarbons are most commonly used clearing agents, but xylene is regularly used in laboratory work. Actually all the three hydrocarbons evaporate at room temperature, they enter in the tissue and harden it, if exposed to longer period. Clearing and dehydration may be checked by observing that there should be no turbidity or milky precipitate on immersing the tissue in it. If any white turbidity appears, it indicates the contamination of water. To overcome this problems return back to absolute alcohol and then again proceed the cleaning agent (Xylene)

9.3.4.2 Chloroform

It is a very good clearing agent as it penetrates the tissue rapidly and never hardness the tissue even if left for long period of time. But it evaporates rapidly at room temperature so it becomes difficult to impregnate tissue with chloroform and wax. Thus it may be used only with big tissues.

9.5.4.3 Cedarwood, clove and Terpinol

These oils are frequently used for big tissue especially for the whole mount. Oils are replaced completely by paraffin so it takes longer time for embedding the tissue in paraffin.

9.5.5 Infiltration

Tissues should be transferred from clearing agent to infiltrating or impregnating agent. Infiltration or impregnation is the process of replacement of clearing agent with paraffin. For this purpose the oven should be adjusted just above the melting point of the paraffin to be used. Now put sufficient amount of paraffin in porcelain disk for melting (leave overnight). Filter the paraffin to remove dust particles and other impurities (which may create problems during section cutting) impregnation or infiltration gives better results, if tissue is transferred first into a mixture of clearing agent and paraffin (1 :1) for 4-6 hours. This is a better method for big and hard tissue. After

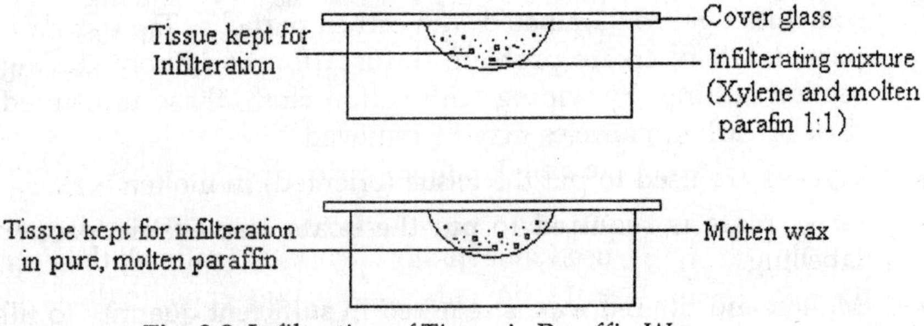

Fig. 9.3. Infiltration of Tissue in Paraffin Wax

infiltration or impregnation the tissue should be transferred to pure molten paraffin for 1 - 2 hours. This helps the tissue to be completely infiltrated with paraffin. Now this tissue is ready for embedding (Fig. 9.3).

9.5.6 Embedding

In this process the tissue is transfered to pure wax. The wax is cooled so that the tissue gets embedded in it. Paraffin should be chosen on its melting point and nature and size of the tissue. Paraffin having melting point 50°C - 52°C and 53°C- 55°C is soft paraffin while paraffin with 56 - 58°C or 60 - 68°C melting point are called hard paraffin. Soft paraffin is good for thick section while hard paraffin is preferred for thin section or tissue. Temperature of working atmosphere also effect the type of paraffin. Warm temperature is good for hard paraffin while soft paraffin is better cut in cold temperature. Before starting the embedding, the following materials should be ready (Fig. 9.4).

1. Spirit lamp
2. Needles - 2
3. Cleaned cotton cloth
4. Fine forceps - 2
5. Glass plate for platform
6. Molten wax for filling the boats
7. Embedding containers or paper (thick) boats.
8. Petridish for cooling the block boats

- Spirit lamp is required to warm the needle or forceps during transfer of tissue to paraffin filled boats.
- Needle and forceps are required to put and set the tissue properly in wax block with the help of warm needle or forceps.
- During transfer of tissue to wax, the needle is warmed which sometimes get contaminated with carbon particles. These carbon particles may create problem (bifurcation of ribbon) during section cutting. By wiping with cotton cloth, these unwanted dust or carbon particles may be removed.
- Forceps are used to put the tissue (oriented) in molten wax.
- Glass plate is required to put the boats and ensure proper labelling.
- Molten and filtered wax is required in sufficient quantity to fill the boats.

- Paper boats are the best embedding containers and may be prepared easily in any size according to the size of the tissue. Any information about tissue may be written on them and they are cooled easily. The length of the boat should never be twice of its height.

9.5.6.1 Orientation of the Tissue in Paraffin

The tissue should be embedded properly i.e. its orientation should be as such that may provide the desired plain of section. The following points should be taken into consideration before embedding the tissue:–

- The tissue should rest in the centre of the block i.e. at least 3 -5 mm wax should be left on all sides of the tissue.
- The wax should be poured in such a way that about 1mm extra paraffin is filled. This will not disturb the tissue after depression (cooling of wax).
- Excess wax should not be poured in the boat because it will overflow from the sides and create problem in cooling and trimming of block.

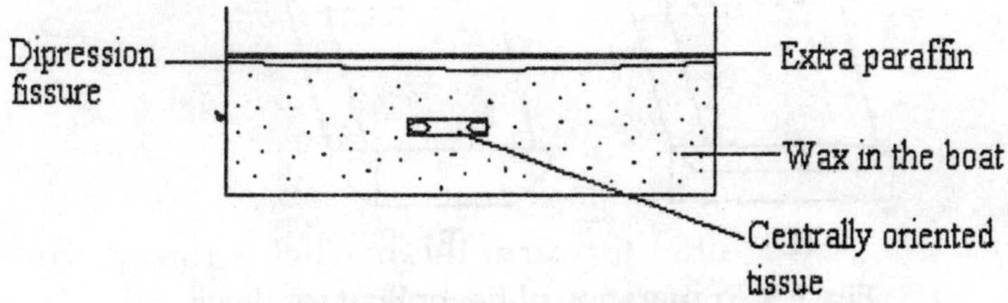

Fig. 9.4. Embedding of the Tissue in Paraffin Wax

9.5.6.2 Block Preparation by Embedding Method

- Arrange the paper boats or L block on glass plate.
- Light the spirit lamp.
- Take out the molten paraffin (should be at melting point) and pour it gently on the boat up to the required mark leaving 0.5 - 1 mm.
- Wait for a few seconds to solidify the wax at bottom side and keep the wax of surface layer molten by touching it with warm needle or forceps.

- Now transfer the tissue from infiltration paraffin to boat with the help of warm forceps. Precaution should be taken at this step that paraffin should not solidify before orientation of the tissue.
- Now keep the tissue in proper orientation by touching it with warm forceps and remove air bubbles if any.
- Gently cool the block in a container of cold water.
- Now remove the block from the paper boat or metal container and trim them (Fig. 9.5).

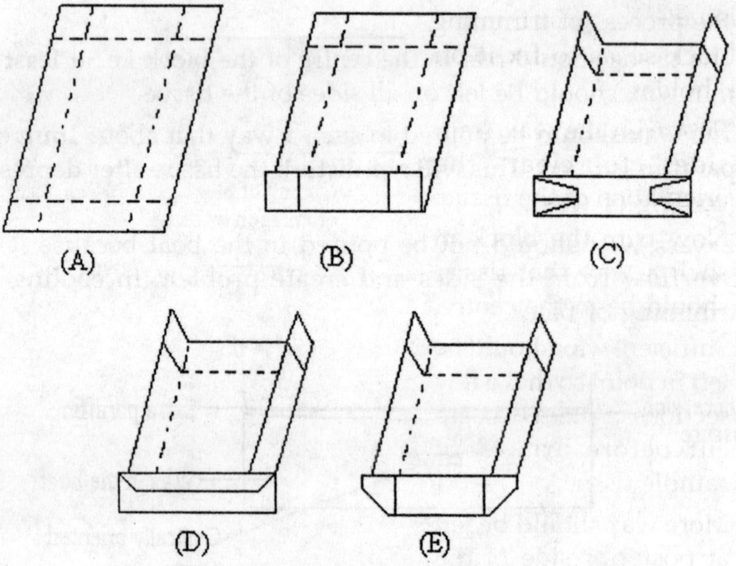

Fig. 9.5. Preparation of Paper Boat for Block

9.5.6.3 General Problems during Embedding

- White fluffy spots appearing in the block are due to slow cooling and crystallization of paraffin. It may also be due to clearing agent (Xylene) left.
- Sharp peaks appearing on the surface are due to rapid cooling of block in cold water.
- Depression in the centre of the block denotes that paraffin used was too hot which showed contraction on cooling. Avoid too hot paraffin for embedding and again embed the tissue.
- Air spaces in the block appear if very hot paraffin is used for embedding and very cold water for cooling. Outer surface of

the block hardens quickly resulting in shrinking of central mass due to which air spaces appear, so paraffin should not be too hot or water too cold.

- Water trapping in block : This happens if freshly prepared blocks are immersed in cold water.
- Fracture appears in cold water: This occurs if paraffin is poured in boats in two layers (after a gap) so always fill the boat up to the mark at a stretch.

9.5.7 Trimming

It is the process of trimming the block so as to fix it on block holder.

- First trim the wax from sides to clear the orientation of the tissue.
- Now trim the block in such a way that tissue should be in the centre.
- Sufficient wax should be left in point so that a few sections of plain wax are cut before arrival of sample tissue.
- More wax should be left at posterior side of the tissue to hold the block holder.
- An equal amount of wax should be left to all sides of the tissue. It gives uniform sectioning (Fig. 9.6).

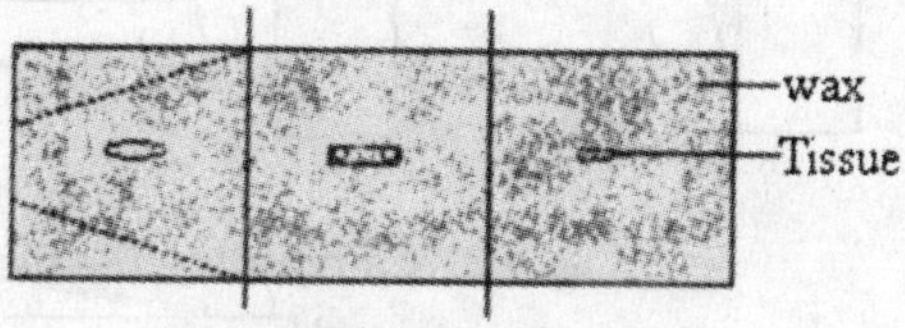

Cutting of block to clear the orientation of tissue

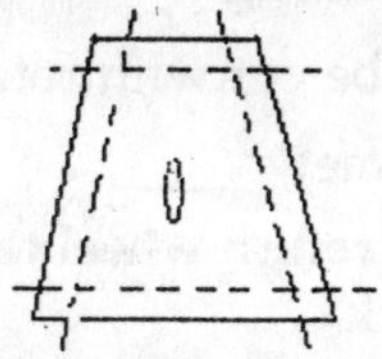

Trimming of block from all sides

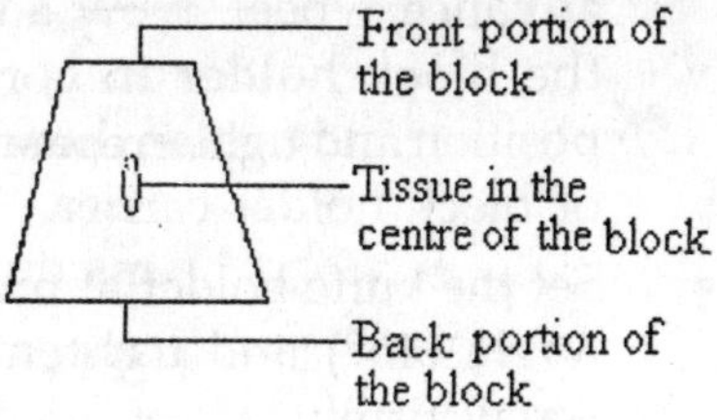

Fig. 9.6. Trimming of the Block

9.5.7.1 Maintaining the Block on Block Holder

Block holder may be wooden or metallic as shown in Fig. 9.6

- Clean the block holder, put few wax chips and melt them with heated scalpel.

- Now stick the paraffin block on molten wax immediately with the help of heated scalpel. Push the block gently on holder.
- Put some molten wax on the side of the block (at base) to stick it firmly.
- Leave the fixed block for few minutes until it is firmly fixed on the holder (Fig. 9.7).

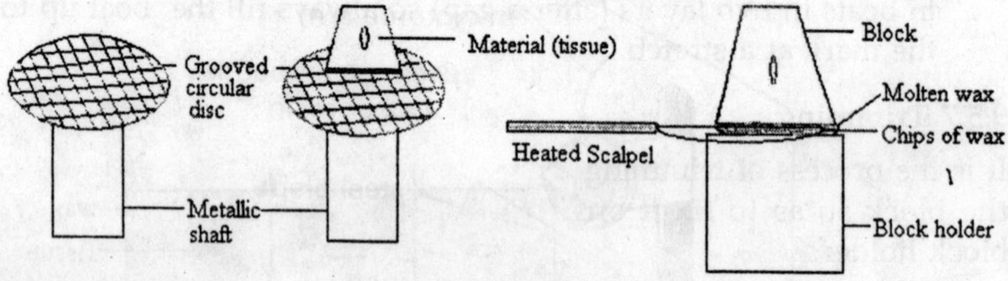

Fig. 9.7. Maintaining the Block on Block Holder

9.5.8 Section Cutting

Section should be cut with rotary microtome.

(See in microtome)

- Adjust the return wheel to provide enough space for cutting the entire block.
- Raise the block holder carriers with the help of advance wheel. Now adjust the block holder in correct position and tighten the screw of block holder carrier.
- Set the knife holder at proper angle (45°) and tighten the screw firmly.
- Now unlock the wheel and move it in order to bring the block just enough, above the knife. Taking care that block should not hit the knife edge.

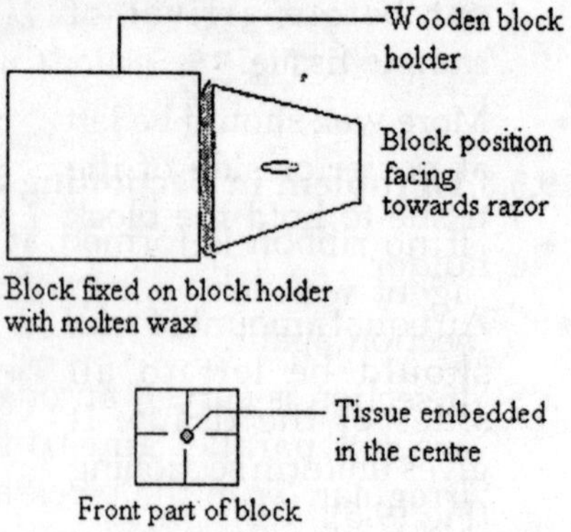

Fig. 9.8. Preparation of Block for Section Cutting

- Move the wheel until the knife is just in front of the block. Then tighten the knife carrier at this position.

- Move the advance wheel to get uniform ribbon of section. Pick and move away the ribbon with the help of dry soft brush and keep the desired length of ribbon on a white paper. Cut the ribbon in small pieces and put them on albumin (Mayer's albumin solution) mounted slide (Fig.9.8 & 9.9).

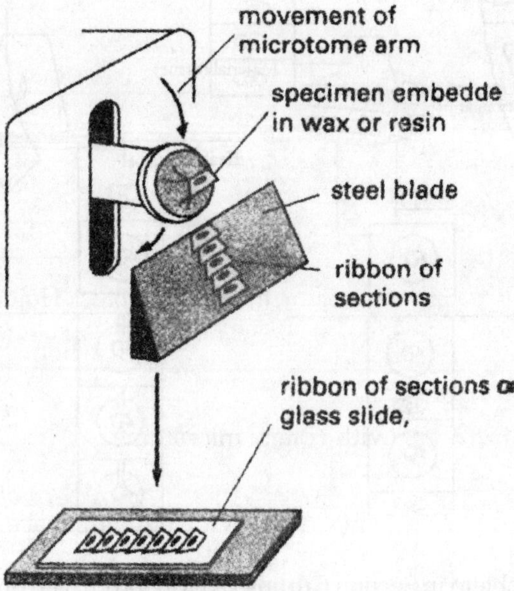

Fig. 9.9. Section Cutting through Microtome

9.5.8.1 Problem in Sectioning and Remedies

- If no ribbon is formed, it may be due to presence of clearing agent wax may get hard. So re-embed in proper paraffin and section again.
- If section is curved on one side, it shows that sides of the block are not parallel and trimmed properly. Knife edge may be irregular. Trim the block again.
- If sections are wrinkled, it shows that the knife is blunt. So sharpen the knife. Wax may be soft, cleaning agent may be left in block, sometimes by tilting the knife problem is solved.
- If ribbon is splitting longitudinally, it indicates the serrated margin. Dirt or carbon particle in wax may cause this problem, remove the particle with warm needle or re-embed the tissue.

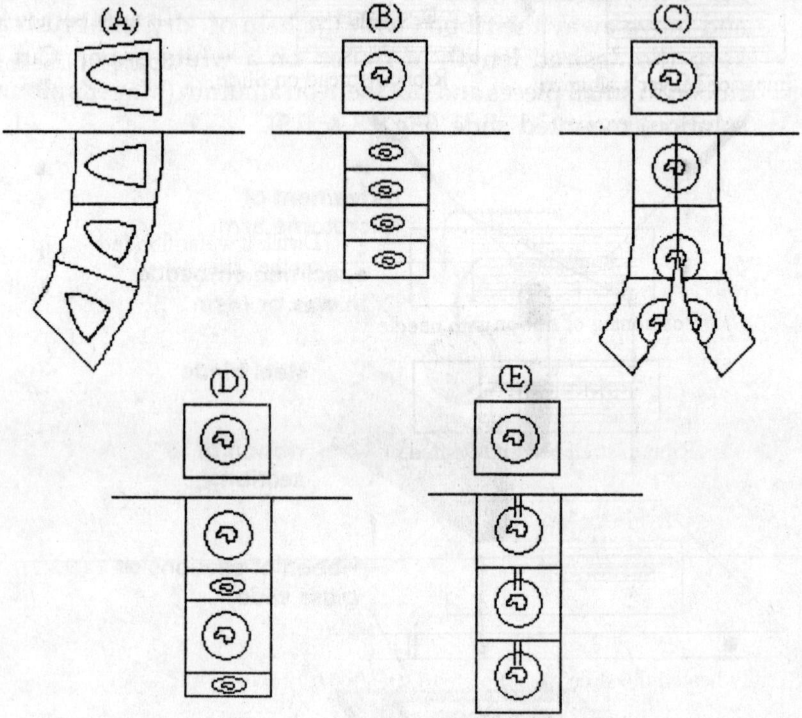

Fig. 9.10. Problem in Section Cutting (A) Ribbon curved on one side (B) Sections are wrinkled (C) Ribbon spliting longitudinaly (E) Sections are not uniform (E) Tissue is bulging from ribbon

- If the tissue breaks away from the ribbon, it shows that infiltration or dehydration is incomplete. Again put the tissue in clearing agent.
- If sections are not uniform i.e. some are thin and others are thick it indicates that knife or block holder is loose, tighten the screw.
- If the tissue is bulging from the ribbon, it shows that infiltration wax is hard and embedding wax is soft. Use the same wax for infiltration and embedding (Fig. 9.10).

9.5.8.2 Mounting of Section (ribbon) on Slide

- Put a very small amount of Mayer's albumin on the clean and marked slide and rub it with your finger to make a uniform smear. Excess albumin interfere with good staining.

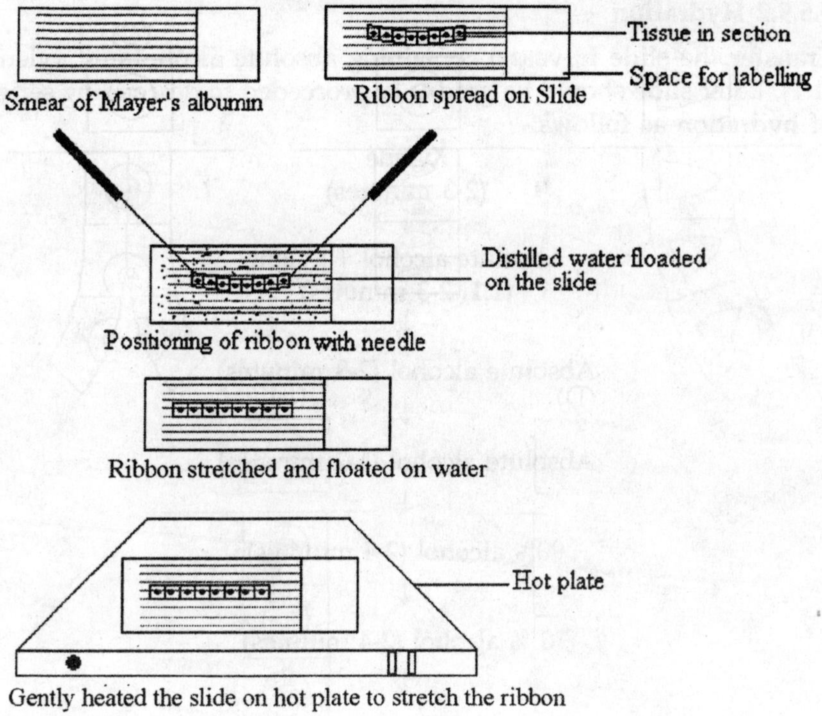

Fig. 9.11. Stretching the Ribbon for Mounting the Slide

- Put the albumin smeared slide on a white paper sheet on a flat platform. Pour few drops of distilled water on it. Now put 1 - 2 pieces of ribbon on it, with the help of forceps or soft brush. Ribbon floats on the slide. (If required add more water).
- Gently warm the slide (intermittently) on spirit lamp or hot plate, till ribbon is stretched completely. Drain excess of water by tilting it or with blotting paper. Properly position the ribbon and leave it to dry (Fig 9.11).

9.5.9 Hydration and Dehydration

It involves the following steps:-

9.5.9.1 Deparaffinization

Put the slide in xylene vessel for 8 - 10 minutes. Xylene will dissolve the paraffin, leaving only sticked section on the slide.

9.5.9.2 Hydration

Transfer the slide to vessel containing absolute alcohol and xylene (1:1). Later slide should be gradually proceeded to descending series of hydration as follows:-

Xylene
(2-3 minutes)
↓
Absolute alcohol + xylene
(1:1, 2-3 minutes)
↓
Absolute alcohol (2-3 minutes)
↓
Absolute alcohol (1-2 minutes)
↓
90% alcohol (2-4 minutes)
↓
70 % alcohol (2-4 minutes)
↓
50 % alcohol (2-4 minutes)
↓
30 % alcohol (2-4 minutes)
↓
Running water (5 minutes)
↓
Stain in Haematoxylin 2 minutes
↓
Proceed for Dehydration

Dehydration
30% alcohol (3-5 minute)
↓
50% alocohol (3-5 minute)
↓
70% alcohol (3-5 minute)

↓

90% alcohol (3-5 minute)

↓

Counter stain
(if it is alocoholic eosine)

↓

Absolute alocohol (2-3 minutes)

↓

Absolute alcohol + xylene
(1:1, 2-3 minute)

↓

Xylene (2-5 minutes)

Mount the slide in DPX mount observe the slide under microscope

9.6 Microtome

Microtomes have a device for advancing the material holder towards the knife. It is designed to cut uniform, thin sections of tissues and other materials, for the histological examination under the microscope. There are various types of Microtomes depending upon the nature of material to be cut and type of sections to be obtained.

1. Rotary Microtome
2. Rocking Microtome
3. Sledge Microtome
4. Freezing Microtome
5. Ultra Microtome
6. Saw Microtome
7. Vibrating Microtome
8. Hand Microtome

9.6.1 Rotary Microtome

Rotary microtome is generally used to cut paraffin wax embedded materials in a continuous ribbon. It can cut semi-thin to thin sections for light microscopy.

The microtome functioning is based upon the rotary action of hand wheel activating the advancement of the block towards knife. As a result the block moves up and down in a vertical plane in relation to the knife and flat sections are cut. In rotary microtome there is a heavy basic part which carries all the parts. The most important part is a circular wheel which is rotated.

Another device is meant for setting the microtome to cut the section of desired thickness. At the distal end, there is an advance wheel which is a circular grooved disc which moves anticlockwise by the exact distance (for which microtome is set). There is a central axle which helps to move the block holder device forward. Front part device carries the block holder in which paraffin block is fixed. The razor is placed on a grooved device at the front base which can be moved forward and backward with the help of screws. The razor is fixed at desired position with the help of locking lever or screw (Fig. 9.12).

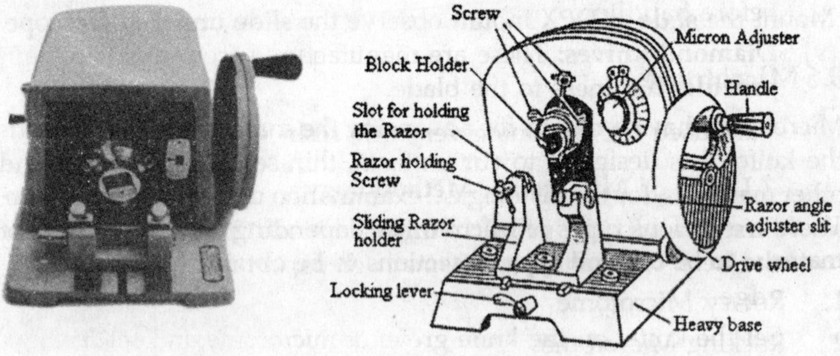

Fig. 9.12. (a) Microtome (b) Different parts of a Rotary microtome

Table 9.4. Types of blades used in Microtome

Types	Specificity	Uses
Plano concave / Biconcave	It has two hollowground surface and very sharp	Used for cutting soft celloiden embedded materials
Wedge-shaped	It is more rigid and extra thick at the tip	Used for cutting harder materials, frozen section, cryostat section, soft plastic wood and textile fibre etc.
Plane-shaped	It is least sharp and has greater stability	Used to cut hard and tough materials such as synthetic resin block, large wax block.

9.6.1.1 Knives of Microtome

The knives of microtome should have uniformly sharp edge on both sides, well greased and not used for a fairly long time. There are basically five types of knives.

(i) **Steel knives:** These are manufactured by high quality tool grade steel and treated by heat to harden the edge. It must be rust resistant and free from impurities.

(ii) **Disposable knives:** These are manufactured from high quality steel and their wedge can be coated with Chromium or Platinum for prolong cutting. It produces high quality section free from compression.

(iii) **Tungsten carbide:** These are manufactured from tungsten carbide and 100 times harder than steel. It is used for cutting section of bone and other hard materials.

(iv) **Glass knives:** These are hard but brittle so care should be taken before handling.

(v) **Diamond knives:** These are manufactured from diamonds and provide hardness to the blade.

These are used for sectioning very thin resin sections.

9.6.1.2 Using of Microtome: Methodology

- First of all fix the properly trimmed block on block holder with the help of molten wax (small chips) on the warmed scalpel edge.
- Set the knife, on the knife grove of microtome and set its angle (20 - 30°)
- Now set the block holder and orient it so that the edge offering least resistant meets the knife edge first.
- Now advance the block until it just touches the knife edge.
- First cut the block 15 μ until the full face has been trimmed.
- Set the advance wheel at desired thickness (3 - 5μ).
- Clean the razor with alcohol to remove any type of dirt (Never use xylene to clean).
- Move the wheel till continuous section (ribbon are obtained).
- Remove the ribbon with the help of moist brush (0 - 2 No.) and put it on a black paper sheet.
- Cut the ribbon of desired length and put them on already

albumin-smeared slide and proceed for stretching (see in microtomy)

References

Baker, J.R., (1958); Principles of Biological technique. Lond. Methuen, John Wiley.

Bancroft, J.D., (1975); Histochemical Techniques. 2nd ed.Lond., Butterworth.

Bancroft, J.D., and Stevens, A., (1982); Theory and Practice of Histological Techniques, Churchill, Livingston.

Carleton, H.M. and Leach, E.H., (1947); Histological Techniques., New York, Oxford Univ. Press.

Culling, C.E.A., (1974); Handbook of Histopathological and Histochemical Technique, London, Butterworth.

Galigher, A.E., (1934); The Essentials of Practical Microtechnique, Philadelphia, Lea, and Febiger.

Glick, D.,(1949); Techniques of Histo-and Cytochemistry, New York., Interscience.

Gray, P., (1958); Handbook of Basic Microtechnique, New York. McGraw Hill.

Griffin, R.L., (1972); In Ultramicrotomy, London, Bailliere Tindall.

Gurr, E., (1958); Method of Analytical Histology and Histochemistry, London, Leonard Hill.

Humason, G.L., (1979); Animal Tissue Techniques 4th ed. W.H. Freeman and Co., San Francisco.

Kraijian, A.A. and Gradwhol, R.B.H., (1952); Histopathological Techniques, St. Louis, C.V. Mosby.

Lillie, R.D., (1954); Histopathological Technique and Practical Histochemistry 2nd ed., New York. Blakiston.

Pearse, A.G.E., (1968); Histochemistry: Theoritical and Applied., Vol I, 3rd ed., London., Churchill.

Walter, F., (1980); The Microtome Mannual of the Technique of Preparation and of Section-cutting. Germany; Ernst Leitz Wetzlar GMBH.

CHAPTER 10

Cryopreservation and Techniques

10.1 Introduction

Cryopreservation is the recent and very useful technique for long-term storage of germplasm. The technique involves cooling of specimen including cells and tissues at very low temperature. At extremely low temperature i.e. -196°C all the genetical activities of the biological material become stable and metabolic activities cease.

Thus cryopreservation involves preservation of biological material such as cells, tissue and organs in liquid nitrogen (at - 196°C). The process aims to minimize ice crystal formation which may damage the cell membrane leading to its death. The process include replacement of water with other compounds that will not form large crystals when frozen. The most commonly used replacement materials are DMSO (Dimethyl sulfoxides) and glycerol. Preservation of cells, tissue, organs or bacteria in living condition is required for a number of reasons as follows:-

- Preservation of accurate cell morphology
- Demonstration of neurological elements
- Demonstration of lipids
- Preservation of antigenic properties for immunocytochemical demonstration
- Preservation of enzyme or diffusable compounds for histochemical demonstration.
- Storage of specimen prior to histological, biochemical or immunological properties.

10.2 Theory of Freezing

In cryopreservation, the tissue is processed for freezing to provide a hardened matrix for section cutting or to preserve the morphological biochemical and immunological properties of the tissue. Actually water is converted into ice at temperature 0 °C and pressure of 1 atmosphere. But at higher rate of cooling the crystal of ice become cubic rather than hexagonal. If cooling rate is increased more, small volume of water is solidified without formation of ice crystals. This solid form of ice is known as vitreous ice. This ice exist in a temperature dependent on irreversible phase transition with cubic ice, hexagonal ice and water. This minimizes the loss.

Actually slow cooling produces an osmotic difference between extracellular and intracellular fluid, which results in a loss of intracellular water. The increased ionic concentration within the cell ruptures the membrane and ice crystals within the cell causing damage to cells. Thus the technique aims to limit ice crystals formation through control of the cooling rates.

10.2.1 Factors affecting the cooling rates

- Cooling limits of the cryogen
- Heat capacity of the cryogen
- Extent of contact between cryogen and sample
- Degree of heat exchange between cryogen and sample
- Diffusion of heat through the sample

Size of the sample also affect its cooling. Cryoprotectants reduce the rate of ice crystal nucleation through freezing point depression.

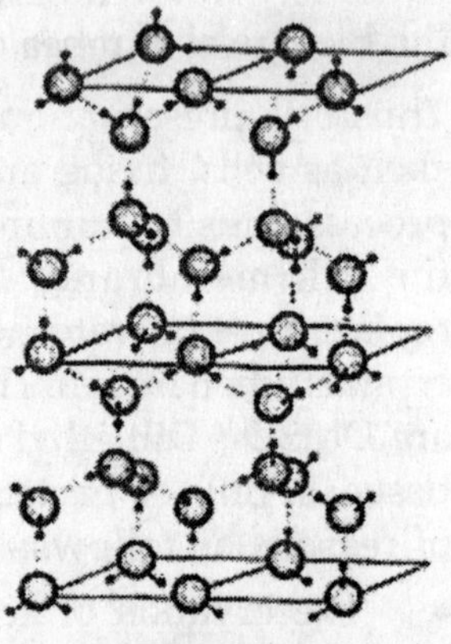

Fig. 10.1. Water molecules in the form of ice

10.3 Cryoprotectants

These are the substances which increase the viscosity of medium at subzero temperature; as a result mobility of water molecules decreases and ice crystals are not formed from water molecules.

Commonly used cryopectants are non-penetrating agents, which protect living cells against freezing injury at extracellular level, cell membrane and intracellular level. It also help to estabilize the intra and inter-molecular arrangment of cellular compound and prevent the removal of water molecules during freezing. There are two types of Cryoprotectants.

10.3.1 Non Penetrating: They cannot move into the cell across the cell membrane. Polyvinyl Pyrrolidone (PVP), dextron, hydroxy ethyl strach and sucrose are commonly used non-penetrating substances. Its large molecule cannot diffuse across the membrane.

10.3.2 Penetrating: They can move into the cell across the membrane. They reduce the injury, but if frozen sample is warmed it causes loss of cells. Commonly used penetrating are dimethyl sulphoxide (DMSO), glycerol, ethylene glycol and dimethyl foramide (DMF), use of 5 % DMSO causes minimum injury to cells.

10.4 Cryogen

These are cooling agents used to decrease the temperature of sample material by heat transfer and diffusion.

10.4.1 Types of Cryogen

There are a number of cryogen recommended which differ in their absolute temperature and heat transfer efficiencies.

10.4.1.1. Liquid Nitrogen (-196°C)

It is used where rapid cooling is recommended. But overcooling may cause cracking and brittleness. To overcome this problem layer of gaseous nitrogen is used which reduces the heat transfer.

10.4.1.2. Liquid Nitrogen Isopentane (-150°C)

Liquid Nitrogen Isopentane or hexane is recommended for histochemical diagnosties. It reduces freezing artifact.

10.4.1.3. Carbon dioxide gas (-70°C)

Carbon dioxide rapidly freezes the sample by heat exchange from the expanding and vaporising gas.

10.4.1.4. Solid Carbon dioxide (-79°C)

It is also known as dry ice and is very useful and effective in rating lab cooling.

10.4.1.5. Mixture of dry ice and hydrocarbon (-79°C)

Mixture of dry ice with isopentane, acetone, hexane or ethanol form slurry. Sample may be kept directly into it.

10.4.1.6. Aerosol Spray (-50°C)

It includes gases liquifies under pressure. It is very effective for routine work. Heat transfer is slow causing freezing artifact.

10.4.1.7. Thermoelectric cooling (-40°C)

In this type of cooling electric current is passed through two metal conductors, which cause absorption heat at the junction. So a sample in contact with this surface freezes due to heat transfer. This device is applied as part of the stage of some frozen microtome.

10.4.1.8. Refrigerated contact (-30ºC)

In most of the cryostat compressure driver refrigerating coils are used to cool the mcabinet but cooling rate is slow.

10.5 Cryopreservation of Cells, Tissues and Micro-organisms

Cells, tissues and micro-organisms are preserved in liquid nitrogen (-196ºC), the process is called cryopreservation. Germplasm of plant and animal material is preserved to get them back in viable condition. It is better to preserve the early stage of tissue or cells. The following steps are involved in cell or tissue culture of plant or animal materials, although process is variable for different types of material.

10.5.1 Procedure

Cells, tissue or organs should be cultured in a medium containing amino acids like proteins, sugar-like sucrose at low temperature. This makes the tissue physiologically fit for freezing and increases membrane fluidity. Cold hardening pretreatment of temperate plants gives better cryopreservation.

- Expand the cell culture to get sufficient number of cells.
- Separate the cells by centrifugation at 200 to 400 rpm for 10 minutes.
- Prepare the necessary volume of cryopreservative media. Generally a mixture of DMSO, glycerol and sucrose is used. For adherent cell types 90 % fresh medium including amino acid and 10 % DMSO is used while for suspension cell type 45 % fresh medium i.e. amino acid, and 10 % DMSO is used.
- Now place the cells again in cryopreservative medium for 30-60 minutes at 0ºC. This preservative makes the cell or tissue hard and improve their survival.
- Now place the desired number of cells into culture vials for cryopreservation.
- Immediately transfer vials to a freezer at -20°C for an hour.
- Later transfer the vials at -80°C for 24 hours.
- At last vials should be transferred to a liquid nitrogen storage (-196°C).

10.6 Freezing

Tissues and cells of different types show different response for cooling. Cooling should be in such a way that damaging ice crystals are not formed. Cooling is in three steps-

1. Slow cooling
2. Rapid cooling
3. Freezing following dehydration

10.6.1. Slow Cooling

0.5 - 4 °C up to - 40°C to - 100°C for 30 - 45 minutes before proceeding to liquid nitrogen.

10.6.2. Rapid Cooling

It ranges from -200 to -900°C and checks the large-sized ice crystal formation.

10.6.3. Freezing Following Dehydration

This step involves vitrification of tissue in highly concentrated aqueous solution of cryoprotective agent followed by liquid nitrogen.

10.7 Thawing or Warming

It brings the cryopreserved material back to normal condition. Culture is removed from liquid nitrogen storage and warmed rapidly at room temperature. Generally the frozen material is plunged into a waterbath at 37 - 40°C for 1-2 minutes. Cell culture is obtained by centrifuging the vial. Replace the culture medium with fresh medium. Thus viable cells will grow normally within 1-2 days.

10.8 Viability

Viability of different biological materials is different for specific procedures. It includes the number of viable cells in the culture. Finally obtained (0.1 ml dilution) cells may be spread on agar and developed colonies are counted for their viability.

10.9 Vitrification

It is the process of conversion of highly concentrated aqueous solution of cryoprotective agents into a meta stable glass state without ice crystal formation at sufficiently low temperature. Big tissues and organs may be compressed in this way.

10.10 Cryostat

It is a device, in which the entire microtome and specimen are enclosed in insulated thermostatically controlled refrigerated chamber. All the controlled system are located outside from this device. Temperature control device is as such that for rapid freezing of the tissue may be done during section. Production of frozen section depends on the following factors:-

Freezing condition of intra and inter cellular water.

Types of Specimen

- Knife of Microtome and its cooling condition
- Environmental temperature.
- Embedding media which provide an inert matrix for sectioning.

Any type of microtome (rotary, rocking, moving knife or ultramicrotome) may be used but it should be equipped with piped carbon dioxide, refrigerated coils and thermoelectric device should be applied.

10.11 Preparation of Frozen section by Cryostat

Section cutting of frozen material is somewhat different from simple microtomy. For the production of frozen section, intra and intercellular water is frozen to produce a hard matrix for slicing of the tissue. For cutting frozen tissue, the sample must be firmly attached to the microtome stage. Here frozen water acts as supporting medium. Sometimes aqueous mixture of glycols and resins are used as inert matrix.

10.11.1 Structure of Freezing Microtome

There is a radial arm attached to a central pivot on this arm, two clamps hold the knife with its cutting edge inclined to horizontal plane. The knife is moved in a horizontal arc over a specimen chuck mounted on central hook. When the knife is moved back and forward the chuck is advanced upwards by a micrometer mechanism. The tissue is mounted on to the freezing stage (hollow metallic block with holes in its side) compresed CO_2, piped into the freezing stage, freezes the tissue. Knife is also equipped with a nozzle supplying CO_2, to lower its temperature. The thermoelectric device maintains the temperature of tissue and knife.

10.11.2 Fixation of Tissue

Tissue may be fresh or fixed. Cut sections of fresh tissue, tend to thaw quickely and are stickly to handle due to presence of unfixed protein. So tissue should be kept in 10 % formaline for 2-5 minutes. But alcoholic fixation should be avoided as alcohol inhibits the freezing point of the tissue.

10.11.3 Infiltration

A specimen or tissue may be infiltered with a protective medium eg: 30 % sucrose in 10 % formaline, 1 % gum acacia in 30 % sucrose, 10 % glycerol + 4 % formaldehyde +2 % dimethyl sulphoxide and an aqueous glycerine- gelatine mixture etc.

Example:

Gelatin infiltration

Gelatin	8 gm
Glycerine	7.5 ml
Distilled water	35 ml
Thymol	pinch for preservation

Dissolve the gelatin in distilled water and add glycerine. Store at 4°C. Melt at 37°C in water bath.

10.11.4 Method

Fix the tissue in 10 % formaline overnight wash throughly in running water for 6-8 hours. Infiltrate in gelatin-glycerine mixture at 37°C for 6-8 hours.

Transfer the tissue to fresh gelatin glycerine mixture, embeded in a suitable mould and freeze for sectioning, trim the block and harden the gelatin glycerine mixture.

10.11.5 Tissue freezing and sectioning

- Put a little volume of water on freezing stage, put the tissue on it, apply pressure on the tissue and freeze it with short application of carbondioxide. The whole tissue looks white frozen block
- Raise the wheel to bring frontal surface of the tissue just in contact with the knife.
- Set the thickness of the section.
- Apply a firm, steady and gental pressure on the wheel.
- Cool the knife with short application of CO_2.

- Cut a number of section until the required thickness is obtained.
- Remove section from the knife with wet brush and put them in a dish of normal saline.

  (If tissue is unfixed, cooled dry knife may be used and section should be picked up directly on a warmed slide. The section will thaw on contact and will adhere to the slide).
- After cutting is completed, the knife should be cleaned and dried.
- Transfer the sections on gelatin or albumin coated slide.
- The section is carefully blotted with filter paper moistened with absolute alcohol.

  "If tissue is fixed the section should be immersed with alcohol, blotted and placed in 0.5% solution of celloidin, slide is drained air dried for 1-2 minutes before being placed into water."
- An unfixed section may be placed into formaline and then washed in water. In both cases after washing in water the section is ready for staining.

10.11.6 Staining of Section

- Transfer the section in a small dish of distilled water.
- Transfer to alum haematoxylin for 1-5 minutes.
- Two changes of distilled water.
- Transfer to alkaline water for 1 minute (to stain nuclei).
- Wash thrice with distilled water.
- Stain with 1% aqueous Eosine for 30-60 seconds.
- Transfer to absolute alcohol for 1 minute.
- Transfer to three changes of absolute alcohol.
- Transfer to xylene twice.
- Mount in mounting media.

References

Angermuller, S. Fahimi, H.D., (1982); Imidazole buffered osmium tetroxide: An excellent stain for the visualisation of lipids in transmission electron microscopy. Histochem J. 14: 825-836

Bancroft, J.D, Stevens, A., (1990); Theory and Practice of histological Techniques. 3rd ed. London: Churchill Livingstone.

Barnard T., (1987); Rapid freezing techniques and cryoprotection of biomedical specimens Scanning Microscopy., 1:1227-1224

Clayden, E.C., (1967); Practical section cutting and staining. Edinburgh: Churchill Livingstone. 16. Hopwood D.(1977) Fixation and Fixatives. In: Bancroft JD & Stevens A, eds. Theory and Practice of Histological Techniques. Edinburgh: Churchill Livingstone.

Disbrey, B.D., Rack, J.H., (1970); Histological Laboratory Methods. London: E & S Livingstone.

Dowell L.G., Rinfret, A.P., (1960); Low temperature forms of ice as studied by x-ray diffraction. Nature 158: 1142-1148

Ishii, T, Kasama K, Kondo M., (1990); Improvement of the quality of frozen sections from formalin fixed tissue. Stain Technol., 65: 43-44

Leong, A.S.Y, Duncis CG., (1986); A method of rapid fixation of large biopsy specimens using microwave irradiation. Pathology. 18: 222-225

Lyon, H., (1991); Theory and strategy in histochemistry. Berlin: Springer-Verlag.

McManus, J.F.A., Mowry, R.W., (1964); Staining methods: histological and histochemical. New York: Harper & Row.

Noble, L., (1981); Impregnation techniques in the preparation of frozen sections from formalin fixed tissue. Histo-logic 11: 55

Pearse, A.G., (1980); Histochemistry: Theoretical and Applied. 4th ed Vol 1. London: Churchill Livingstone.

Pearse, A.G.E., (1980); Histochemistry. Theory and applied. 4th ed. Edinburgh: Churchill Livingstone.

Preece, A., (1972); A manual for histologic technicians. Boston: Little, Brown and Company.

Ralis, H.M., (1973); Beesley R.A., Ralis, Z.A. Techniques in Neurohistology. England: Butterworths.

Rasmussen, D.H., (1982); Ice formation in aqueous systems. J Microsc., 128: 167-174.

Surrey, E. Quinn P., (1990); Successful ultrarapid freezing of unfertilized oocytes. J in Vitro Fert Embryo Transfer., 7: 262-266

Vacca, L., (1985); Laboratory manual of Histochemistry. New York: Raven Press.

CHAPTER 11

Biosensor

11.1 Introduction

The word Biosensor consists of two words "Bio"- means biological materials i.e. enzyme, cell organalles, harmones or antibodies and sensor is a "Physicochemical transducer". Thus Biosensor is an electronic analytical device using biological material as immobilized layer closely associated with a physical component (sensor). The physicochemical or transducing microsystem may be optical, electrochemical, thermometric or magnetic. The biological materials associated with the physical component react with the analyte and produce a biological signals which are further converted into an electric signal. In biosensor the biological material such as enzyme, cell organalles, nucleic acid, harmones or antibodies are immobilized as a layer on the physicochemical component which may be a single carbon electrode, oxygen electrode, an ion sensitive electrode or photocell.

11.2 Basic Principle

The analyte (sample) when passed through an immobilized layer of biological materials interacted with it and forms some detectable products in the form of gas, heat, electrons, hydrogen ions or ammonium ions. These products (signals) further pass through transducing microsystem (transducer) and are converted into an electric signals. Now the electrical signals are amplified by an amplifier.

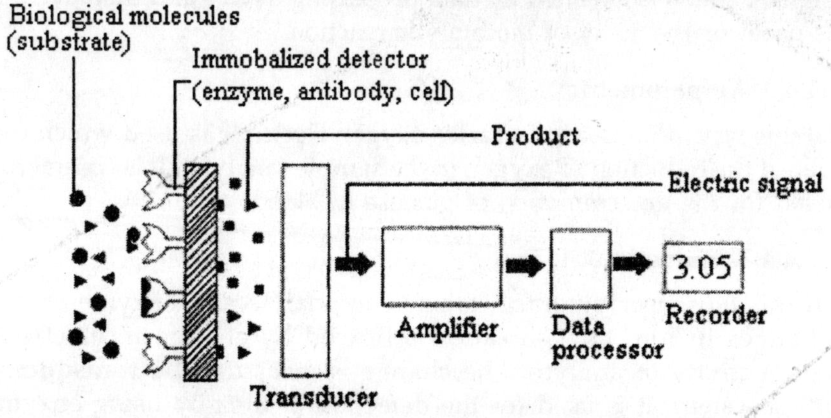

Fig. 11.1. A Typical Process of Biosensor

The amplified signal is passed into data processing device and displayed on the recorder (Fig. 11.1).

11.3 Types of Biosensor

On the basis of interaction between analyte and biological materials, it is of two types:

11.3.1 Catalytc biosensor

When catalytic enzymatic reaction converts the analyte into new chemical compound, it is termed as catalytic biosensor.

11.3.2 Affinity biosensor

When the analyte binds with the biological materials present on the biosensor, it is termed as affinity biosensor.

11.4 Transducing microsystem in Biosensor

11.4.1 Thermometric

It is also known as colorimetric biosensors, used for coloured solution of analyte. At the time of analysis the interaction between analyte and enzyme synthesize product in the form of heat. This change in temperature of analyte is detected by the transducer.

11.4.2. Potentiometric

In this type of biosensor ion selective electrode such as pH meter glass electrode, NH_3 sensitive electrode or CO_2 sensitive electrode are used. They convert biological signal (gas or ions) into electric signals which is detected by data processing device and displayed. It is used for the assay of biocatalytic reaction.

11.4.3. Amperometric

In this type of biosensor, Clark's oxygen electrode is used which can detect the reduction of oxygen in the sample (analyte). It is commonly used for the determination of glucose in blood.

11.4.4. Conductimetric

In this biosensor, interaction between analyte and enzyme causes changes in ion concentration followed by change in electrical conductivity of analyte. The change is measured by transducing microsystem. It is used for the detection of urea by using enzyme urease.

11.4.5. Optical

It is based on the detection of radiolabelled enzyme or fluorescence labelled substance formed by the interaction of analyte and biological membrane. It is used for the detection of bacteria in food or pathological sample by using enzyme luciferase.

11.4.6. Piezoelectric

It is based on the piezoelectric effect (when charged crystals under stress produce electrical field). Piezoelectric crystals are used for the detection of mass of analyte, that interact with the biological materials. It is used for the detection of cocaine by using antibodies and piezoelectric crystals.

11.4.7. Whole Cell Act as Transducer

In this biosensors the whole cell of an organism or their organalles are used instead of enzyme. It provides longer response and lower selectivity.

Presently cellulose strips precoated with enzyme and reagents are available for the detection of glucose in blood or urine of diabetic patients. When strips are dipped in analyte solution, they show change in colour, which is compared with standard to detect the amount of analyte present in the sample.

11.5 Application of Biosensor

- It is very useful due to the small size, easy handling, greater sensitivity and selectivity.
- It is used for detecting glucose in the blood of diabetic. It is extremely sensitive and can measure the glucose concentration in a single drop of blood and display the results within 20 seconds.
- It is used for the detection of mutagenicity of chemicals and toxic substances produced in the body due to infections or disease.
- Biosensors are also used in environmental monitoring and pollution control.
- It is used in the measurement of L - amino acid, alcohol, phenol, methane, various sugars, ethanoic acid (vinegar) and antibiotics.
- It is useful to measure the odour and freshness of food materials.
- It is also used to measure cholesterol level in blood.

- In patients with ovarian cancer, biosensor technology is being used to characterize the function of therapeutic antibodies.
- It is useful for determination of antigen antibody reaction.
- Biosensor technology is also used in vaccine development.

11.6 Advantages

It includes the following advantages:-

- These are highly specific so we can analyze the substrate from mixture of chemicals without purification.
- These are very sensitive hence may be used for the detection of very low concentration of analyte in a very small amount of sample.
- They provide accurate, rapid response and can be made very small.

11.7 Disadvantages

- They are not sterilizable and stable.
- They require careful handling.

References

Bartlett, P.N. , Biosensors: A Practical Approach (AEG Cass- Editor) IRL Press.

Class, A. E. G., (1990); Biosensors : A practical approach. IRL Press, Oxford.

Giardi, M.T., Koblizek, M., Masojidek, J., (2001); Photosystem II-based biosensors for the detection of pollutants. Biosensors and Bioelectronics. 1027-1033.

Hall, E.A.H., (1990); Biosensors. Open University Press, Milton Keynes.

Murphy, L., J., and Galley, P., T., (1991); Accurate measurement of human Plasma glyceraol with H2O2 detecting microdialysis enzymes electrodes.

Glossary

Abrasive media: Extremely hard materials (Diamond, SiC, Al_2O_3 etc.) usually in a very fine particulate form used to grind or polish specimen to desired thickness or finish.

Adjuvant: The substance capable of inducing immune response, when mix with antigen.

Albumin: A blood protein that is made in the liver and helps to regulate water movement in the body

Alkaloid: A nitrogen containing organic compound isolated from plants.

Alpha Particle: A specific particle ejected from a radioactive atom. It has low penetrating power and short range.

Antibodies: These are sepecific glycoproteins produced by B lymphocyte cells in response to the infection by an antigen.

Antigen: A susbstance capable of inducing immune response in the host cell is known as Antigen.

Antiserum : Serum of an animal that contains antibodies aganist a particular antigen.

Aperture: A thin (<100 micrometer thick) disk or strip of metal (usually Pt) with a small (2-100 micrometers) circular hole used to restrict electron beams and filter out unwanted scattered electrons before image formation.

Atom: The smallest piece of an element that cannot be divided or broke up by chemical means.

Autoradiograpy: It is a method of detection of radioactivity of test sample with the help of photographic emulsion and radioactive tracer.

Auxochrome: It is any group which does not itself act as a chromophore but whose presence brings about a shift of the absorption band towards the red end of the spectrum (longer wavelength).

Backscatter Electrons: Produced by an incident electron colliding with an atom in the specimen which is nearly normal to the incident's path. The incident electron is then scattered "backward" 180 degrees with no appreciable loss of energy, an elastic collision.

Base Peak : The largest peak in a mass specrum is known as base peak. It has highest intensity.

Bathochromic shift: It is an effect due to which the absorption maximum is shifted towards longer wavelength due to the presence of auxochrome or by the change of solvent.

Beta Particle : A small particle ejected from a radioactive atom. It has a moderate penetrating power and a range of upto a few meters in air.

Bright Field Imaging: A imaging mode in a TEM that uses only unscattered electrons to form the image. Contrast in such an image is due entirely to thickness and density variations in a sample.

Buffer: Solution of weak acid and one of its salt. It resist change in H^+ and OH^- ion concentration and maintains pH.

Camera: A light tight box that receives light from an object or scene and focuses it to form an image on a light sensitive material or a detector.

Characteristic X-Ray: An X-ray having a unique energy that is emitted by an atom during its de-energization after ionization of one of its electron.

Chopper : It is a wheel like structure used for the breaking of steady light into pulsating light.

Colorimetery : It is the method of measurement, the colour intensity of a solution.

Column : It is a device placed between injector and detector. It facilitates separation of sample mixture.

Composition: The elements that a specimen is composed of and their relative ratios.

Cosmic rays: These are high energy radiation that orginates outside the earth's atmosphere.

Cryogenics: A branch of physics concerned with study of cause and effects of extremely low temperature.

Cryonics: A branch of cryopreservation deals with the preservation of dead human body or an organ (brain) with the help of medical technologies.

Crystal Structure: The order in which atoms are arranged in a material. These arrangements have a direct effect on the physical properties of the material. These arrangements commonly take the form of cubes, rectangular solids, hexagonal solids etc.

Dark Field Imaging: Using a single diffracted beam to form the image in a TEM. This causes all regions of the specimen not of the same crystal structure and orientation as the region which produced the diffracted beam to be represented as very dark in the final image, allowing phase differentiation visually in the TEM.

Detector : A device that is sensitive to radiation and can produce a response signal for analysis.

Diffraction: Periodic scattering of moving objects when they collide with an orderly pattern of fixed objects.

DNA Probe: The DNA fragemnt used to detect a target DNA molecule known as DNA probe.

Dyes: Coloured organic compounds that binds with suitable substrate and impart colour to it.

ECP: Electron Channeling Patterns: A pattern formed by the periodic backscattering of electrons by the specimen lattice in SEM. It allows determination of crystal structure and lattice parameters in crystals >20 micrometers diameter.

EDS: Energy Dispersive Spectroscopy: A technique that is based on the characteristic X-ray peaks that are generated when an energetic electron beam interacts with the specimen.

Electron Gun: A cathode or anode device intended to produce a stream of electrons.

Electron: A subatomic particle which allows the atom to react with its environment and form bonds with other atoms. Electrons and their orbits around the nucleus of an atom account for most of the physical properties of the element.

Electrophoresis: A technique for separating various blood fractions by running an electric current through gel containing a blood sample.

EMR : A travelling wave motion that results from changing electric and magnetic fields.

Emulsion : A coating on potographic film or paper, mainly consisting of silver halide grains uniformely suspended in gelatin.

Epitops: These are sites either on or within the antigen with which antibody react.

Exposure : A quantity used to indicate the amount of ionization in air produced by X-ray or Gamma ray radiation.

Exposure: The amount of light allowed to strike the film or paper.

Filter : A piece of glass or other transparent medium is used to change the colour or density of the scene.

Free atom: A free atom means an atom not combined with other atoms.

Frequency: The total number of waves which can pass through a point in one second.

G.M. Counter : It is an instrument that is used to detect and measure radiation.

Globulins: A group of proteins in blood plasma whose levels can be measured by electrophoresis in order to diagnose a variety of serious illness.

Gradient elution : When two or more solvents are used for the separation of sample component then it is known as Gradient elution.

Haematein : Active ingredient of Haematoxylin dye obtained from a tree *Haematoxylon compechianum.*

Haptoglobin: A protein in blood plasma that binds haemoglobin.

Hypsochromic shift: Due to this, absorption maximum is shifted to shorter wavelength. It is due to reduction in conjugation or change in polarity of solvent.

Immunoglobulin: Any of several types of globulin that function as antibodies.

Incadescent Source: The light or glowing produce by heating an electric filament.

Ion : An atom in a charged state, either having a deficiency (a positive charge) or a surplus (having a negative charge).

Khymograph: It is an instrument used to record the temporal variation in heart beat and muscular twitch (Physiological processes).

LASER: Light amplification by stimulated emission of radiation. It is highly monochromatic.

Lattice: An orderly arrangement of atoms in a material, usually thought of as an infinite series of cells forming a lattice work of atoms in 3-dimensions.

Lens: A homogenous transparent medium bounded by two curved surfaces or one curved and plane surface.

Macrophotography: The photographic recording of image of magnification near 1:1.

Magnetic Lens: Circular electromagnets capable of projecting a precise circular magnetic field in a specified region. The field acts like an optical lens, having the same attributes (focal length, angle of divergence etc.) and errors (spherical aberration, chromatic aberration etc.). They are used to focus and steer electrons in an Electron Microscope.

Magnifying Power: The ability of an optical system to make an object appear larger.

Microphotography : This is the technique of taking photograph of large object in greatly reduced size.

Monochromatic: All objects in a group (electrons, light, X-rays etc.) have the same energy/wavelength.

Monochromator : It is an optical device used for isolating a single resonance line from the emitted light spectrum

Morphology: The shape and size of the particles making up the object, direct relation between these structures and materials properties (ductility, strength, reactivity etc.).

PCR: Polymerase Chain Reaction is an in vitro method of Nucleic Acid synthesis by which a small amount of DNA can be amplified into millions of copy.

pH: It is defined as the negative common logarithm of hydrogen ion concentration.

Phase: A specific crystal structure, known as phase.

Photomicrograpy: It is the technique of taking image of very small object with the help of a compound or stereomicroscope.

Pumps: These are specific device to flow the solvent into the column with pressure and constant flow rate.

Radioactivity : The spontaneous emmission of radiation from the nucleus of an unstable atom. As a result the radioactive atom converts into other atom.

Resolution : The ability of a mircoscope to distinguish two closely related points.

Retention : It is the measure of speed of sample at which it move in chromatographic system.

Secondary Electrons: Each incident electron when falls on a metallic surface can produce several secondary electrons.

SLR Camera : The camera in which the scene is viewed through the same lens which takes the picture.

Specimen Interaction Volume: The volume inside the specimen in which all specimen interaction occur during electron beam irradiation.

Specimen Interaction: When a beam of energetic electron struck on specimen the interaction occur inside the specimen is known as specimen interaction.

Spectroscopy: Study of interation between material and electromagnetic radiation.

Topography: The surface features of an object i.e. texture, hardness, reflectivity, etc.

Torr: A unit of pressure, 760 Torr is standard pressure at sea level.

Wave number: The total number of wave which can pass through a space of 1 cm. It is reciprocal of wavelength.

Wavelength: The distance between two peaks in a light wave is termed as wave length. It is denoted by λ.

X-Rays : These are penetrating electronic radiation whose wavelength are shorter than those of visible light.

Zoom Lens : A lens whose focal length can be adjusted over a wide range.

Index